The History of Technologic Advancements in Urology

Sutchin R. Patel • Michael E. Moran
Stephen Y. Nakada
Editors

The History of Technologic Advancements in Urology

Springer

Editors
Sutchin R. Patel
Department of Urology
University of Wisconsin School of Medicine and Public Health
Madison, WI
USA

Michael E. Moran
William P. Didusch Center for Urologic History
Linthicum, MD
USA

Stephen Y. Nakada
Department of Urology
University of Wisconsin School of Medicine and Public Health
Madison, WI
USA

ISBN 978-3-319-61689-6 ISBN 978-3-319-61691-9 (eBook)
DOI 10.1007/978-3-319-61691-9

Library of Congress Control Number: 2017953444

Printed on acid-free paper

This Springer imprint is published by Springer Nature
The registered company is Springer International Publishing AG
The registered company address is: Gewerbestrasse 11, 6330 Cham, Switzerland

This text is dedicated to the spirit of innovation. To all those that have contributed to technology in medicine and whose creativity and perseverance serve to inspire the next generation of urologists, scientists and inventors.

– Sutchin R. Patel, Michael E. Moran and Stephen Y. Nakada

This text is also dedicated to the memory of Dr. Manoj B. Patel (1967–2017), a dear friend, colleague and inventor.

– Sutchin R. Patel

Contents

Chapter 1
Introduction

Sutchin R. Patel, Michael E. Moran, and Stephen Y. Nakada

We live in exciting times and in our lifetime we have seen tremendous changes in science and technology. These changes have affected all aspects of our life, from communication to transportation to health care.

The field of urology has always been at the forefront of technology in medicine and has been able to adapt to as well as pioneer many of these changes. Advances in optics and Edison's incandescent lightbulb helped lead to the development of better cystoscopes. The work of Clayman and Kavoussi in performing the first laparoscopic nephrectomy ushered in the field of minimally invasive surgery. Chaussy's ingenuity in using shock waves lead to a disruptive technology that changed how we treated stones.

Clio, the muse of history, has a lot to teach us (Fig. 1.1). Understanding the history and evolution of our field is important, as it shows us the big picture, giving us perspective, and allows us to realize the work of those that came before us to give us the tools that we use today. It teaches us that not all new innovations last and that only time will judge which technologies are validated and adopted. It teaches us not to be over confidant, not to become too comfortable and that we must always strive to improve because "change is the only constant in life" (Heraclitus of Ephesus).

Thomas Edison summed up the most important traits in an inventor when he stated "There is a way to do it better—find it." and in one of his most famous quotes "Genius is one percent inspiration and ninety-nine percent perspiration."

In our text we share the stories of how many of the technologies we use today were developed. We hope these stories will inspire you and help you to appreciate

S.R. Patel, M.D., F.A.C.S. (✉) • S.Y. Nakada, M.D., F.A.C.S.
Department of Urology, University of Wisconsin School of Medicine and Public Health, Madison, WI 53726, USA
e-mail: sutchin_patel@yahoo.com

M.E. Moran, M.D.
American Urological Association, William P. Didusch Center for Urologic History, Southwest Urology, 1015 Delaware Ave., Suite B, McComb, MS 39648, USA

S.R. Patel et al. (eds.), *The History of Technologic Advancements in Urology*,
DOI 10.1007/978-3-319-61691-9_1

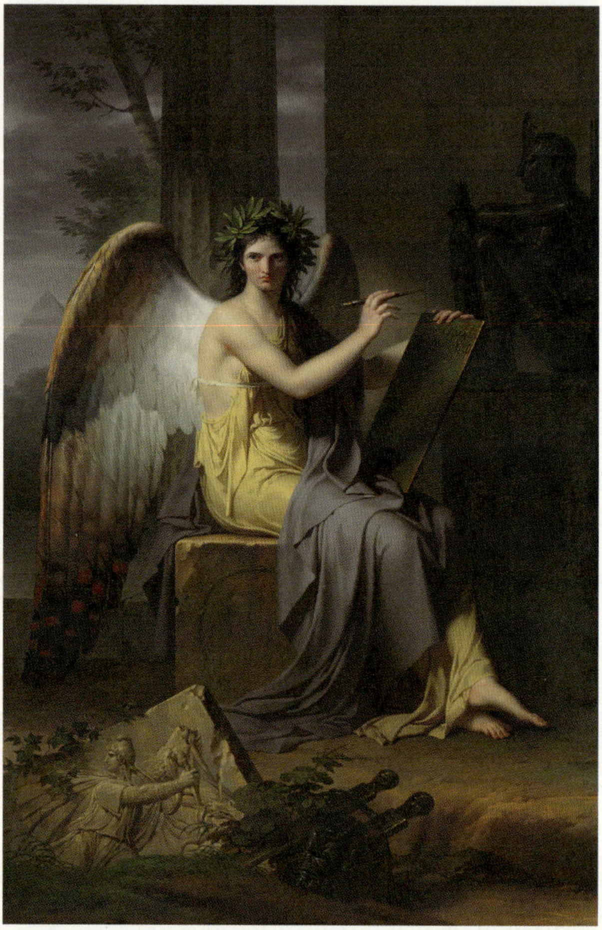

Fig. 1.1 *Clio, Muse of History*, 1800. Charles Meynier (French, 1768–1832). Oil on canvas; framed: 290 × 192.4 × 6.9 cm $\left(114\frac{1}{8} \times 75\frac{11}{16} \times 2\frac{3}{4}\text{in.}\right)$; unframed: 273 × 176 cm $\left(107\frac{7}{16} \times 69\frac{1}{4}\text{in.}\right)$. The Cleveland Museum of Art, Severance and Greta Millikin Purchase Fund 2003.6.5

the ingenuity, creativity and the countless hours of work and perseverance (which unfortunately we will never be able to fully appreciate) that it took to develop these technologies. Despite the technologic achievements of the past, our field continues to push the envelope in terms of innovation and creativity.

Chapter 2
History of Cystoscopy

Michael E. Moran and Friedrich H. Moll

Introduction

Light allows the physician to peer into the interstices of body cavities, with organs and organ systems [1, 2]. The development of light-guided devices underscores the history and development of the cystoscope [3]. The very beginnings of urology saw the introduction of increasingly sophisticated methods of looking into the lower urinary tract. On May 2, 1868 a little known surgeon who had arisen during the American Civil War to become the Surgeon General of the Navy wrote a seminal work in *The Medical and Surgical Reporter*. Philip S. Wales would go on to devise and develop his own cystourethroscope which he used on multiple occasions in his private practice. He stated, *"the endoscope, from ενδον "within" and the word σχοπεω "I examine" to become an instrument that but recently introduced to the notice of the profession"* [4]. More than one of the founding fathers of the specialty of urology declared that this new and burgeoning technology was the founding stone of the specialty. It is now difficult as a urologist to even imagine a time when we were not able to not only visualize the bladder but have almost complete access to the upper tracts as well, but this was not the case till rather recently. At the dawn of the twentieth century, one early investigator of urologic applications who is better known as the "father of gynecology," Howard A. Kelly demonstrated the potential of endoscopic evaluation of the urinary tract. Kelly and Curtis F. Burnam from Johns Hopkins published *Diseases of the Kidneys, Ureters and Bladder* in 1914 [5].

M.E. Moran, M.D. (✉)
American Urological Association's William P. Didusch Center for Urologic History, Carolina Urology, 720 Jefferson St., Whiteville, NC 28472, USA
e-mail: memoran2@juno.com

F.H. Moll, M.D.
Department of the History, Philosophy and Ethics of Medicine and Department of Urology, Heinrich-Heine-Universitat, Kliniken der Stadt Koln, Düsseldorf, Germany
e-mail: friedrich.moll@uni-koeln.de

S.R. Patel et al. (eds.), *The History of Technologic Advancements in Urology*,
DOI 10.1007/978-3-319-61691-9_2

On page 270 of his classic textbook, Kelly noted that *"It is our habit in catheterizing ureters in practically all cases to wax the catheter tip before its introduction"*. This is the era prior to x-rays, there was no fluoroscopy, and only the hopes for illuminated endoscopes could provide the much needed information for expanding the diagnostic as well as therapeutic potential much need in the primitive specialty. Yet the need for knowledge about what pathology lies within visceral structures existed and the ability of physicians to anticipate pathology rose as autopsies (the word *autopsy* means "personal observation") increased in numbers and were correlated to clinical symptoms. The scratches on the freshly waxed catheters were critical to identify the presence and location of a potential ureteral calculus before other imaging strategies existed.

In this historical sojourn on the development of the cystoscope, we will not recapitulate the histories of the past, but will begin by discussing how the cystoscope impacted the development of urology as a specialty, discuss the earliest beginnings with the founding fathers, and then present the findings of these primordial investigations that led to the twentieth century and an explosion of cystoscopes and the proliferation of modern urology. First we begin with the development of direct and indirect light-guides which forms the basis of all types of urethroscopes followed by cystoscopes. This is followed by the methods for delivering better illumination which is closely related to the improved development of image improvement from the rod-lens systems, to the modern utilization of fiber optics. Next came camera systems which allowed the urologist to multitask which is so fundamental to modern or historically more accurate, current cystourethroscopy [6]. Finally, to simplify this rather complex historical overview- I will present the reader with a simplified outline of the historical development of the cystoscopy, which is a modification of that of Bransford Lewis, 8th President of the A.U.A. and a huge proponent of cystoscopy in early American urology. The history of the writings about the origins of cystoscopy would make an admirable topic unto itself, since most of the major urologic historical authors have attempted this topic and so too has the William P. Didusch Center for Urologic History with one of its first exhibits being this topic. But these writings, like so much of history itself is spread about like the diaphanous web of glimmerings that tempt the historian mightily to seek, to present, to clarify the past and a true and accurate history of cystoscopy would evolve into a mighty tome indeed.

Cystoscopy and Urology

The history of cystoscopy has been largely written about by many authors and historians and there is precious little left to be included in the burgeoning literature. There has been little appreciation of the ability to visualize the lower urinary tract and the truly revolutionary implications that this newfound and precious information allowed urologist and perhaps might have been the key technology that allowed the development of urology as a specialty. The first lighted examinations were external openings to the gastroenteral tract and the female introitus. Early Greek specula have been unearthed that record the foundations of primitive endoscopy. Early practitioners of medicine realized that to view a viscus from the inside should provide valuable information in the management of illnesses and applications were devised for their use in the urethra of both males and females [6]. But before advances in genitourinary medicine and surgery could proceed, the visualization of the lower urinary tract was essential and well recognized by the founding fathers. In Ramon Guiteras's founding remarks at the First Annual Meeting of the American Urological Association held in Saratoga, New York on June 13, 1902 he stated, "*The use of artificial illumination by means of tubes and reflected light was an important step in the advance of modern urology*" [7]. Guiteras continued with a very brief historical overview in the founding document of the A.U.A. It was an early American proponent of cystoscopy that we will next turn for the truly monumental role, then perceived by the cystoscope to come to an appreciation of how revolutionary it was to the nascent profession of urology.

Bransford Lewis was another of the primordial American urologists and the 4th President of the American Urological Association in 1907. His Presidential Address is most illuminating in the annals of the history of cystoscopy, ***The Dawn and Development of Urology*** [8]. This is worth reading from many historical perspectives, but we will focus upon the comments he made regarding Max Nitze first and then his longer comments that followed, "*…how shall I adequately express the esteem in which the father of cystoscopy, Max Nitze, is held? The one who did more than any other to pave the way to precision in urological diagnosis and therapy as they exist to-day*" [8]. Heady praise indeed, but he is just warming to the topic of the historical significance of cystoscopy. "*If there has been one reason to explain the substantial progress along broad and scientific lines that has been made by this department of medicine in late years, the cystoscope is the reason. It has transferred the study of urinary diseases from an inexact, intangible, shifting basis to one of definite and established proportions. Together with ureteral catheterization, the cystoscope has been the means of bringing within the definite diagnostic reach all of the upper urinary tract- the bladder, the ureters and kidneys. Through this instrument, the world is ours, now, for the taking. A world of diseases and disorders is now placed lucidly before us- conditions that have hitherto been inaccessible and remote, or even unrecognizable. This field has therefore been noted as one of speculation and argumentation, a diagnostic shuttle-cock, dancing from point to point in accordance with the strength or weakness of theoretical contention. It was the mind of Nitze that materialized to practical use the idea of direct inspection of the bladder; his hand guided the growth of this wonderful instrument from its infancy to its maturity; from the cumbersome and dimly-lighted mechanism of the early days to the graceful and effective instrument of the twentieth century; and, fortunately, he lived to see the fruition of his hopes, the world-wide recognition of his instrument, as a blessing to humanity, and its use in all civilized countries*" [8]. Now lest the perceptive reader believe that the cystoscope was the last word on the development of urology as a specialty, let's be thorough in the comments from Hugh Cabot, the 8th President of the A.U.A. just to temper the argument with a just rebuttal, "*The assistant who spends his days with his eye glued to the butt of a cystoscope would probably be admitted to be a specialist, and as such he has my deepest sympathy, for a specialist he must remain to the end, and that of the narrowest type*" [9]. Krotoszyer from San Francisco went even further in his address stating that "*The history of* *urology is best divided into two parts: the pre-cystoscopic and cystoscopic era"* [10]. Hugh Hampton Young was the 5th President of the American Urological Association and he was more enamored with the instruments that followed from the development of the cystoscope stating, "*Truly marvelous are the instruments which followed in steady succession*" [11]. He added that the people who are attracted to training as a urologist should also be interested in the equipment.

Now what is the purpose of all of this investigative knowledge that was pouring out of cystoscopist's findings? How would it make the difference in care and management of urinary troubles? Let's look at several early examples- one in females, one on general endoscopic potential and one from Leo Buerger, one of the founding fathers of American cystoscopy. A truly unheralded work was published in 1872 by a physician in New York City, Robert Newman entitled, *The Endoscope: Considered Particularly in Reference to Diseases of the Female Bladder and Urethra* [12]. He begins apologetically to his audience stating, "*I need not at the present time offer an apology for presenting to this honorable body the recent discovery of an instrument which, added to the repertoire of medical science, promises to be of incalculable benefit to a very large class of sufferers"* [12]. Here we have the allusion to the fact that urinary pathology is common and that people will have benefit from correct diagnoses. Newman waxes philosophical implications to urinary disease, "*…we must hail with enthusiastic welcome any aid by which the veil can be more and more lifted, or the obstacles further removed from a direct and palpable certainty in regard to our treatment of these classes of disease"* [12]. He then demonstrates the Desormeaux device which he utilized in seven cases, and presents the patients' symptoms in which it was used, the findings and therapies. He concludes by stating the obvious, that finding the true pathologic process absolutely relates to the physician's ability to treat it as follows, "*My opinion is not based upon theory, but upon evidence derived from close observation of clinical facts, and is valuable only as the result of careful investigation upon many cases, not only those occurring in my immediate practice, but in the greater field of inquiry and facilities afforded me by hospital practice"* [12].

The findings of cystoscopy were vigorously applied by early urologists. E. Hurry Fenwick was one such practitioner in London who was the President of the Section on Urology at the XVIIth International Medical Congress in 1914. *"With so many ardent disciples of Nitze, the symptomatology of diseases of the lower urinary tract has been entirely reconstructed. Facts have replaced unstable supposition. Each phase in the life-history of each vesical disease has been studied by means of the cystoscope and so accurately described that there are now few bladder or prostatic complaints- if we except those of nerve origin, which are not recognizable to the expert, merely on enumeration of their complexus of clinical features: but in most the final diagnosis is referred to the cystoscope for confirmation"* [13]. At the very same meeting, David Newman from Glasgow presented his findings with photographs of renal and vesical tuberculosis demonstrated by cystoscopy. Newman has several findings summarized as follows: "*(1) when the orifice of the ureter is strictly normal no serious disease exists in the corresponding kidney; (2) when the kidney is normal the orifice of the ureter is also normal; (3) when there is evidence of tuberculosis at the orifice of the ureter there is always associated with it tuberculosis of the corresponding kidney; (4) in tuberculosis of the bladder the ureter does not become involved if the corresponding kidney is free from disease"* [14]. His treatise was accompanied by 12 illustrations of the progression of tuberculous lesions by cystoscopy.

Leo Buerger was a prolific urologist at Mount Sinai Hospital in New York City and the major designer of what became the Brown-Buerger cystoscope by Wappler [15]. He wrote extensively about cystoscopy and urethroscopy which now described in many of the findings we take for granted today. In January, 1911 one of his articles discussed the normal and pathologic findings of the posterior urethra and bladder neck. He states, *"In the exposition of my subject I shall devote myself to the following thems: first, anatomical landmarks; second, elementary principles underlying the use of the instrument, and technic; third, the normal pictures of the neck of the bladder and urethra; and fourth, pathological lesions"* [16]. This work was followed by his *Cysto-urethroscopy. A Study of the Normal and Pathological Posterior Urethra* [17]. This was a major paper including 50 illustrated figures on the normal and abnormal urethra. He would later publish works correlating his cystoscopic findings with actual stained pathologic specimens showing clear correlation of anatomy and histology. Modern urologic interventions were on the threshold of achieving everything modern urology could accomplish. One final hallmark contribution cannot be overlooked prior to proceeding with this history, that is the work of the very controversial Abraham L. Wolbarst on his wax models of pathologic lesions in the male posterior urethra which were utilized in training and teaching [18]. Others of course, would develop simulators or phantom trainers that could be utilized to help the neophyte cystoscopist develop proficiency in handling the cystoscope [19].

Light Guides and the Urinary Tract

Vision and sight are humans' most dominant sense and particularly the sense that physicians utilize the most for discerning subtle signs of pathology. Light has long since fascinated mankind, but our ability to manipulate it and refine its intensity is a relatively late event. Sunlight was the dominant source up to and including the nineteenth century, but burning animal fats and vegetable oils were utilized. Since the beginnings of medicine as a profession the ability to utilize light to aid in diagnosis has been documented at least as soon as the Hippocratic period when the speculum was described. Most likely, the first instrument described for peering into the recesses of the human body was a rectal speculum. Hippocrates' treatise on fistulas clearly mentions this technique and later, Galen's *Levicom* refers to the catopter which is an anal speculum [20]. Long-fingered urethral specula were devised and utilized by the 16th and 17th centuries. The limitation only being the amount of sunlight that could be directed into the visual field, usually only for a few centimeters, but innovative urethroscopists devised reflecting mirrors to aid in visualization

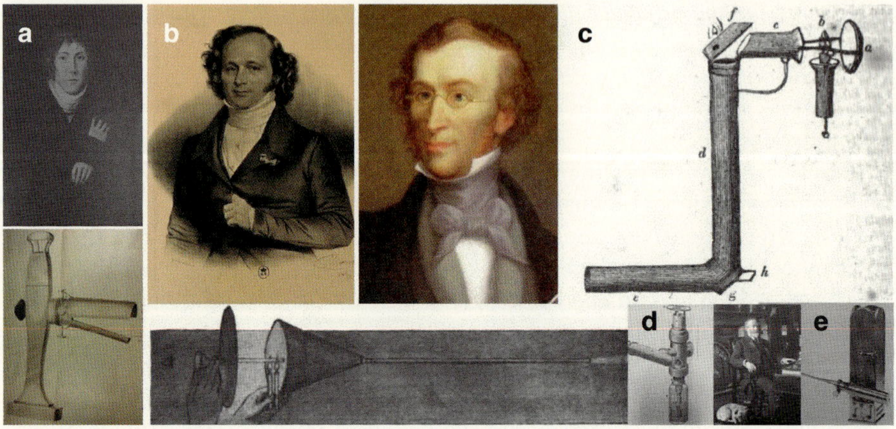

Fig. 2.1 The founding fathers of endoscopy. (**a**) Philipp Bozzini and his Lichtleiter, (**b**) Pierre Salamon Ségalas and his speculum urethra-cystique, (**c**) John Dix Fisher and his early American endoscope, (**d**) Antonin Jean Desormeaux's endoscope (**e**) Francis R. Cruise and his modified Desormeaux scope

which were then applied to general cystoscopes of the late nineteenth century. Bee's wax candles would work when finally mineral oils with additions such as turpentine added to the light intensity with the side-effect of more heat. Finally, heated platinum wires which produced incandescence were investigated following William Hyde Wollastan's breakthrough in isolating and purifying platinum in London almost single-handedly as well as devising methods for generating fine platinum wires [21, 22]. Julius Bruck, who was a dentist, picked up on the potential augmented illumination by the brilliance of incandescent platinum wires to visualize within body cavities, though these early prototypes required complex water-cooled irrigating systems [23]. In 1880 Thomas Edison presented his incandescent electric light bulb and the Scottish physician, David Newman in Glasgow placed and incandescent bulb in the distal end of a rather large cystoscope [24]. Charles Preston followed, an electrician from Rochester, New York devised a 'cold' low amperage mignon bulb in 1898 and Ferdinand Valentine in New York City devised an air-cystoscope that utilized these newest innovations [25].

Waxed candles and mirrors provided the illumination for the first endoscope. Phillip Bozzini (Germany) in 1805 constructed an instrument called "lichtleiter" for the viewing of the openings in the human body (Fig. 2.1a) [26]. Bozzini's insight into the potential for direct visualization of the body is as amazing as the harsh criticism of his peers regarding his endoscopic adventures utilizing his device. Bozzini's light guide consisted of a housing in which a candle was placed. Open tubes of various sizes and configurations could be placed on one side [27]. He then devised a reflecting mirror between the visual tract and the candle light, so that the light would be reflected only toward the targeted organ and not backward into the examiner's eye. The opposite side of the system was the eyepiece. He had published his results in 1806 and began to lecture in 1807 and even tried to have prospective studies of the instrument performed in military hospitals of the time [26, 27]. This development was remarkable in that it was the first use of reflected light as an illumination source. Unfortunately he was censured for his ingenuity since the intended use of the instrument was considered an unnatural act under contemporary mores. Bozzini died at the age of 35 after contracting typhus probably acquired during house calls [26].

In 1824 an ingenious physician in Boston, John Dix Fischer, almost replicated Bozzini's attempts with virtually the same outcomes (Fig. 2.1c). He published his only paper on his endoscope in 1827 as "an instrument for the illumination of dark cavities" [28]. He utilized higher illuminating burning oil as well as integrated telescopic lenses from a periscope. In his paper he even mentions that illumination with a galvanized wire might be possible (incandescence) [28] (Fig. 2.1b). Two years later, in Paris before the Academy of Sciences, Pierre Salomon Ségalas presented his 'urethrocystic speculum' for examination of the urethra and the bladder [29]. Daniel Colladon demonstrated light guiding at the University of Geneva in 1841 [30]. Total internal reflection of light made for a spectacular demonstration and this mechanism was quickly artificially simulated by fellow physicist, Auguste de la Rive using an electric arc light [3]. Jacques Babinet also took the method to use bent glass rods to examine difficult regions of the oral cavity in 1840 [3]. The Paris Opera began to use the same methods for spectacular stage effects in 1849 "*Elias et Mysis*" and again in 1853 for Gounod's *Faust* [3]. In England, John Avery also toyed with a version of a cystourethroscope and apparently Sir Henry Thompson was given a demonstration by 1840. Thompson stated, "*very little could be seen in the bladder.*" Other external illumination sources followed, however the next major innovation was to be the development of an independent light source that could be transported into the body cavity being inspected. Julius Bruck (Poland) in 1860 examined the mouth using illumination provided by a platinum wire loop heated by an electric current within a water jacket [23]. This was the first galvanic endoscope and preceded the invention of Edison's filament globe by 20 years. There were numerous other descriptions throughout the remainder of the late nineteenth century on open tube endoscopy procedures including Kussmaul's description of removal of a foreign body from the esophagus using reflected sunlight. Killian in 1898 employed a tube endoscope with illumination via a reflecting head mirror with the assistance of topical cocaine to inspect the bronchus [31].

Antonin Jean Desormeaux in 1867 developed "open tube" endoscopy for examination of the genitourinary tract and was the first to identify that lenses serve to condense the light source beam to a narrower brighter region that allows for more intricate observations [32] (Fig. 2.1d). He is considered by many to be the father of endoscopy because his work was so influential to the others that followed. In his popular book, he stated triumphantly "Nos quoque oculos eruditos habemus" [32]. Hacken in 1862 and Cruise in 1865 directly picked up the work of Desormeaux and began to investigate small modifications and improvements (Fig. 2.1e). Bevan in 1868 utilized such a device to remove foreign bodies in the esophagus using a ¾ inch diameter, 4 in. length tube with a reflecting mirror [6]. Waldenburg in 1870 lengthened these instruments and referred to them as "telescopes." Furstenheim in Berlin substituted gas for the petroleum light and Andrews then Stein utilized a magnesium light. In 1881, American entrepreneur William Wheeler developed a "light pipe" which he hoped to deliver light to every household, but the incandescent bulb would become his chief rival [3]. The International Health Exhibition held in South Kensington of 1884 displayed a giant "illuminated fountain" created by Sir Francis Bolton [3]. Stoerk in 1887 designed a right angled endoscope to allow greater manipulation away from the ocular [13]. In that same year, Charles Vernon Boys developed a method of creating small stretched almost pure silica fibers that could transmit light [6]. Rosenheim in 1895 employed a flexible rubber obturator for safer introduction and easier handling of endoscopes [6]. Kelling in 1897 designed a true flexible scope with small interdigitating metal rings covered by rubber on the outside [6].

Killian in 1898 first used cocaine anesthesia during bronchoscopy [31]. Nitze in 1879 pioneered the first modern endoscope for cystoscopy [33]. He worked with an optician (Beneche), an instrument maker (Leiter), and a dentist (Lesky) to create a 7 mm. deviating prismed endoscope with a liquid cooled glowing wire of platinum [34]. He followed this later with a separate light source, a miniature electric globe (Mignon Lampchen) [25]. In the United States, Otis designed a new cystoscope with telescopic lenses and a distal electric globe. The instrument maker for this scope was Reinhold Wappler (1900) and clearly became the premier optical system of that time. In 1936 Schindler worked with Wolf (an optical physicist) to design the first working flexible endoscope with steel spiral construction and 48 lenses [6]. As early as 1893, Albert Musehold described an apparatus to photograph the endoscopic appearance of the pharynx [35]. Nitze published the first photographic atlas of the pathology of the urinary bladder in 1893 [36]. On December 30, 1926 Clarence Weston Hansell, an RCA engineer wanted to view images from a distance using fiberoptic bundles [37]. Henning and Keihack published the first color photographic pictures of the stomach in 1938 (Rudolf Schindler developed a rigid, then a semi-rigid gastroscope and Heinrich Lamm tried to reproduce Hansell's findings with fiberoptics as a third year medical student using commercially available optical fiber) [38, 39]. Lejeune produced the first endoscopic motion pictures of the larynx in 1936.

Abraham Cornelius Sebastian van Heel noted that cladding improved the light transfer and image quality of fiberoptics and speculated that it could be used for cystoscopy in a letter he published in *Nature* [40]. Harold Horace Hopkins also published in the same volume of *Nature* with a young graduate student named Narinder S. Kapany, but their fibers were unclad [41]. Basil Hirschowitz (a physician) and Lawrence E. Curtiss (a physics student, later transferring to the American Cystoscope Makers, Inc.) working at the University of Michigan produced a fiberoptic gastroscope which was first tried on Hirschowitz and then presented at the annual meeting of the Optical Society of America in October 1956 in Lake Placid (site of the first digital televised sporting event using fiberoptics) [42]. Numerous modern advances have contributed to our modern arsenal of endoscopic equipment (fiber optic bundles, super-heated halide element light sources, electronic charged-coupled devices, CCD, and others) [43, 44]. The need to be able to visualize and eventually operate with tiny endoscopic manipulators is increasingly apparent [45].

Early Endoscopic Developments

Maximilian Carl-Fridrich Nitze (1848–1906) was a general practitioner who thought that if an instrument could be introduced with ease, minimal pain, and relative safety that the endoscopes must be smaller [34] (Fig. 2.2d). His idea was to place lenses into the tubes at prescribed distances to focus the image at an ocular. In addition, his early version used a platinum wire in a glass jacket with water cooling methods. He began clinical investigations with this cystoscope in 1877. By 1879, Nitze's design team was aware of Edison's invention of the filament globe and they immediately miniaturized it to fit into the tip of the cystoscopes [46]. But Nitze's reputation not only included his brilliance and dedication to the development of the cystoscope, he was also well known for his dark side, biting sarcasm and intolerance for any modifications that were not his own. In telling statements by Hugh Hampton Young, the fifth President of the A.U.A in 1908, "*And I decided to go to Berlin for study and experience. I spent two months at the clinic of Dr. Leopold Casper who had devised the most practical cystoscope for ureter catheterization. It was not difficult to learn to use his instrument, and I profited greatly by his lectures and the large number of cases I saw at his clinic. Nitze had devised a retrograde cystoscope with a complicated system of lenses and a mirror to look backward and view the neck of the bladder. He had never been successful, because the mirror became clouded. Working with a lensmaker, I constructed a four-sided prism with which we could replace Nitze's mirror. A cystoscope was constructed with a prism in place gave an excellent retrograde view of the bladder. Casper was delighted that I had been able to improve an instrument made by Nitze. When I proposed to take it to the father of cystoscopy, Casper said: 'Don't do it. He will insult you.' Nitze had broken with almost everyone with whom he worked. He brought lawsuits against Leiter, who constructed his first cystoscope, Hartwig who made several others for him, and Heinemann who had also worked with him. When Casper brought out his catheterizing cystoscope, Nitze had sued him for a large sum*" [47]. The first actual use of the Edison incandescent lamp for cystoscopic application was by Newman

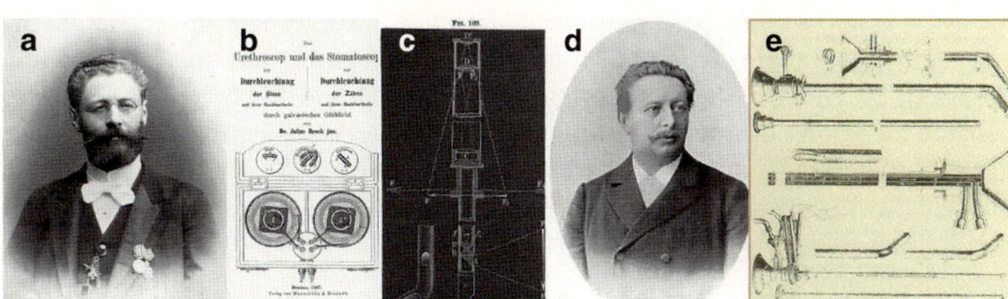

Fig. 2.2 Early modern cystoscopes. (**a**) Julius Bruck, (**b**) Bruck's modification of Wollaston's fine platinum wires for incandescensce, (**c**) du Rocher's cystoscope, (**d**) Maximilian Carl-Friedrich Nitze, (**e**) Some of Nitze's first cystoscopes

(Glasgow, 1883), followed by Nitze (1887), Leiter (1887), and Dittel (1887) [25]. Modern methods of cystoscopic development and utilization would now follow the pathway to its current utilization in urology- the extension of the urologist, and now often times by physician-extenders as a diagnostic and therapeutic in everyday practice (Fig. 2.2e). Nitze stated, "*The writing presents only a framework, the complete construction of which will be accomplished over the course of years through the joint work of numerous researchers. We are dealing here with a large new field of work which assuredly harbors untold treasures of knowledge*" [46].

The modern instrument was now only steps away from both development as well as utilization and innumerable workers in the field of urology entered into a frenzied developmental cycle of creation and improvement utilizing now the major manufacturers of instruments in Germany, France, England and the United States. Just following the turn of the twentieth century urology as a specialty was ready for full fledged speciality status. Rapid advances in radiology improved upon the ability of X-rays to image the urinary tract. Listerian antiseptic methods of surgery allowed the virtual unlimited potential of surgery to intervene on the entire genito-urinary system. Anesthesia made tremendous strides for patient management during ever more complex surgical interventions. Now the full potential for the cystoscope was poised to bring the next phase to the complex pathway for the development of modern urology. We will utilize one relatively obscure hospital, not Johns Hopkins, to make this point about the potential of the cystoscope and its profound impact on the direction of urology- the Mount Sinai Hosptial in New York City [48]. This was originally the Jew's Hospital founded in 1852 on West 28th Street by Israel Moses and Alexander Mott. No coincidence was the fact that one of the early specialists in New York City, William Holme Van Buren married Mott's daughter and became one of the first urinary specialists at Bellvue Hospital where F. Tilden Brown would eventually emigrate. A dermatology/venereal disease clinic began at Mt. Sinai in 1890 with Sigmund Lustgarten and Hermann Goldenberg who became chief of urology, when this service was started in the Department of Surgery in 1895 [49]. William Fluhrer took the reigns after joining the Hospital in 1880. The chief of surgery was Howard Lilienthal, himself to bcome famous also practiced cystoscopy. George Brewer was the first to use rubber gloves in surgery in 1899 at Mt. Sinai. Hermann Goldenberg utilized the cystoscope to diagnose and treat urethral polyps [49]. F. Tilden Brown did his internship at Mount Sinai but Leo Buerger became the young urologist of note by 1908, considered the protégé of Emanuel Libman the premier clinician of his time in New York [50, 51]. Buerger developed his own modified cystoscope in 1908 and began extensive investigations and writing from this time onward [51]. Edwin Beer joined the team and developed a pediatric cystoscope in 1911 and then went on to become chief as well as develop new methods of treating bladde cancer by electrodessication and then resection [52, 53]. Maximillian Stern was appointed in 1910 and developed the Stern-McCarthy resectoscope by 1926. He was the Chief of Urology from 1911 to 1937 [54]. Moses Swick joined the house staff in 19924 after working in

Berlin on fellowship funds gifted by Libman to work in Berlin with von Lichtenberg and modern urinary tract radiology developed following the perfection of intravenous pyelography. By the time the Hospital upgraded its primitive cystoscopy suite in 1933, 1800 cystoscopies were performed annually [48]. In 1939 this increased to 2900. In 1935 the urology group was performing about 1000 transurethral prostate resections annually [15]. Modern urology had come into existance.

The Cystoscope

The role that cystoscopy was about to have can also be seen by reference again to Hugh Young, who describes the use of the cystoscope in clinical practice at Johns Hopkins, "*Before long the American Surgical Society met at the Johns Hopkins Hospital. I was invited to appear before the meeting in the amphitheater and to catheterize the ureters of a male patient. Dr. Howard A. Kelly was to do the same in a female. Kelly's patient, under deep anesthesia, was brought in; she was in the knee-chest position. He introduced his cystoscope, which was an open tube with external illumination from a head mirror, but without lens system. The bladder was distended with air; Dr. Kelly quickly inserted a catheter first up one ureter and then up the other amid the applause of the audience. I was nervous when I brought in my patient, who was not anesthetized. Introducing Casper's cystoscope, I too had little difficulty finding the ureters and promptly catheterized them. The audience had their watches out. The contest was close, and each of us required only two or three minutes*" [47].

Throughout this time, urologists have managed to extend the limits of visualized access to the recesses of the urinary tracts though early cystoscopes were expensive and did not give an adequate view (Fig. 2.3a). There have been improvements in optical imaging systems, both rod-lens and fiber optic. Illumination systems provided unprecedented color and brightness secondary to halide lamps. Minimization of the trauma of access is the result of smaller and smaller endoscopes. Finally, by moving the surgeon's eye away from the ocular, video camera

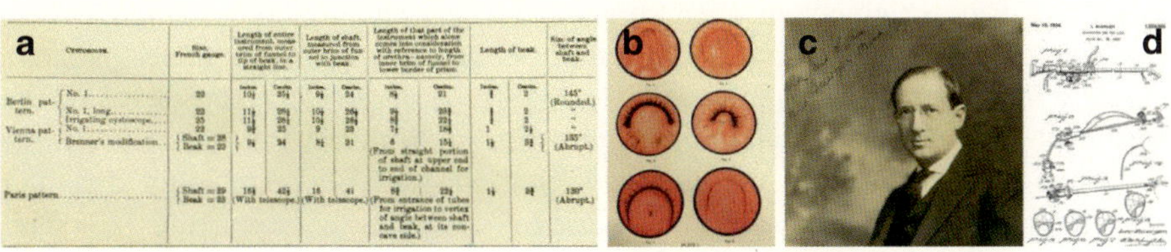

Fig. 2.3 First commercial cystoscopes. (**a**) Comparison from Willy Meyers chapter on "Cystoscopy" from Prince Morrow's textbook, *A System of Genito-Urinary Diseases* 1893, (**b**) Luy's colored illustration of cystoscopic view of the verumontanum, from *A Treatise on Cystoscopy and Urethroscopy*, C.V. Mosby, St. Louis 1918, (**c**) Leo Buerger from about 1934, (**d**) One of several of Buerger's patents for cystoscopes

systems allow the urologist the freedom to control complex endoscopic interventions. Electronics is now the key to many of these newer innovations. The charged coupled device was invented by George Smith and Willard Boyle at the Bell Laboratory on October 17, 1969 for electronic video recording. This was rapidly applied to fiber optic technology initially by Welch Allyn in 1983. Japanese makers Olympus, Fuji and Pentax all introduced video-endoscopy in the early 1980s [55]. The digital cystoscope that are now almost universally utilized by many modern urologists makes the performance of this task even easier on our patients. Though initially perceived as having a longer learning curve than rigid cystoscopy, the fact that skilled secondary medical providers are now capable of performing some routine cystoscopic tasks probably represents the future. Virtual reality cystoscopy is undoubtedly possible by newer imaging modalities, but the lower urinary tract remains complex and there is some distinct probability that some sort of direct imaging system might still need to be deployed for compete visualization for some time to come [56].

This has been a revised history of the cystoscope primarily focusing upon the technology itself and the impact that this technology has had upon the burgeoning field of urology. It would be fitting to conclude with a nearly forgotten saga that so typifies history, yet serves as the punctuation to conclude this tale as it involves one of the major players, Leo Buerger. As we have seen, the Mount Sinai Hospital in New York City, heralded some of the very first innovations in urology at the turn of the twentieth century [48, 51, 57] (Fig. 2.3c). Sarah Bernhardt was at the peak of her international reputation considered by many to be the first superstar diva of the modern era who bridged between the stage and early silent films. She was touring the U.S. when she became ill with obstructive pyohydronephrosis just following her appearance for the 4th of July festivities in New York City. Ms. Bernhardt was admitted to Mount Sinai under the care of Dr. Emanuel Libman, whose archives at the National Library of Medicine are indebted for maintaining the records of this specific encounter. Leo Buerger, the urologist was asked to see and evaluate the starlet and he proceeded to operate upon Ms. Bernhardt on Saturday July 14th and he recorded that a "*large amount of pus washed out from left kidney.*" Her vital signs during the ensuing post-cystoscopic period reflect that she remained unwell. She had five attending physicians including her own private French physician that met again on the evening of Tuesday, July 17th when her condition had become critical enough to warrant emergent open surgery. Buerger again records, "*Incision was made into the kidney and six ounces of foul smelling pus obtained. Large irregular calculus in the pelvis, which was removed.*" Her post-operative records revealed that her hospital vital signs showed rapid improvement. With no available antibiotics it is almost miraculous that she survived. She adopted Buerger's only daughter, Yvonne and as her godmother became close to Germaine Schnitzer, Buerger's wife. Of the five attending physicians who cared for Ms. Bernhardt, she kept in contact with both Buerger and Libman in her final years [58]. She was a dynamo of activity working on another silent movie in her final year, dying on March 26, 1923 in Paris. Dr. Buerger's life apparently fell to pieces following this surgery, becoming a footnote only in the history of urology.

Cystoscopy rapidly expanded with the development of newer and cheaper endoscopes in the arly part of the twentieth century as did the specialty of urology with rapid progression, in fact, this explosion of technology is quite complex to fully chronicle since so many investigators were involved [59] (Figs. 2.4 and 2.5). The cystoscope has changed to include both flexible cystourethroscopes as well as digital flexible cystourethroscopes. Already histories of these flexible cystoscopes are becoming rapidly antiquated by even more advanced technologies [60]. No longer does it appear necessary that the urologist be the person performing the cystoscopy, at least in non-complex situations [61]. Capsular endoscopy has also been developed for GI utility and it is probable that such technology can and will be adapted for cystoscopy in the future [62]. The ability of radiographic imaging to better visualize the lower urinary tract might also result in "virtual cystoscopy" [63].

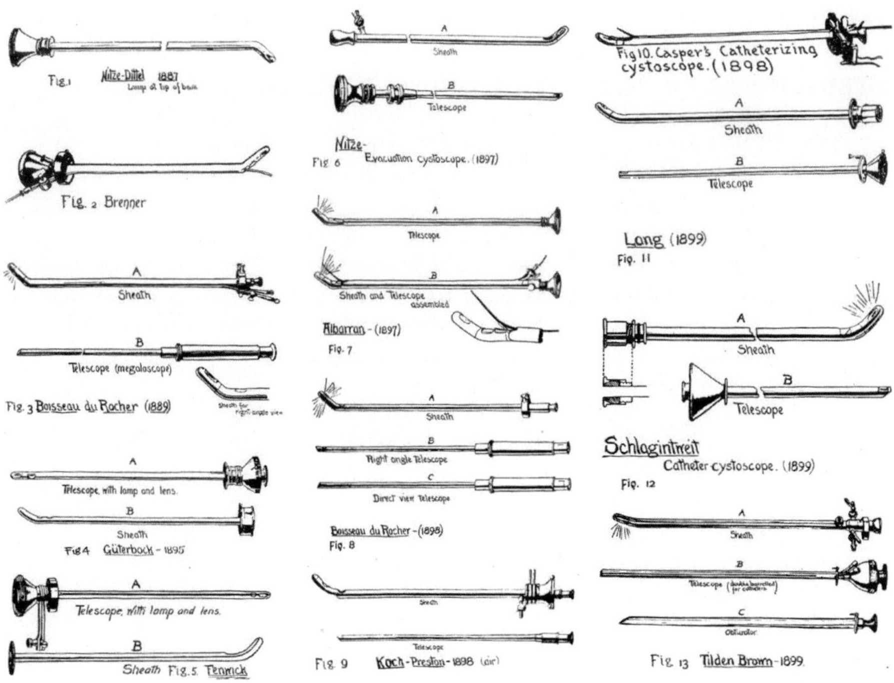

Fig. 2.4 Summary of modern cystoscopes via Bransford Lewis's ***Illustrated Résumé*** from his 1908 paper (Illustrations 1–13)

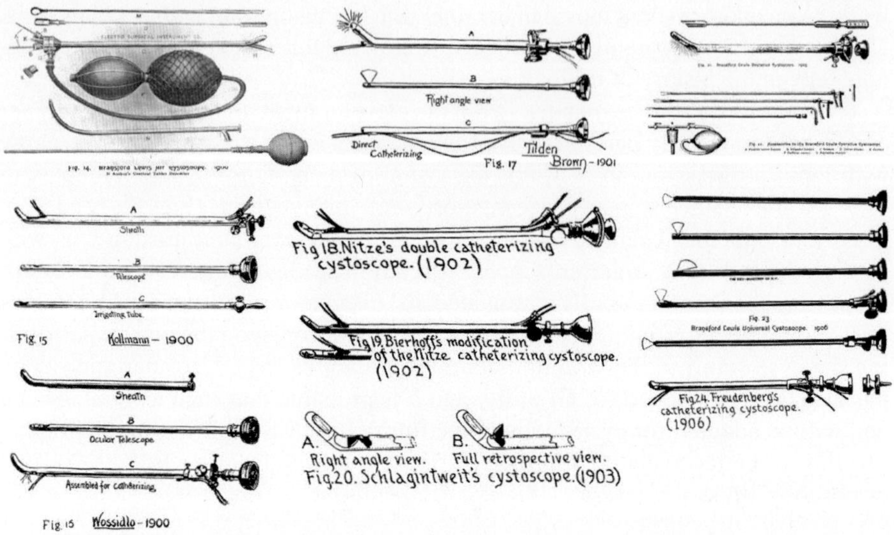

Fig. 2.5 Summary of modern cystoscopes via Bransford Lewis's ***Illustrated Résumé*** from his 1908 paper (Illustrations 14–24)

Bransford Lewis Tabulated History (Modified) [64]

1806	Philipp Bozzini of Frankfurt presents Lichtleiter to Josephine Academy
1824	John Dix Fisher wrote about his telescopic endoscope but it was published in 1827
1826	Pierre Salamon Ségalas presents his "Speculum urethra-cystique" to Academy of Sciences of France
1826	M. Bombolzini an illuminated speculum supposedly utilized on the urinary bladder
1853	Antonin J. Desormeaux- presented to Imperial Academy of Medicine in 1855 utilizing spirit lamp; first real descriptions of bladder pathology; published book in 1865
1862	August Haken- used dilation and direct vision scope in women's urethra and bladder, head mirror
1865	Francis R. Cruise utilizes a modification of Desormeaux's device
1867	E. Andrews modifies Desormeaux's device but uses magnesium wire incandescence for urethroscopy
1867	Julius Bruck- platinum-wire glow-lamp
1868	Philip Skinner Wales- publishes on endoscopy Figure 2.6c. and d.
1870	Furstenheim substituted combustion from gas to illuminate urethroscope
1872	Robert Newman- New York presented modifications and expanded series Figure 2.6a. and b.
1874–1876	Grünfeld- endoscopic inspection of bladder; introduction of ureteral catheter outside and along the endoscope, first successful endoscopic ureteral catheterization; external mirror illumination (rapidly modified by Steurer and then Klotz)
1875	Gustav Simon- first ureteral catheterization, "fishing method" via anatomical landmarks and touch
1876	Rutenberg, Vienna, used forced air-inflation for distension of bladder
1877	Maximilian Carl-Friedrich Nitze- first application of telescopic lenses for cystoscopes, uses Bruck's glow-lamp (incandescent platinum filament), wrote book on cystoscopy in 1889

1880	Dittel- applied glow-lamp to tip of beak
1883	David Newman- first to use incandescent lamp in cystoscopy
1885	Boisseau du Rocher- incandescent lamp with indirect-view with megaloscopic lenses
1886–1888	Karl Pawlik- air-distension, knee-chest cystoscopy in females and ureteral catheterization, external illumination
1887	Max Nitze- application of Edison bulb to two models of cystoscope, direct and indirect views with telescopic lenses, Lehrbuch der Kystokopie 1889
1887	Leiter- indirect-view telescopic lens cystoscope (similar to Nitze 1)
1887	Dittel- application of incandescent lamp to tip of beak, indirect view
1889	Alexander Brenner- addition of single ureteral catheter channel to Nitze's direct-view cystoscope (James Brown, 1st urologist at Johns Hopkins uses his scope to catheterize a male's ureter)
1889	Boisseau du Rocher- composite cystoscope; first of sheath-and-telescope plan; first to give synchronous double ureteral catheterization through two channels; two models for direct and indirect views
1891	F. Tilden Brown develops a bivalved-wire urethral speculum, indirect illumination (first a mirror then developed an electric light delivery system)
1891	W. K. Otis modifies Leiter and Nitze's instruments for urethroscopy, in 1892 calls it the 'perfected urethroscope"
1892	E. Hurry Fenwick also modifies Nitze device called aero-urethroscope
1893	Howard A. Kelly- air-distension, direct-view, similar to Pawlik's (complains that Nitze device though ideal for males is too "*elaborate, delicate and expensive for examining females*")
1894	Leopold Casper- first model of catheterizing cystoscope, indirect-view
1894	Friedrich Nitze- single tube ureter-catheterizing cystoscope, indirect-view
1895	Güterbock- sheath-and-telescope, both lamp and lens on telescope, indirect-view, non-catheterizing, irrigation through sheath
1896	E. Hurry Fenwick- sheath-and-telescope, both lamp and lens on telescope, indirect-view, non-catheterizing, irrigation through sheath, writes Electric Illumination of the Bladder and Urethra in 1904
1897	M. Nitze- evacuation cystoscope, sheath-and-telescope, indirect-view, non-catheterizing, free irrigation for evacuation through sheath
1897	Joaquin Albarrán- sheath-with-telescope, indirect-view, irrigation and ureteral catheterization, movable lever-system to direct catheter
1898	Boisseau du Rocher- improved 2nd system, multi-telescopes for direct and indirect views, irrigation
1898	Koch-Preston- cold lamp, air cystoscope, sheath and multiple telescopes, for direct and indirect-views, extra tube for ureteral catheter
1898	Leopold Casper- double catheterization cystoscope
1899	Lang- sheath-and-telescope, indirect-view, non-catheterizing
1899	Schlagintweit- evacuation, sheath-and-telescope, indirect view, non-catheterizing
1899	F. Tilden Brown- sheath-and-telescope, double catheter channel, direct view
1900	Bransford Lewis- air cystoscope, fixed ureter catheter channel (first single, then double)
1900	Kollmann- sheath-and-indirect telescope, irrigating, non-catheterizing
1900	Wossidlo- sheath-and-indirect telescope, double catheterizing, non-irrigating
1900	F. Tilden Brown- composite sheath, multiple telescopes, direct and right-angle view, double catheterizing, irrigation, lamp at tip of beak (Dittel's plan)
1902	M. Nitze- double catheterizing cystoscope

1902	Bierhoff- modified Nitze, sheath-and-scope
1903	Schlagintweit- retrograde cystoscope by movable lens, non-catheterizing
1903	Hugh H. Young- retroscpective fixed-prism cystoscope
1903	Bransford Lewis- operative air-distension cystoscope
1903	Le Für posterior urethroscope
1904	Kolischer-Schmidt- sheath-and-telescope, distal window, direct-view, double catheterizing using Casper's arrangement
1904	Follen Cabot- composite cystoscope, direct-view, double catheterizing, lamp on beak, irrigation
1904	Bransford Lewis- set globular-lens for retrospective view
1904	Baer- universal cystoscope, sheath-and-multiple telescopes, catherizing, irrigation, and operative features
1904	Freudenberg- direct-view double catheterizing (altered in 1906)
1904	Georges Luys- direct-view, air cystoscope for females only
1905	G. Luys- direct-view, air cystoscope for males, textbook A Treatise on Cystoscopy and Urethroscopy translated into English by Abraham Wolbarst in 1918
1905	Cathelin- direct-view air cystoscope
1905	W. K. Otis- sheath and close-fitting telescope, wide-angle indirect-view, non-catheterizing
1906	Goldschmidt irrigation cystoscope
1906	Bransford Lewis- universal cystoscope, sheath with multiple telescopes, double catheterization, irrigation, protected inverted lamp
1906	Freudenberg- seath-and-telescope, double catheterizing, irrigation, movable-cath lever
1907	Freudenberg- multiple sheaths, single telescope, indirect-view, non-catheterization, irrigation
1907	Kreissl- sheath, direct-view, double catheterizing
1909	Leo Buerger- modified Goldschmidt, Brenner and Brown's instruments and makes device with Reinhold Wappler (Wappler Electric Co, NYC) Brown-Buerger cystoscope

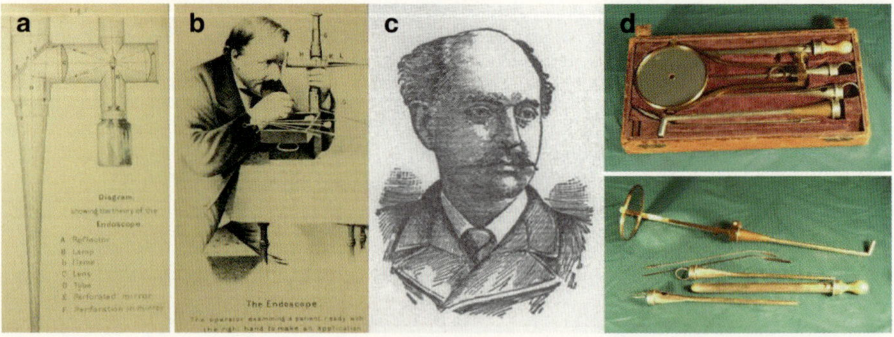

Fig. 2.6 Early cystoscopes. (**a**) Robert Newman's 1872 modification of Desormeaux's scope, (**b**) The Endoscopist, (**c**) General Philip Skinner Wales of Washington, DC, (**d**) The Wales cystoscope

References

1. Moran ME. The law of accelerating returns. J Endourol. 2006;20(6):1–8.
2. Bragg W. The universe of light. New York: Macmillan Co.; 1933.
3. Hecht J. City of lights: the story of fiber optics. New York: Oxford University Press; 1999.
4. Wales PS. Instrumental diagnosis. Med Surg Rep. 1868;18(18):377–81.
5. Kelly HA, Burnam CF. Diseases of the kidneys, ureters and bladder. New York: D Appleton & Co.; 1914.
6. Moran ME. In: Monga M, editor. History of ureteroscopy. Ureteroscopy: indications, instrumentation & technique. New York: Springer; 2013. p. 3–12.
7. Guiteras R. The evolution of urology. N Y Med J. 1902;76(15):617–22.
8. Lewis B. The dawn and development of urology. Trans Am Urol Assoc. 1907;1:9–19.
9. Cabot H. Is urology entitled to be regarded as a specialty? Trans Am Urol Assoc. 1911;5:1–20.
10. Krotoszyer M. Urology-past, present, and future. Am J Urol Sex. 1911;10:292–6.
11. Young HH. The Renaissance of urology. South Med J. 1916;9(2):146–53.
12. Newman D. Cystoscopic appearances of renal and vesical tuberculosis in the early stages demonstrated by the projectoscope. Am J Urol Vener Sex Dis. 1914;10(8):401–10.
13. Fenwick EH. Presidential address to the section on urology of the XVIIth international medical congress in London. Am J Urol Vener Sex Dis. 1914;10(8):355–68.
14. Newman R. The endoscope: considered particularly in reference to diseases of the female bladder and urethra. Albany: Weed, Parson & Co.; 1872.
15. Brendler H, Ferber WLF. Early days of urology at Mount Sinai. Urology. 1974;3(2):246–50.
16. Brueger L. The normal and pathological posterior urethra and neck of the bladder. Am J Urol Sex. 1911;7(2):1–10.
17. Buerger L. Cysto-urethroscopy. A study of the normal and pathological posterior urethra. Trans Am Urol Assoc. 1911;5:130–68.
18. Wolbarst AL. Demonstration of wax models of pathologic lesions observed in the posterior male urethra by means of the posterior urethroscope. Trans Am Urol Assoc. 1915;9:470–5.
19. Fenwick EH. A handbook of clinical electric-light cystoscopy. London: J&A Churchill; 1904.
20. Peters L. The evolution of modern cystoscopic instruments and methods. Am J Obstest Dis Women Child. 1906;54:486–501.
21. Wollaston WH. The Bakerian lecture: on a method of rendering platina malleable. Philos Trans R Soc Lond. 1829;119:1–8.
22. Wollaston WH. A method of drawing extremely fine wires. Proc R Soc Lond. 1800;1:455–6.
23. Bruck J. Das Urethroscop und StomatoscopDurchGalvanischesGluhlict. Breslau: Marushke and Berendt; 1867.
24. Newman D. Lectures to practitioners on the diseases of the kidney amenable to surgical treatment. Glasgow Med J 1883;131.
25. Moran ME. The light bulb, cystoscopy and Thomas Alva Edison. J Endourol. 2010;24(9):1395–7.
26. Figdor PP. Philip Bozzini: the beginnings of modern endoscopy. Tuttlingen: Verlag Endo-Press; 2002.
27. Bozzini P. Lichtleiter, eineEnfindungzurAuschschauunginnere Theiler und Krankheiten. J der PractischenArzneykunde und Wunderartzneykunst. 1806;24:107–24.
28. Fisher JD. Instruments for illuminating dark cavities. Phil J Med Phys Sci. 1827;14:409.
29. Segalas PR. Un moyend'eclairer 'uretre et la vessie de maniere a voirdansl'interieur de ces organs. Revue MedicaleFrancaise et de L'etrangere. 1827;1:157–8.
30. Colladon D. On the reflections of a ray of light inside a parabolic liquid stream. Comptes Rendus. 1842;15:800.
31. Killian G. ZurGeschicnte der Oesophago und Gastroskopie. Deutsche Zeitschrift fur Chirirgie. 1900;59:499–512.
32. Desmoreaux AJ. The endoscope and its application to the diagnosis and treatment of affections of the genitourinary passages. Chicago Medizinhist J. 1867;24:177–94.
33. Nitze M. Eineneue Beleuchtungs und Untersuchungs method fur Harnrohre, Harnblase, und Rektum. Wiener Med Wochen. 1879;24:649.

34. Nitze M. Beitragezur Endosckopie der mannlichen Hamblase. Arch fur KlinishceChirurgie. 1881;36:661–732.
35. Musehold A. Stroboskopische und Photographische Studien. Ann des Mal du Larynx Jan 1893.
36. Nitze MCF. Kystophotograpischer atlas. Wiesbaden: JF Bergmann; 1894.
37. Sircus W, Flisk E, Craigs Z. Milestones in the evolution of endoscopy: a short history. J R Coll Physicians Edinb. 2003;33:124–34.
38. Brittain JE. Scanning the past. Hansell, CW and Carter, PS. Proc IEEE 1996;84(4).
39. Henning N, Keilhack H. Die gezielteFarbenphotographie in der Magenhohle. Deutsche Med Wschr. 1938;64:1392–3.
40. van Heel ACS. A method of transporting optical images without aberrations. Nature. 1954;173:39.
41. Hopkins HH, Kapany NS. A flexible fiberscope, using static scanning. Nature. 1954;173:39–41.
42. Hirschowitz BI. A personal history of the fiberscope. Gastroenterology. 1970;36:864–7.
43. Kieser CW. Introduction of cold light endoscopy. Aktuelle Urol. 2008;39(2):130–4.
44. Vilardell F. Digestive endoscopy in the second millennium: from Lichleiter to endoscopy. Madrid: Thieme; 2006.
45. Lang P. Candles to computers: the story of minimally invasive procedures. UWOMJ. 2011;80(1):34–6.
46. Newell OK. The endoscopic instruments of Joseph Leiter of Vienna and the present development of endoscopy. Boston Med Surg J. 1887;117:528–30.
47. Young HH. A Surgeon's autobiography. New York: Harcourt, Brace & Co.; 1940.
48. Aufses AH Jr, Niss B. This house of noble deeds: the Mount Sinai hospital, 1852–2002. New York: New York Univ Press; 2002.
49. Lilienthal H. The Mount Sinai hospital and its surgeons of the middle eighties; a few recollections. J Mt Sinai. 1937;3:229–40.
50. Brown TH. The cystoscope and ureteral catheter in the diagnosis of surgical disease of the kidney and ureter. Med News. 1905;86:442–4.
51. Buerger L. A new indirect irrigating observation and double catheterizing cystoscope. Ann Surg. 1909;49:225–37.
52. Beer E. Cystoscopy and utereral catheterization in young children. Am J Surg. 1911;25:79–81.
53. Beer E. Removal of neoplasms of the urinary bladder: a new method, employing high-frequency (Oudin) current through a catheterizing cystoscope. JAMA. 1910;54:1768–9.
54. Stern M. Minor surgery of the prostate gland; a new cystoscopic instrument employing a current capable of operation in a water medium. Int J Med Surg. 1926;39:72–7.
55. Samplaski MK, Jones JS. Two centuries of cystoscopy: the development of imaging, instrumentation and synergistic technologies. BJU Int. 2008;103:154–8.
56. Schultheiss D, Machtens SA, Jonas U. Air cystoscopy: the history of an endoscopic technique fromt the late 19th century. BJU Int. 1999;83:571–7.
57. Buerger L. Intravesical diagnosis and treatment. N Y Med J. 1913;8:57–62.
58. Moran ME. Obstructive pyohydronephrosis and life saving intervention of the greatest starlet of all time- Sarah Bernhardt. Abstract presented at 2017 American Urological Association Annual Meeting, Boston.
59. Reuter MA, Reuter HJ. The development of the cystoscope. J Urol. 1998;159:638–40.
60. Radhakrishnan S, Dorkin TJ, Johnson P, Menezes P, Greene D. Nurse-led flexible cystoscopy: experience from one UK Centre. BJU Int. 2006;98(2):256–8.
61. Wuilleumier J, Point D, Fooks H, Zaslau S. The history of cystoscopy in urology. Internet J Urol. 2015;14(1):1–8.
62. Gomella LD. From the Lichleiter to capsule cystoscopy. Eur Urol. 2009;55:1034–6.
63. Karabacak OR, Cakmakci E, Ozturk U, Demirel F, Dilli A, Hekimoglu B, Altug U. Virtual cystoscopy: the evaluation of bladder lesions with computed tomographic virtual cystoscopy. Can Urol Assoc J. 2011;5(1):34–7.
64. Lewis B. Résumé of progress in the development of modern cystoscopes. Trans Am Urol Assoc. 1908;2:215–24.

Chapter 3
History of Optics in Endourology

Kimberly A. Maciolek and Sara L. Best

Optics is the branch of physics that studies the behavior and properties of light, including its interactions with matter and the construction of instruments to detect it. From its earliest days, physicians have found the urinary tract to be a tempting target for intervention since it lies so tantalizingly close to the surface and has a natural aperture. This accessibility allowed urologic procedures to be among the earliest attempted by practitioners, with interrogation of the bladder first occurring thousands of years ago. While lithotomists made their diagnosis based on history and the transurethral "sounding" of the bladder to identify bladder calculi, the actual surgery was traumatically transperineal as the technology to *see* in the urethra and bladder did not yet exist.

The birth of endoscopy, or the ability to see inside the human body, did not occur until the nineteenth century. Dr. Phillip Bozzini in 1806 points out that in the study of the internal workings of the human body, "it is necessary that (1) a sufficient amount of light be introduced; and (2) the light rays be reflected back to the eye" [1]. Thus Bozzini, the father of endoscopy, succinctly defines the "problem" facing the developers of technology. The rest of this chapter will describe the innovations developed to address these problems.

First-Generation Endoscopy: Extracorporeal Light Sources

Bozzini began designs for his "lichtleiter," translated to "guided light," in the early 1800s (Fig. 3.1). In his 1806 publication, Bozzini describes a "vase" containing a wax candle. The tube had two apertures, one through which the user could look and

K.A. Maciolek, B.S. • S.L. Best, M.D. (✉)
Department of Urology, University of Wisconsin School of Medicine
and Public Health, Madison, WI 53705, USA
e-mail: best@urology.wisc.edu

S.R. Patel et al. (eds.), *The History of Technologic Advancements in Urology*,
DOI 10.1007/978-3-319-61691-9_3

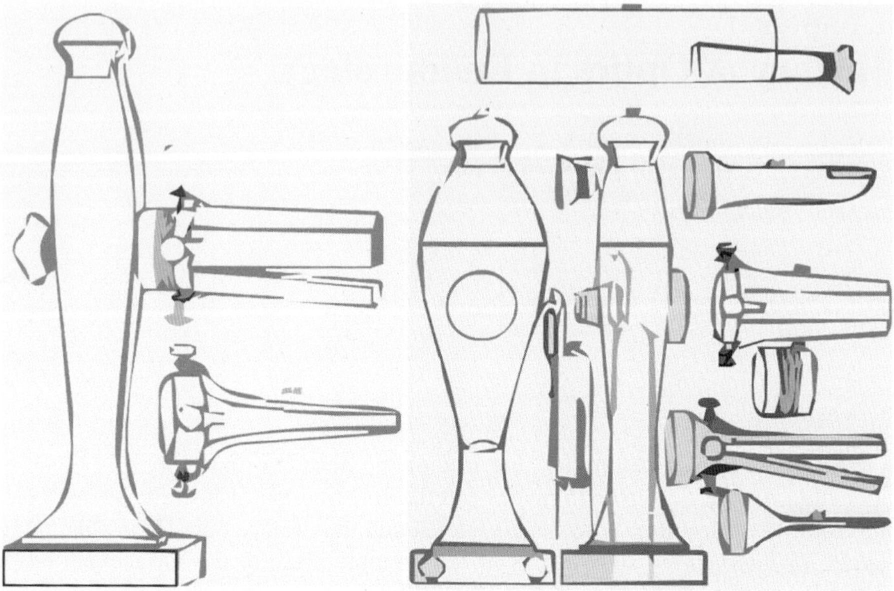

Fig. 3.1 Bozzini's Lichleiter with one aperture for the user and one for light conductors (By Philipp Bozzini (1773–1809) [Public domain], via Wikimedia Commons; By Countincr at en.wikipedia (Transferred from en.wikipedia) [Public domain], from Wikimedia Commons)

the other to which a variety of sizes of "light conductors" could be attached, some of which are strikingly similar to modern specula. The light would pass through the conductor into the target anatomy and allow the physician peering through the eyepiece to see inside [2, 3]. With this device, Bozzini successfully observed a stone within the bladder of a female cadaver. The litchtleiter, however, had limited urologic utility as it only allowed inspection of a small area of bladder mucosa and illumination was poor with weak extracorporeal lighting. Bozzini and the lichtleiter became the victim of medical politics of the day and his untimely death shortly thereafter left his invention forgotten. Despite this setback, future investigators would go on to find numerous ways to solve the bi-fold problem of endoscopy, namely to deliver light to the internal cavity and to return a useful image to the human eye [2, 3].

Decades would pass before the literature revealed new forays into the endoscopy problem. Two physicians, Pierre Salomon Segalas and John Fischer, are generally given credit for simultaneously and independently improving Bozzini's cystoscope. Segalas introduced his invention, the "urethro-cystique" in 1826, which incorporated a double lens system and mirror to improve the lighting and black coating on the viewing tube to reduce light scatter [4]. Fischer used the same principle as Segalas but used hollow tubing with two right-angled turns to form a Z-shape to visualize the urethra and bladder [5]. Like Bozzini's lichtleiter, Segalas and Fischer's inventions improved visualization but similarly failed to enable effective inspection of the bladder due to limited delivery of light.

The term 'endoscope' was coined in 1853 by French urologist Antonin Desormeaux. He reported the use of *gazogène* (a mixture of alcohol and turpentine) instead of a candle to illuminate his "l'endoscope" device based on Bozzini's lichtleiter. This new light source provided a much brighter yet clearer flame than candlelight. He also adjusted the angle of his lenses to better focus the light, providing a clearer image [4]. Désormeaux used his device to perform the first endoscopic surgery, an endoscopic excision of a urethral papilloma, and is heralded as the "father of cystoscopy." Unsurprisingly, the major complication of his procedure was burns [4]. Despite this improvement, Desormeaux's endoscope was only able to inspect a very narrow field of view and still lacked sufficient illumination [6].

Second Generation Endoscopy: The Advent of Electricity, Intracorporeal Light Sources, and Increased Field of Vision

Advances in the techniques of illumination were intimately coupled with the discovery of electricity. Bozzini's successors concentrated primarily on visualizing the urethra and bladder via speculum examination and an external light source. The next major breakthroughs came with German urologist Maximilian Nitze (Fig. 3.2). Nitze was uniquely credited with achieving a sweeping revolution in the diagnosis, treatment and photographic documentation via cystoscopy and is appropriately titled the father of modern urology [5, 7].

Nitze is credited with the first use of intracorporeal electric light sources. Aware of the limitations plaguing endoscopes of the time, Nitze is famously quoted stating that, "in order to light up a room one must carry the lamp inside" [7]. Nitze was inspired by the early works of Julius Bruck, a young dentist in Breslau, to overcome "insufficient illumination of objects" [8]. Bruck used incandescent platinum wires,

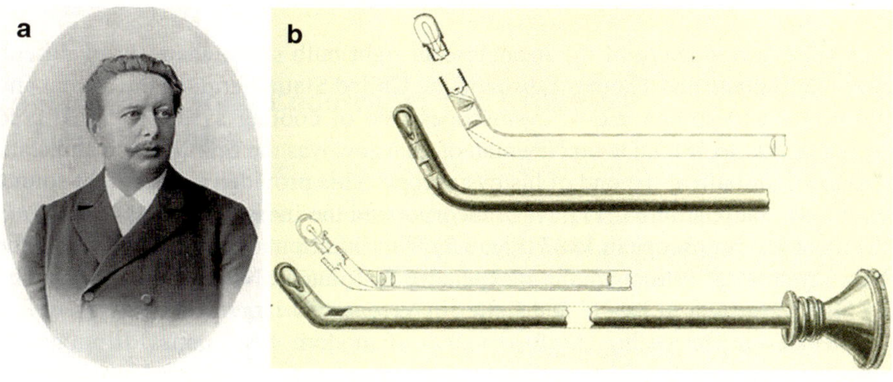

Fig. 3.2 (**a**) Maximilian Carl-Friedrich Nitze (1848–1906). (**b**) Prototype of Nitze's cystoscope including the hot platinum filament at the tip (By Internet Archive Book Images [No restrictions], via Wikimedia Commons)

14. Goodman TM. Ureteroscopy with pediatric cystoscope in adults. Urology. 1977;9(4):394.
15. Lyon ES, Banno JJ, Schoenberg HW. Transurethral ureteroscopy in men using juvenile cystoscopy equipment. J Urol. 1979;122(2):152–3.
16. Pérez-Castro E, Carbonero M, Mancebo JM, Massarra J, Iglesias JI. Treatment of benign prostatic hypertrophy using transurethral thermotherapy. Initial experience. Arch Esp Urol. 1991;44(5):637–45.
17. Hecht J. City of light. Cary: Oxford University Press; 2004.
18. Gow JG. Harold Hopkins and optical systems for urology—an appreciation. Urology. 1998;52(1):152–7.
19. Hirschowitz BI, Curtiss LE, Peters CW, Pollard HM. Demonstration of a new gastroscope, the fiberscope. Gastroenterology. 1958;35(1):50. discussion 51-53
20. Hopkins HH. Optical system having cylindrical rod-like lenses. June 28, 1966. Patent US3257902.
21. Cockett WS, Cockett AT. The Hopkins rod-lens system and the Storz cold light illumination system. Urology. 1998;51(5A Suppl):1–2.
22. Marshall VF. Fiber optics in urology. J Urol. 1964;91:110–4.
23. Takagi T, Go T, Takayasu H, Aso Y, Hioki R. Small-caliber fiberscope for visualization of the urinary tract, biliary tract, and spinal canal. Surgery. 1986;64(6):1033–8.
24. Bush IM, Whitmore WF. A fiberoptic ultraviolet cystoscope. J Urol. 1967;97(1):156–7.
25. Tsuchida S, Sugawara H. A new flexible fibercystoscope for visualization of the bladder neck. J Urol. 1973;109(5):830–1.
26. Wilbur HJ. The flexible choledochoscope: a welcome addition to the urologic armamentarium. J Urol. 1981;126(3):380–1.
27. Burchardt P. The flexible panendoscope. J Urol. 1982;127(3):479–81.
28. Wagenknecht LV. Inspection of the urinary tract by flexible instruments (author's transl). Urologe A. 1982;21(2):112–4.
29. Fowler CG. Fibrescope urethrocystoscopy. Br J Urol. 1984;56(3):304–7.
30. Clayman RV, Reddy P, Lange PH. Flexible fiberoptic and rigid-rod lens endoscopy of the lower urinary tract: a prospective controlled comparison. J Urol. 1984;131(4):715–6.
31. Fowler CG, Badenoch DF, Thakar DR. Practical experience with flexible fibrescope cystoscopy in out-patients. Br J Urol. 1984;56(6):618–21.
32. Boyle W, Smith GE. Buried channel charge coupled devices. February 12, 1974, US 3792322 A.
33. Boyle W, Smith GE. Three dimensional charge coupled devices. February 16, 1970, US 3796927 A.
34. Berci G, Paz-Partlow M. Electronic imaging in endoscopy. Surg Endosc. 1988;2(4):227–33.
35. Quayle SS, Ames CD, Lieber D, Yan Y, Landman J. Comparison of optical resolution with digital and standard fiberoptic cystoscopes in an in vitro model. Urology. 2005;66(3):489–93.
36. Andonian S, Okeke Z, Anidjar M, Smith AD. Digital nephroscopy: the next step. J Endourol. 2008;22(4):601–2.
37. Andonian S, Okeke Z, Smith AD. Digital ureteroscopy: the next step. J Endourol. 2008;22(4):603–6.
38. Shibuya K, Hoshino H, Chiyo M, Iyoda A, Yoshida S, Sekine Y, Iizasa T, Saitoh Y, Baba M, Hiroshima K, Ohwada H, Fujisawa T. High magnification bronchovideoscopy combined with narrow band imaging could detect capillary loops of angiogenic squamous dysplasia in 2008;heavy smokers at high risk for lung cancer. Thorax. 2003;58(11):989–95.
39. Yoshida T, Inoue H, Usui S, Satodate H, Fukami N, Kudo SE. Narrow-band imaging system with magnifying endoscopy for superficial esophageal lesions. Gastrointest Endosc. 2004;59(2):288–95.
40. Bryan RT, Billingham LJ, Wallace DM. Narrow-band imaging flexible cystoscopy in the detection of recurrent urothelial cancer of the bladder. BJU Int. 2008;101(6):702–705; discussion 705-706.
41. Naito S, Algaba F, Babjuk M, Bryan RT, Sun YH, Valiquette L, de la Rosette J, Group CNBIGS. The clinical research office of the endourological society (CROES) multicentre

randomised trial of narrow band imaging-assisted transurethral resection of bladder tumour (TURBT) versus conventional white light imaging-assisted TURBT in primary non-muscle-invasive bladder cancer patients: trial protocol and 1-year results. Eur Urol 2016;70(3):506–15.
42. Traxer O, Geavlete B, de Medina SG, Sibony M, Al-Qahtani SM. Narrow-band imaging digital flexible ureteroscopy in detection of upper urinary tract transitional-cell carcinoma: initial experience. J Endourol. 2011;25(1):19–23.
43. Lipson RL, Baldes EJ, Gray MJ. Hematoporphyrin derivative for detection and management of cancer. Cancer. 1967;20(12):2255–7.
44. Burger M, Grossman HB, Droller M, Schmidbauer J, Hermann G, Drăgoescu O, Ray E, Fradet Y, Karl A, Burgués JP, Witjes JA, Stenzl A, Jichlinski P, Jocham D. Photodynamic diagnosis of non-muscle-invasive bladder cancer with hexaminolevulinate cystoscopy: a meta-analysis of detection and recurrence based on raw data. Eur Urol. 2013;64(5):846–54.
45. Grossman HB, Stenzl A, Fradet Y, Mynderse LA, Kriegmair M, Witjes JA, Soloway MS, Karl A, Burger M. Long-term decrease in bladder cancer recurrence with hexaminolevulinate enabled fluorescence cystoscopy. J Urol. 2012;188(1):58–62.
46. Davidovits P, Egger MD. Scanning laser microscope. Nature. 1969;223(5208):831.
47. Hoffman A, Goetz M, Vieth M, Galle PR, Neurath MF, Kiesslich R. Confocal laser endomicroscopy: technical status and current indications. Endoscopy. 2006;38(12):1275–83.
48. Sonn GA, Jones SN, Tarin TV, CB D, Mach KE, Jensen KC, Liao JC. Optical biopsy of human bladder neoplasia with in vivo confocal laser endomicroscopy. J Urol. 2009;182(4):1299–305.
49. Tavora F, Fajardo DA, Lee TK, Lotan T, Miller JS, Miyamoto H, Epstein JI. Small endoscopic biopsies of the ureter and renal pelvis: pathologic pitfalls. Am J Surg Pathol. 2009;33(10):1540–6.
50. Wang JK, Tollefson MK, Krambeck AE, Trost LW, Thompson RH. High rate of pathologic upgrading at nephroureterectomy for upper tract urothelial carcinoma. Urology. 2012;79(3):615–9.
51. Smith AK, Stephenson AJ, Lane BR, Larson BT, Thomas AA, Gong MC, Jones JS, Campbell SC, Hansel DE. Inadequacy of biopsy for diagnosis of upper tract urothelial carcinoma: implications for conservative management. Urology. 2011;78(1):82–6.
52. Bui D, Mach KE, Zlatev DV, Rouse RV, Leppert JT, Liao JC. A pilot study of in vivo confocal laser endomicroscopy of upper tract urothelial carcinoma. J Endourol. 2015;29(12):1418–23.
53. Huang D, Swanson EA, Lin CP, Schuman JS, Stinson WG, Chang W, Hee MR, Flotte T, Gregory K, Puliafito CA. Optical coherence tomography. Science. 1991;254(5035):1178–81.
54. Lerner SP, Goh AC, Tresser NJ, Shen SS. Optical coherence tomography as an adjunct to white light cystoscopy for intravesical real-time imaging and staging of bladder cancer. Urology. 2008;72(1):133–7.
55. Manyak MJ, Gladkova ND, Makari JH, Schwartz AM, Zagaynova EV, Zolfaghari L, Zara JM, Iksanov R, Feldchtein FI. Evaluation of superficial bladder transitional-cell carcinoma by optical coherence tomography. J Endourol. 2005;19(5):570–4.
56. Miladi M, Peyromaure M, Zerbib M, Saïghi D, Debré B. The value of a second transurethral resection in evaluating patients with bladder tumours. Eur Urol. 2003;43(3):241–5.

Chapter 4
Development of the Ureteroscope

Demetrius H. Bagley

Ureteroscopy has grown from single incidental episodes to its present role as the major interventional approach to the upper urinary tract. The first endoscopes used as ureteroscopes were capable solely for visualization. Only as endoscopes were developed with channels for irrigation and mechanisms for deflection as well as appropriate working instruments did ureteroscopy become a practical and useful procedure. The process has been dependent on the materials and the instrument designs available.

In 1912, Hugh Hampton Young performed the first ureteroscopy when he unintentionally passed a rigid pediatric cystoscope into a severely dilated ureter of a pediatric patient with posterior urethral valves. This episode was not reported until 1929 in a review article on congenital urethral valves [1].

The next period of purposeful ureteroscopy began with the development and then application of fiberoptic imaging [2]. The potential of fiber optics began in the 1840s when Colodon introduced the concept of internal reflection and "light guiding" or fiber optics [3]. Babinett showed that light could be guided along bent glass rods. Baird and Hansell patented fiber bundles which could provide image transmission through internal reflection in 1927 and 1930, respectively [4]. In 1957 Curtiss developed fibers with glass cladding that improved the reflection and subsequently light transmission. In that same year, 1957, Hershkowitz used glass fibers with cladding to develop the first flexible gastroscope which he used on himself [5]. This provoked particular interest in endoscopy in other specialties [6].

In 1960 Marshall used a 9Fr flexible fiber-optic scope without a channel or deflection. It was placed through a ureterotomy during an open operation to inspect for calculi. Two years later, the first transurethral flexible ureteroscopy was performed by MacGovern and Walzak and reported by Marshall [2]. The 9Fr fiberscope

D.H. Bagley, M.D., F.A.C.S.
Department of Urology, Sidney Kimmel Medical College, Thomas Jefferson University, 1025 Walnut Street, Suite 1100, Philadelphia, PA 19107, USA
e-mail: Demetrius.bagley@jefferson.edu

S.R. Patel et al. (eds.), *The History of Technologic Advancements in Urology*,
DOI 10.1007/978-3-319-61691-9_4

was inserted through a 26Fr McCarthy endoscope into the left ureter to visualize a calculus.

Takagi et al. (1968) described the first purposeful efforts to develop flexible fiberoptic ureteroscopes [7]. They used a 70 cm 8Fr fiber-optic scope to visualize the renal pelvis and papillae in cadavers and patients. They could not manipulate the tip and identified the need for a deflectable instrument. They also identified the difficulty inserting the endoscope from the bladder into the ureter and the deficiency of irrigation. They first used a cystoscope sheath for insertion and later a flexible introducer sheath which was also used for irrigation [8]. Adequate deflection and irrigating channels could not be added because of the limits of size.

Nearly a decade later rigid ureteroscopy was introduced. Initially pediatric and then juvenile cystoscopes were used before specific rigid endoscopes became available.

Goodman and Lyon had independently reported using pediatric endoscopes for transurethral ureteroscopy in women [9, 10]. As longer instruments became available, Lyon reported using them in males (1979) [11]. Some were up to 13Fr and required dilation of the ureter and development of instruments and techniques.

It was only with the development of working instruments that more therapeutic procedures were possible. In 1981, Das performed the first transurethral ureteroscopy with basket retrieval of a calculus under direct vision [12]. In 1982, Huffman used the 23 cm ureteroscope to treat 16 distal ureteral calculi [13]. The success rate was 69% but the technique was limited to the distal ureter because of the length of the endoscope.

Perez-Castro and Martinez-Piniero reported a longer, 41 cm, rigid ureteroscope which could also be passed to the level of the renal pelvis in some patients [14]. At the same time others were developing endoscopes of various lengths and diameters as well as models with interchangeable lenses. These ureteroscopes also had working channels of 4 to 5Fr which could accept working instruments such as stone baskets, biopsy forceps and wires.

In 1983, a report by Huffman et al. confirmed the safety of the long ureteroscope and also, more importantly, reported the first ureteroscopic ultrasonic lithotripsy of large ureteral and renal pelvic calculi [15]. Ultrasonic lithotripsy was possible only with the development of a long ultrasonic probe 2.5 mm in diameter. It could be placed through the sheath of a long ureteroscope with removable/interchangeable lenses.

In order to treat a stone, the scope was passed to visualize the calculus. After it was engaged in a basket, the telescope was removed. The ultrasound was then placed through the lumen and advanced to contact the stone. Using a "tactile technique" the operator could feel the probe touch the stone and also feel the resistance as he held the basket. The probe was activated to fragment and remove that portion of the stone. The operator could feel the probe pass through the stone. The ultrasonic probe was removed and the telescope replaced again to visualize and reposition the stone. The lithotripsy was then repeated. This pattern continued in order to remove enough of the stone to allow it to be removed. Huffman noted and stated that "any stone that can be visualized can be extracted using a combination of stone basket or forceps and the ultrasonic transducer" (Fig. 4.1).

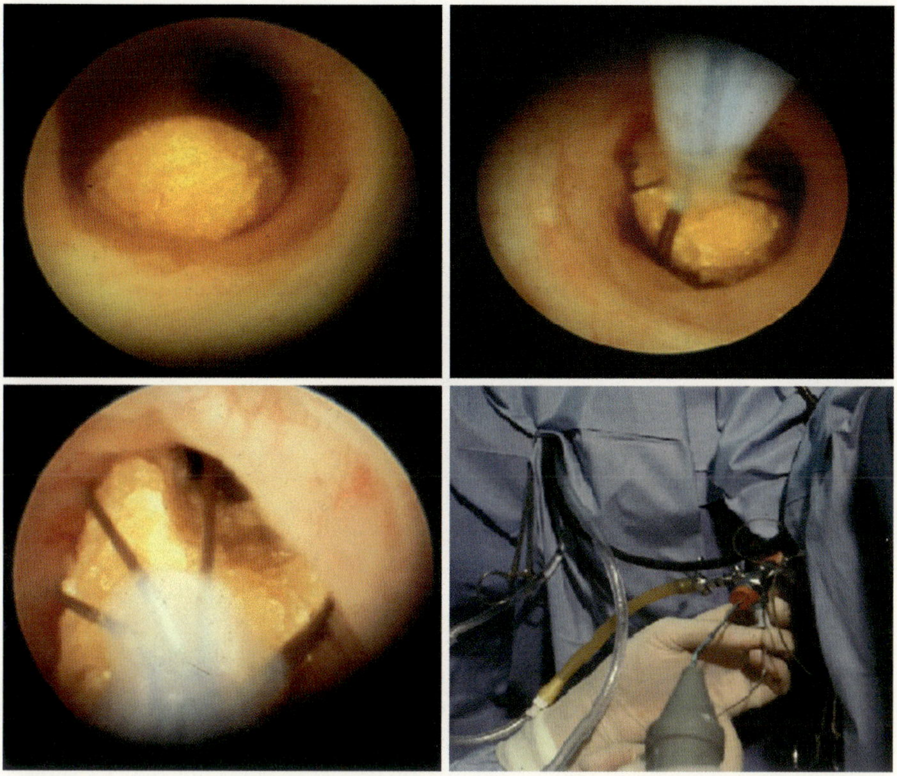

Fig. 4.1 Stones could be broken ureteroscopically using the tactile technique. The stone was visualized, grasped in a basket and pulled to the tip of the ureteroscope. The ultrasound probe was felt against the stone and then as it cleared the stone with fragmentation

The next step included downsizing the ultrasonic transducer to 4Fr and development of a rigid ureteroscope with a straight channel. The design of the ureteroscope included an angled eyepiece so that the working channel passed straight through the endoscope. There was a side port to introduce a basket through the scope. The ultrasound probe was reduced to 4Fr. With these devices, the stone could be engaged in the basket and the probe passed under direct vision to touch and fragment the stone. Only tiny fragments could be removed through the probe but the stone could be treated to be cleared (Fig. 4.2).

Another endoscopic device to fragment stones is the electrohydraulic lithotripter (EHL). Developed in the 1970s, it had been used successfully to fragment bladder stones with probes as large as 7 and 9Fr [16]. When these were used blindly in the ureter there was significant damage with resultant stricture. After the probes were downsized to 3Fr they could be placed through the channel of the ureteroscope to fragment stones under direct vision. The safety of this combination was well documented [17, 18]. The probes have been downsized even further to 2.5, 1.9 and 1.7Fr and have the advantage of being very flexible. They could be used with flexible ureteroscopes as they became available.

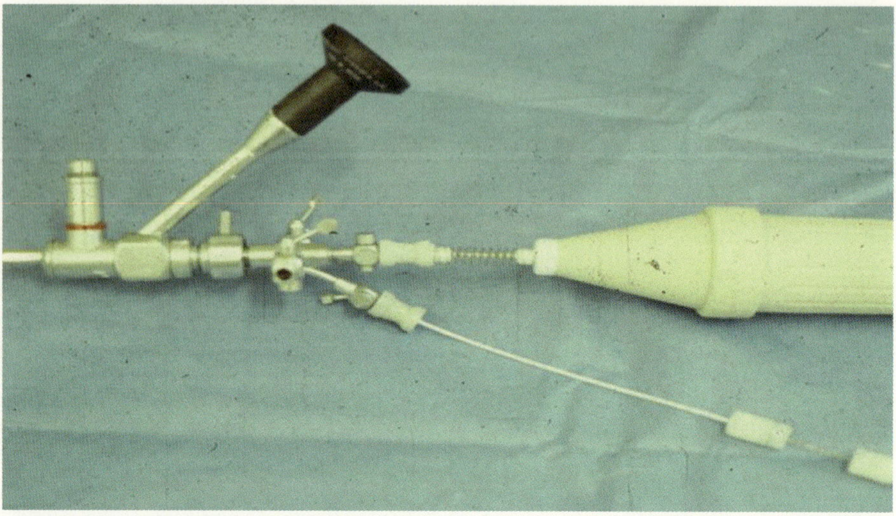

Fig. 4.2 An endoscope with an off angle lens, a straight channel and a side channel permitted visual ultrasonic lithotripsy

The development of these instruments allowed routine access to the distal ureter and frequently access to the proximal ureter and even the renal pelvis. Thus it became evident that there was a need for a flexible instrument which could give visualization and access to the entire intrarenal collecting system.

Initial attempts with the non-deflecting or passively deflecting scopes showed their in-adequacies. Even attempts to place them through deflecting and irrigating sheaths were unsuccessful. Similarly, small ureteroscopes which could be passed through the rigid ureteroscope sheath experienced inadequate irrigation and deflection [19].

In the 1980s, deflectable flexible ureteroscopes became a reality. These instruments had a channel and could be inserted over a wire. They did not require the stabilizing sheath needed with the earliest models. Active primary and passive secondary deflection were used to gain access to the lower pole. Deflection of 175° was used as the benchmark to reach the lower pole. This was based on observations from contrast radiographs [20]. However, deflection is often limited by instruments in the channel or the pattern of the collecting system itself. Deflection has been further enhanced with active secondary deflection or continuous controlled deflection which allows the tip to advance further into the lower pole [21] (Fig. 4.3).

The first practical, deflectable flexible ureteroscope was a prototype from Olympus. One unit in the USA in the early 1980's was shared between Robert Kahn in San Francisco and D. Bagley in Philadelphia and made two trips weekly via Federal Express to be available at both sites. This was a modification of a pediatric bronchoscope. It was designed with maximum deflection in the upward direction with downward movement of the control lever activated by flexion of the thumb.

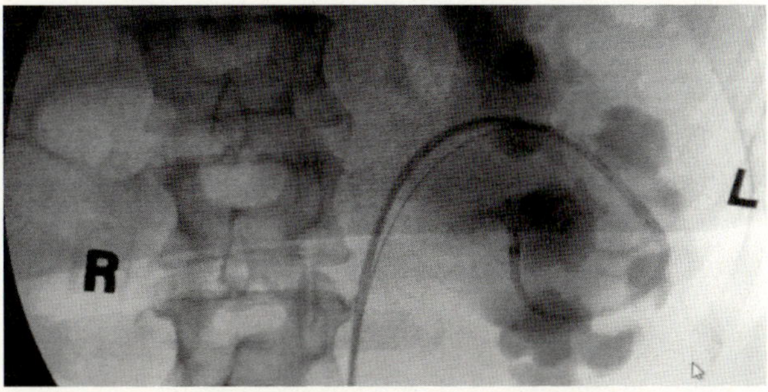

Fig. 4.3 Fluoroscopic image of a flexible ureteroscope entering an anterior lower pole calyx in a dilated collecting system

The next entry was the AUR series from ACMI. The AUR8 was 8.5 French with a 2.5Fr channel while the AUR9 was 9.8 with a 3.6Fr channel. They both had deflection in a single direction. Downward deflection of the thumb lever gave downward deflection of the tip of the endoscope. This was chosen because most attempts at deflection would be to get the tip down into the mid to lower calyces of the kidney. It also uses the most efficient movement of the thumb, flexion, to activate downward deflection. It was considered logical deflection. Down is down. Another innovation in these endoscopes was angulation of the optical system at approximately 8° toward the working channel. In this way, the device exiting the working channel could appear in the center of the field of view. With a 0° angle, the device would be parallel to the imaging axis and would never enter the center of the field.

The next entry in the series was the AUR7 which had 2 way deflection and a 7.4Fr shaft throughout the 30 cm working length. This size was much easier to place into the ureter. Initially, the shaft was slightly tapered from the tip proximally to the handle. It was very difficult to manufacture and a change was made to put a step down segment at approximate 30 cm. It thus became unstable at that point and the shaft tended to twist as the endoscope was advanced and rotated. Only larger diameter flexible ureteroscopes were produced by any manufacturer after that point with a hope for durability.

Fiberoptics remained the optical system for visualization until the introduction of the first digital flexible ureteroscope. These were also termed videoscopes or chip on a stick [22]. The early versions suffered from their large size (nearly 12Fr) and high cost. After Storz first introduced their video ureteroscope with a shaft of 8.4Fr, other companies gradually decreased the size to approximately 8.5Fr currently used. Most of the video endoscopes have been filtered and shielded to allow use of the Homium laser. Most are not equipped to use the Neodynium:YAG laser and lose the image to white out when it is activated. In one disposable version, we noted that activation of the electrocautery unit also caused loss of the image. Although these endoscopes remain expensive, there is considerable competition and the cost of chips has been falling significantly. This may be reflected in the cost of the endoscopes in the near future (Fig. 4.4).

Flexible ureteroscopes suffer from expense and fragility. The longevity of scopes in clinical use has been reported to be from 10 to 100 uses before breakage. Most reports indicate a range of 20–40. The single report showing 100 uses was in

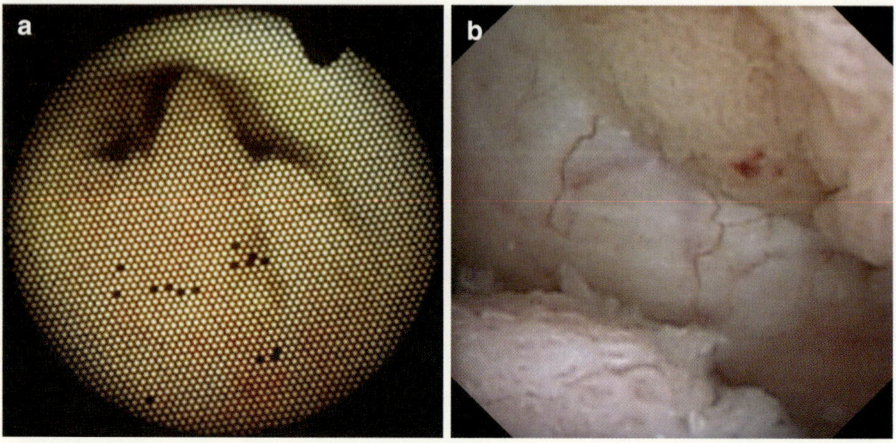

Fig. 4.4 Urinary neoplasms shown with (**a**) a fiber optic endoscope showing broken fibers and the fiber pattern (**b**) image with a digital endoscope

a limited practice of only two urologists where the instruments are cleaned and then soaked for disinfection in the endoscopy suite [23].

One solution proposed for the problem of sterilization and breakage has been single use, "disposable" endoscopes. In the early models available from two different companies, the flexible portion of the scope was disposable while the handle containing the optics was reusable. These were both fiber optic instruments. The first practical disposable ureteroscope was produced by VanTec. There were two designs with flexible but nondeflectable tips of 7 and 8.5 French with a working channel (Fig. 4.5). They also created a small rigid endoscope at 7Fr. The entire project was discontinued after the company was acquired by Boston Scientific.

Bard presented a flexible but deflectable ureteroscope with a similar modular tip and reusable eyepiece/handle. The deflecting mechanism used a turn knob which was slow and difficult to use. The production models presented an image which was upside down and backward. The endoscope was not clinically useful.

Other entries have been seen and each has failed because of design flaws. In some, the deflection mechanism was difficult or impossible to use and in one model the shaft was not torque stable so that it could not be rotated.

The latest entry (2016) is the single use LithoVue (Boston Scientific, Marlborough, MA) which is a fully deflectable digital ureteroscope. The shaft is 9.5 French and is torque stable with a firm durometer which allows it to be placed into and advanced within the ureter. The image has the typical superior quality of the digital instruments.

During the 1980's, rigid endoscopy was improved with the development of smaller, multi-channel scopes. The overall size was reduced by replacing the rod lens system with fiber optic imaging bundles. These have been referred to as "semi rigid" ureteroscopes. They are composed of metal and are truly rigid but have some

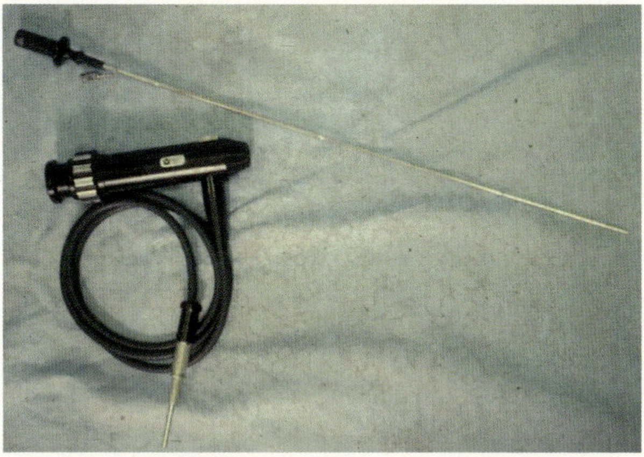

Fig. 4.5 The modular VanTec ureteroscope with interchangeable disposable tips

ability to flex without breaking. The first semi rigid scope had two working channels each 2.3F and the distal tip at 7.2F [24]. This scope could be passed directly into the ureteral orifice without dilation. It was designed specifically for the pulsed dye laser. The small channels were adequate for laser fibers but not for any retrieval devices available at the time. A similarly sized endoscope with a 3.4 and 2.3F channels was adequate for laser fibers and 3F working instruments soon became available [25].

This latter endoscope (the ACMI MR-6) became very popular because 3Fr working devices had become available and could fit through the larger channel. It was also available to any customer and not just laser owners. Both of these ureteroscopes had a flat tip. Their acceptance and widespread use demonstrated the capabilities of the design. Another design with a beak or a lip was a holdover from the tip of a cystoscope adapted from the Timberlake obturator. That curve at the tip had been made for the male urethra and is clearly not necessary for ureteral endoscopy.

Changes in endoscopes would have been meaningless without changes in working instruments, endoscopic lithotriptors and ablative devices. Size and effectiveness were the two factors resulting in true progress. Baskets and graspers were available in sizes of 5Fr and greater before the endourology revolution. As the limits of size for ureteroscopic instruments was recognized, they gradually decreased in overall diameter. As Jim Vance of VanTec stated in the 1980s when a 4Fr basket was requested, “that’s really small.” Now baskets and other devices have gradually decreased to 3Fr, 2.5 and even sub 2Fr sizes.

The initial baskets were helical, or Dormia design made in stainless steel. A major step was the introduction of the Segura or flat wire basket composed of two perpendicular loops. It offered a greater area between the wires so that larger stones could be captured. It was particularly useful percutaneously but still had a role in ureteroscopy for biopsy. Another, even greater, advance was the introduction of nitinol wires for the construction of baskets. This material had memory for shape and did not kink. This property in contrast to stainless steel, which can kink thus trapping the stone, allowed for baskets which could be used in the ureter [26].

The ultrasonic lithotriptor was the first endoscopic device for breaking stones. Its major advantage was that it could remove fragments. However, it was not very powerful and the probe was rigid. It still has a major role for percutaneous procedures but has not been useful for ureteroscopy. Impact devices for breaking stones date from their use in the nineteenth century for bladder stones. The development of small powerful probes made these devices very useful in ureteroscopy and percutaneous nephroscopy. The effect of the impactor is directly at the tip of the probe and there is no lateral scatter of energy. It is a very effective lithotriptor but the fragments remain in place to pass or to be removed. There are several impact devices available in the market now and they all have very high success rates [27, 28].

Lasers have gained a dominant role in ureteroscopy. The small fibers are perfectly suited to the small ureteroscopic instruments. The first practical laser for lithotripsy was the pulsed dye laser [29]. As the instruments became more powerful they became effective even for the very hard calcium oxalate monohydrate stones [30]. The disadvantages were that they were expensive and difficult to maintain and could only break stones.

As soon as the holmium laser became available, its many advantages were recognized. Johnson and Webb reported the capabilities of the laser including ureteroscopic lithotripsy [31, 32]. It could break stones, cut and ablate tissue. Despite these mixed capabilities, it was safe because its action was only at the end of the activated fiber. There was minimal penetration of approximately 0.5 mm in water. The laser energy could be delivered through fibers ranging from 100 to 1000 μm in diameter. It can be used throughout the ureter and the intrarenal collecting system. It can be positioned through a flexible ureteroscope into the lower pole. Despite its cost, it has become the dominant intracorporeal lithotriptor. The major concerns and reports have shifted to variations in techniques. These include dusting versus fragmenting stones, multiple pulse applications, pulse duration, optimal fiber size and shape, and fiber shielding.

Ureteroscopy can be used for more than just calculi. Among Lyon's first patients in the late 1970s was one who had a distal ureteral tumor that could be visualized and removed ureteroscopically. He followed her for several years, treating recurrences intermittently. She died of unrelated causes with both kidneys intact [33]. Other early reports included neoplasms incidentally. Later, more substantial series appeared suggesting the true value of local endoscopic treatment of upper tract neoplasms [34, 35]. There are clearly many long-term survivors who have benefited from ureteroscopic treatment. The controversy continues over the appropriate selection of patients and the application of these techniques.

Another major application has been for the incision of narrow areas within the ureter or intrarenal collecting system. The most prominent and most common application was endopyelotomy for ureteropelvic junction obstruction. Reports of short-term success appeared as early as 1986 [36]. Although it was possible to do the procedure with rigid ureteropyeloscopes in some patients, it was facilitated with the introduction of flexible endoscopes [37]. After the introduction of laparoscopic pyeloplasty, long-term comparative studies demonstrated the marked inferiority of endoscopic pyelotomy, thus ending the widespread application of that technique for primary obstruction and limiting it to special patients [38].

Current Innovations

Robotic ureteroscopy has been considered as a solution for some of the difficult and repetitive manual maneuvers for ureteroscopic procedures. It might offer a shortcut over extended experience and could alleviate some of the ergonomic risks to the surgeon [39]. The first presentation was a totally robotic ureteroscope which was controlled from a console. The scope itself was too large and the concept was considered to be too limited [40]. The next concept proposed was a platform which could be used with an existing flexible ureteroscope. This model could achieve the advantages of robotic manipulation with endoscopes that were already in use and of an acceptable size. It has been carried into clinical studies [41]. Some companies are now approaching robotic ureteroscopy as one part of a platform of robotic capabilities.

With the advent of digital cameras in ureteroscopes, the opportunity is presented for manipulation of the images. The first practical application has been through narrow band imaging. This technique emphasizes certain wavelengths and enhances visualization of small vessels in the wall of the bladder, ureter or kidney without the introduction of any medicines or chemicals [42]. It uses blue and green light to emphasize blood and makes visualization of tumors more prominent and easier. It has been suggested that NBI makes it easier to visualize tumors and to detect them initially and determine their extent. KarlStorz has a visual management system (Image IS) which enhances darker areas and can also emphasize vascular tissue. The true value and applicability of the systems has yet to be proven but the FDA has approved it for use in the bladder.

Today and the Future

After 30–40 years, ureteroscopy holds a major role in the upper tract. Just as cystourethroscopy gives vision in the urethra and bladder, ureteroscopy provides vision and access to the entire upper tract for diagnosis and treatment. The endoscopes, both rigid and flexible, are functional and reliable, yet, they remain imperfect. The small rigid scopes are very good but the image depends on a relatively small fiber optic bundle. Chips are becoming small enough to fit on these endoscopes. Flexible scopes remain fragile despite their size and they can certainly be downsized to reach the 7.4Fr seen in the 1980s. We have yet to see the end of innovation and development and can hope for better instruments in the future (Table 4.1).

Table 4.1 Landmarks in ureteroscopes

Early history	
1929	Transurethral ureteral endoscopy in patient with valves [1]
1964	Flexible ureteral endoscopy [2]
Purposeful ureteroscopy	
1968	Flexible urinary endoscopy [7]
1974	Ureteral guidetube [8]
1977	Distal ureteroscopy with rigid endoscope [9, 10]
1981	Ureteroscopic basket retrieval of calculus [12]
1983	Ureteroscopic ultrasonic lithotripsy [15]
1986	Ureteroscopic treatment of UPJ obstruction [36]
1987	Pulsed dyed laser [29]
1989	Holmium laser [31, 32]
1990	Small diameter rigid scope [24, 25]
1998	Nitinol basket [26]
2008	Flexible robotic ureteroscope [40]
2011	Narrow band imaging flexible ureteroscope [42]
2016	Single use digital flexible ureteroscope [43]

Acknowledgements The author wishes to thank Kelly A. Healy, MD for her contributions to the Figures.

References

1. Young HH, McKay RW. Congenital valvular obstruction of the prostatic urethra. Surg Gynecol Obstet. 1929;48:509.
2. Marshall VF. Fiber optics in urology. J Urol. 1964;91:110.
3. Colladon D. On the reflections of a ray of light inside a parabolic liquid stream. Comptes Rendus. 1842;15:800.
4. Hecht J. City of lights: the story of fiber optics. New York: Oxford University Press; 1999. p. 13–27.
5. Hirschowitz BI, Curtiss LE, Peters CW, Pollard HM. Demonstration of a new gastroscope, the fiberscope. Gastroenterology. 1958;35:50.
6. Barlow DE. Fiberoptic instrument technology. In: Small animal endoscopy. St Louis: C.V. Mosby; 1990. p. 1.
7. Takagi T, Go T, Takayasu H, Aso Y. A small-caliber fiberscope for visualization of urinary tract, biliary tract, and spinal canal. Surgery. 1968;64:1033.
8. Takayasu H, Aso Y. Recent development for pyeloureteroscopy: guide tube method for its introduction into the ureter. J Urol. 1974;112:176.
9. Goodman TM. Ureteroscopy with pediatric cystoscope in adults. Urology. 1977;9(4):394.
10. Lyon ES, Kyker KS, Shoenberg HW. Transurethral ureteroscopy in women: a ready addition to the urological armamentarium. J Urol. 1978;119:35.
11. Lyon ES, Banno JJ, Shoenberg HW. Transurethral ureteroscopy in men using juvenile cystoscopy equipment. J Urol. 1979;122:152.
12. Das S. Transurethral ureteroscopy and stone manipulation under direct vision. J Urol. 1981;125:112.

13. Huffman JL, Bagley DH, Lyon ES. Treatment of distal ureteral calculi using rigid ureteroscope. Urology. 1982;20(6):574.
14. Perez-Castro EE, Martinez-Piniero JA. Transurethral ureteroscopy-a current urological procedure. Arch Esp Urol. 1980;33(5):445–60.
15. Huffman JL, Bagley DH, Schoenberg HW, Lyon ES. Transurethral removal of large ureteral and renal pelvic calculi using ureteroscopic ultrasonic lithotripsy. J Urol. 1983;130:31–4.
16. Raney AM. Electrohydraulic ureterolithotripsy-preliminary report. Urology. 1978;12:284–5.
17. Green DF, Lytton B. Early experience with electrohydraulic lithotripsy of ureteral calculi using direct vision ureteroscopy. J Urol. 1985;133:767.
18. Willscher MK, Conway JF, Babayan RK, Morisseau P, Sant GR, Bertagnall A. Safety and efficacy of electrohydraulic lithotripsy by ureteroscopy. J Urol. 1988;140:957–8.
19. Bagley DH, Huffman JL, Lyon ES. Combined rigid and flexible ureteropyeloscopy. J Urol. 1983;130:243–4.
20. Bagley DH, Rittenberg MH. Intrarenal dimensions: guidelines for flexible ureteropyeloscopes. Surg Endosc. 1987;1:119–21.
21. Grasso M, Bagley DH. A 7.5F actively deflectable, flexible ureteroscope: a new plateau in both diagnostic and therapeutic upper urinary tract endoscopy. Urology. 1994;43(4):435–41.
22. Lusch A, Abdelshehid C, Hidas G, et al. *In vitro* and *In vivo* comparison of optics and performance of a distal sensor ureteroscope versus a standard fiberoptic ureteroscope. J Endourol. 2013;27(7):896–902.
23. Defidio L, DeDominicis M, DiGianfrancesco L, Fuchs G, Patel A. Improving flexible ureterorenoscope durability up to 100 procedures. J Endourol. 2012;26(10):1329–34.
24. Dretler SP. An evaluation of ureteral laser lithotripsy: 225 consecutive patients. J Urol. 1990;143:267–72.
25. Abdel-Razzak OM, Bagley DH. The 6.9F semi-rigid ureteroscope in clinical use. Urology. 1993;41(1):45–8.
26. Honey RJ. Assessment of a new tipless nitinol stone basket and comparison with an existing flat-wire basket. J Endourol. 1998;12:529–31.
27. Languetin JM, Jichlinski P, Farre R, van Niederhausern W. The Swiss Lithoclast. J Urol. 1990;143:179A.
28. Chew BH, Arsovska O, Lange D, et al. The Canadian StoneBreaker trial: a randomized, multicenter trial comparing the LMA StoneBreaker™ and the Swiss LithoClast® during percutaneous nephrolithotripsy. J Endourol. 2011;25:1415–9.
29. Dretler SP, Watson G, Parrish JA, Murray S. Pulsed dye laser fragmentation of ureteral calculi. Initial clinical experience. J Urol. 1987;137:386–99.
30. Bagley DH, Grasso M, Shalaby M, Abass El-Akkad M. Ureteral laser lithotripsy using the pulsolith. J Endourol. 1989;3:91–8.
31. Johnson PE, Crameens DM, Price RE. Use of the holmium: YAG laser in urology. Lasers Surg Med. 1992;12:353–63.
32. Webb DR, Kocklburgh R, Johnson WF. The versapulse holmium:YAG laser in clinical urology: a pilot study. Minim Invas Ther. 1993;2:23–6.
33. Lyon ES. The birth of modern ureteroscopy: the Albona Jaybis story. J Endourol. 2004;18:525–6.
34. Pak R, Moskowitz E, Bagley DH. What is the cost of maintaining a kidney in upper tract transitional cell carcinoma. J Endourol. 2009;23:341–6.
35. Grasso M, Fishman AI, Cohen J, Alexander B. Ureteroscopic and extirpative treatment of upper urinary tract urothelial carcinoma: a 15 year comprehensive review of 160 consecutive patients. BJU Int. 2012;110:1618–26.
36. Inglis JA, Tolley DA. Ureteroscopic pyelolysis for pelviureteric junction obstruction. Br J Urol. 1986;58:250–2.
37. Conlin MJ, Bagley DH. Ureteroscopic endopyelotomy at a single setting. J Urol. 1998;159:727–31.

38. Yanke BV, Lallas CD, Pagnani C, McGinnis DE, Bagley DH. The minimally invasive treatment of ureteropelvic junction obstruction: a review of our experience during the last decade. J Urol. 2008;180:1397–402.
39. Healy KA, Pak R, Cleary R, Colon-Herdman A, Bagley DH. Hand problems among endourologists. J Endourol. 2011;25:1915–20.
40. Desai MM, Aron M, Gill IS, et al. Flexible robotic retrograde renoscopy: description of novel robotic device and preliminary laboratory experience. Urology. 2008;72:42–6.
41. Saglam R, Muslumanoglu AY, Tokatliz Z, et al. A new robot for flexible ureteroscopy: development and early clinical results (IDEAL stage 1-2b). Eur Urol. 2014;66:1092–100.
42. Traxer O, Geavlete B, deMedina SG, et al. Narrow band imaging digital flexible ureteroscopy in detection of upper urinary tract transitional cell carcinoma: initial experience. J Endourol. 2011;25:19–23.
43. Silvia Proietti, Laurian Dragos, Wilson Molina, Steeve Doizi, Guido Giusti, Olivier Traxer, (2016) Comparison of New Single-Use Digital Flexible Ureteroscope Versus Nondisposable Fiber Optic and Digital Ureteroscope in a Cadaveric Model. Journal of Endourology 30 (6):655–659

Chapter 5
Development of Transurethral Resection of the Prostate (TURP)

Richard K. Babayan

For nearly three quarters of a century the transurethral resection of the prostate (TURP) has been a mainstay of urologic surgery. Initially developed as an alternative to open surgery, many consider TURP to be the first minimally invasive urologic procedure. It has withstood the test of time, evolving with adaptation of new optical and electrosurgical technologies and remains the gold standard for the surgical treatment of benign prostatic hyperplasia (BPH). TURP has withstood the challenges of a variety of newer minimally invasive technologies. Transurethral resection remains a technically challenging procedure to master, but it is still essential for all urologists to have in their armamentarium, as it has important value not only in treating BPH but also in the diagnosis and treatment of bladder tumors.

The TURP of today is a far cry from its rudimentary origins in the 1930s. As with most surgical procedures which have survived for many decades, the TURP continues to evolve and adapt to and incorporate technological advancements. Better optics, illumination, instrument design, accessories, working elements, electrosurgical generators and the transition from mono-polar to bi-polar technology have all contributed to making the TURP a better, safer and more versatile technique, with a much wider range of application than was possible with first or second generation resectoscopes. It is not uncommon today for a well-trained and experienced resectionist to remove 100 g or more tissue, during a 60 min TURP, whereas with prior instrumentation few urologists would attempt to remove more than 50 g of tissue transurethrally in a short period of time.

R.K. Babayan, M.D.
Department of Urology, Boston University School of Medicine, Boston Medical Center, Shapiro Center, Suite 3B, 725 Albany St., Boston, MA 02118, USA
e-mail: rbabayan@bu.edu

S.R. Patel et al. (eds.), *The History of Technologic Advancements in Urology*,
DOI 10.1007/978-3-319-61691-9_5

TURP developed as a natural progression from prior blind transurethral incisions and punch resections of the prostate, which had little long-term success and were fraught with bleeding and other morbid complications. As optics improved and electrosurgical generators became more readily available, investigators began to combine the two technologies, which would allow for more precise removal of obstructing prostate tissue while providing sufficient hemostasis. The history of development of the TURP is a testament to the ingenuity and resourcefulness of pioneering urologists of the last century.

The surgical management of BPH in the early twentieth century consisted of a variety of open enucleations of the BPH adenoma performed either via a transabdominal or perineal approach. To avoid the morbidity of the open surgical procedures, attempts were made at transurethral incisions of the prostate with cold knives or punch resections of obstructing adenomas largely involving bladder neck or median lobe tissue. The evolution of the current TURP has involved a few seminal events, which will be outlined in this chapter.

Early Development of the Resectoscope

The concept of transurethral access to the prostate had been a challenge to physicians due to lack of instrumentation to allow both visualization and surgical treatment simultaneously. Prior to the development of the resectoscope, early urologists depended on modified sounds to dilate and later incise the bladder neck and prostatic urethra in an attempt to relief outlet obstruction. Ambrose Pare is credited with performing and reporting the first of these blind procedures within the prostatic urethra in the 1634 [1]. In the late 1800s, Bottini modified a male sound by adding a platinum wire and then applying an electric current to burn and incise the bladder neck and anterior prostate [2]. Unfortunately this was also a completely blind procedure with little long-term success. Practical cystoscopies allowed direct visualization of the urethra, but manipulation was limited to crude incisions or punch resections, which were largely limited to the bladder neck and were fraught with difficulty in controlling hemorrhage.

Hugh Hampton Young described his prostatic punch operation in JAMA in 1913 [3]. This involved a sliding blade that blindly trapped and removed obstructing prostate tissue largely located at the bladder neck. There was no means of controlling the hemorrhage, which often resulted from these punch resections. Braasch modified Young's procedure in 1918 by adding direct vision cystoscopy but hemorrhage remained a problem [4] It was not until 1935 when Thompson added a coagulating electrode to the cutting blade of the punch instrument that bleeding began to be controlled. By that time, the TURP was already gaining popularity and the punch resection had lost its general appeal.

A major breakthrough came when mono-polar electrosurgical current was combined with the insulated inner shaft of a cystoscopic instrument to allow for removal

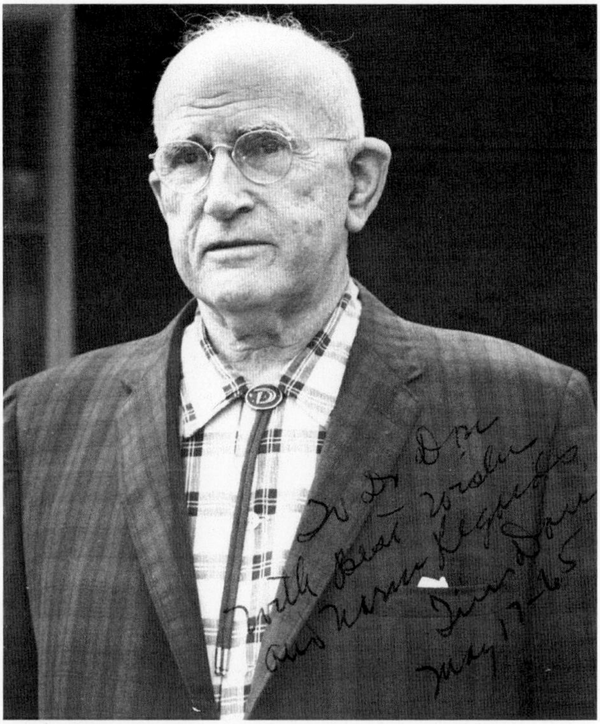

Fig. 5.1 Theodore M. Davis (1889–1973) (Picture from the William P. Didusch Center for Urologic History, Linthicum, MD)

of chips of tissue as well as control of bleeding resulting from the sequential removal of obstructing prostatic tissue. Stern reported on his early resectoscope in 1926 [5].

His initial instrument allowed a rudimentary high voltage diathermy current to run through a tungsten wire and this was very efficient in cutting tissue but had little ability to coagulate and control bleeding. In 1931 Theodore Davis, who had worked as an electrical engineer before becoming a urologist, improved on Stern's initial design by substituting a more sophisticated diathermy, which would allow the sequential use of both cutting and coagulating current (Fig. 5.1). He further improved the design by developing a foot pedal, which enabled the operating urologist to alternate between cutting and coagulation current as needed [6].

The Stern resectoscope was further modified by McCarthy and Wappler who designed the fore-oblique lens for better visualization and also provided better insulation for the resectoscope by adding a Bakelite sheath [7]. By the late 1930s, a practical resectoscope was readily available for the performance of the TURP. Further modifications came over the next half century including: improvements in the fiber-optic lighting and lens systems, the introduction of the wide angled Hopkins rod lens, the Nesbit and Iglesias modifications of the working element (which allowed for a single handed operation), the application of video technology and refinements in electrosurgical energy.

Evolution of the Electrosurgical Generator and TUR Loop

The ability to apply electrosurgical energy via a fluid medium was essential to the development of the functional TURP. The original tungsten wire loop utilized by Stern was coupled to rudimentary spark gap radiofrequency generators developed by Wappler. Davis modified both the design of the loop as well as the generator used to supply the energy (Fig. 5.2). All of these early electrosurgical generators were adaptations of William T. Bovie's basic design [8]. This was a mono-polar electrosurgical unit, which required the use of a grounding pad. Cutting current incorporates high current and high power in the form of continuous alternating radiofrequency in a sinusoidal wave pattern, which is ideal for cutting tissue but provides minimal coagulation or heating of surrounding tissue. The basic principle is to heat tissue

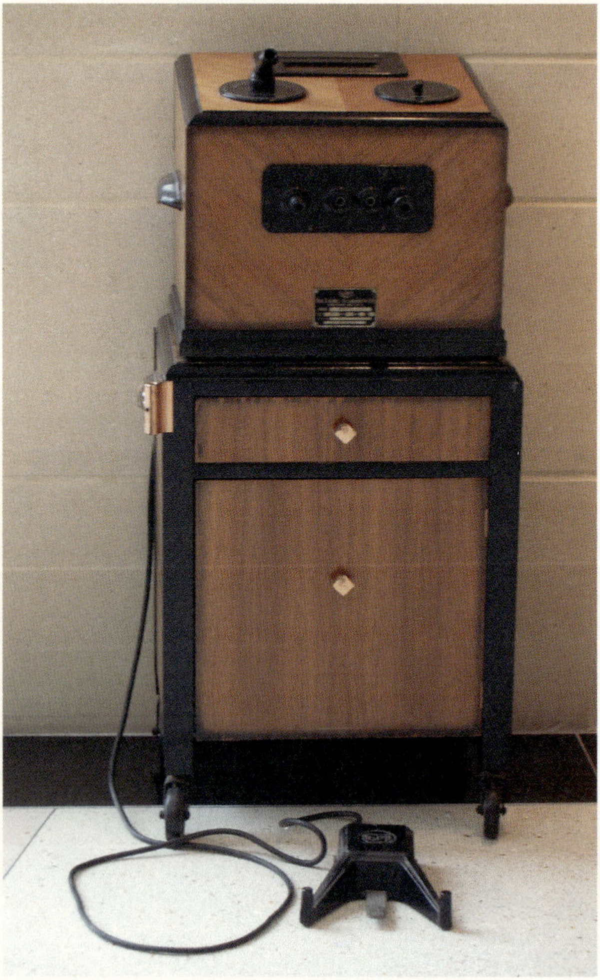

Fig. 5.2 Davis-Bovie Generator (Picture from the William P. Didusch Center for Urologic History, Linthicum, MD)

using rapid high temperatures (>100 °C). This results in vaporization of intra and extracellular fluids and hence the smooth cutting of prostatic tissue.

On the other hand, coagulation or fulguration occurs when short bursts of high voltage radiofrequency results in greater depth of penetration of the tissue.

Temperatures generated for coagulation are generally in the 70–100 °C range. Water was initially used as the irrigation of choice, but water is hypotonic and causes hemolysis and potential electrolyte changes. Water was replaced by fluids of higher osmolality such as glycine or sorbitol, which decreased the deleterious consequences of fluid absorption but did not eliminate the potential for TUR syndrome. TUR syndrome is most often the result of such issues as prolonged resection time, over distention of the bladder and deep resection beyond the capsule of the prostate. High intravesical pressure, from over distension of the bladder has been somewhat mitigated by the introduction of continuous flow resectoscopes. None-the-less TUR syndrome with mono-polar TURP remains a risk in 1–2% of cases.

In the last 50 years many improvements have been made in electrosurgical generators, most notably the advent of solid-state bi-polar systems, which have increased the efficiency of resection while minimizing the risks. There is no longer a need for grounding pads and resections can been done with conductive normal saline irrigation further decreasing the risk of TUR syndrome. These new solid-state generators incorporate a microprocessor feedback system allowing for constant adjustment of power output. Improvement of loop design made bipolar resection possible by allowing return of the current from "smart" generators to occur within the loop itself. The resulting active bipolar electrode produces a localized plasma and actually cuts tissue at a lower thermal temperature and a radio frequency output far less than monopolar generators. The resulting low frequency and low voltage used in bipolar TURP markedly decreases electrical interference with cardiac pacemakers. Depending on the configuration of the electrode, modern bipolar systems can both resect and vaporize prostatic tissue with minimal coagulation artifact.

Optics

No other technologic improvement has had a greater impact on the evolution of the TURP than the revolutionary improvements in endoscopic optics, including fiberoptics and video technology, which have largely occurred in the last 30 years.

For the first 30 years of TURP, performance was impeded by poor visualization and poorly illuminated monocular visualization. The original resectoscopes utilized small incandescent light bulbs for illumination. Not only were these small and dim but required frequent replacement. The advent of cold fiberoptic light cables and the elimination of the light bulb illumination was another significant advancement. Although early lenses came in a variety of angles ranging from 0 ° to 120 °, the 15 and 30 ° lenses provided the best field of view for TURP. The early lenses, however, were hampered by poor clarity and narrow angles. The Hopkins rod lens system was a major technological advancement, which replaced the old system of bulky air filled tubes with relay and field lenses with long glass rods which significantly decreased the lens profile while increasing the size and clarity of the image [9] An added benefit of the rod lens system was a ninefold increase in light transmission. This advance greatly helped urologists to better see and more efficiently resect and coagulate prostate tissue. The advent of CCD video camera technology and the use of high definition TV monitors brought urologists out of the dark ages of monocular vision to a more ergonomic and comfortable posture. Not only was binocular visualization achieved, but resectionists no longer needed to contort their bodies, especially their necks, in order to adequately complete their resections.

Monitor based images are larger, brighter and clearer than monocular endoscopic images. An added benefit of fiberoptic, camera and monitor technology was an enhancement of endoscopic resident and medical student education. The video TURP allowed for a better understanding of the anatomic landmarks critical for the performance of the TURP as well as the ability of real time teaching with instantaneous alteration of surgical technique. Urologists who trained after the mid-1980s would find it difficult to conceive of a monocular TURP without the benefit of monitor based binocular visualization.

Resectoscope Design

The design of the resectoscope has changed dramatically over the last 80 years.

First generation resectoscopes were of large caliber and often required routine urethral dilation using such antiquated instruments as the Otis urethrotome prior to insertion of the scope. The evolution of resectoscope design has incorporated a multitude of mechanical, material and technologic changes. Modern resectoscopes are of a smaller profile with better optics, irrigation channels and better accessories. The Timberlake obturator, which was classically used for initial blind passage of the resectoscope has been largely replaced by visual obturators which enable passage of the resectoscope sheath with minimal risk of urethral trauma. Continuous flow technology is now universally available. Not only does this diminish intravesical pressure but also speeds the process of resection, allowing the urologist to resect for longer periods of time without the need for as frequent emptying of the bladder. The original Stern-McCarthy resectoscope utilized a two-handed design, requiring the urologist to steady the resectoscope with one hand while using the second hand to manually move the loop in and out (Figs. 5.3 and 5.4). The spring loaded single hand design largely popularized by Iglesias has resulted in a more ergonomic simpler mechanism. The continuous flow resectoscope has allowed for better visualization with lower intravesical pressures and less risk of complications. No longer do urologists need to consider placement of supra-pubic tubes to vent the bladder during a TURP.

As previously mentioned, mono-polar TURP has been largely replaced by bipolar technology, which has resulted in a safer, more efficient instrument capable of larger tissue removal in a shorter period of time with marked decrease in the potential

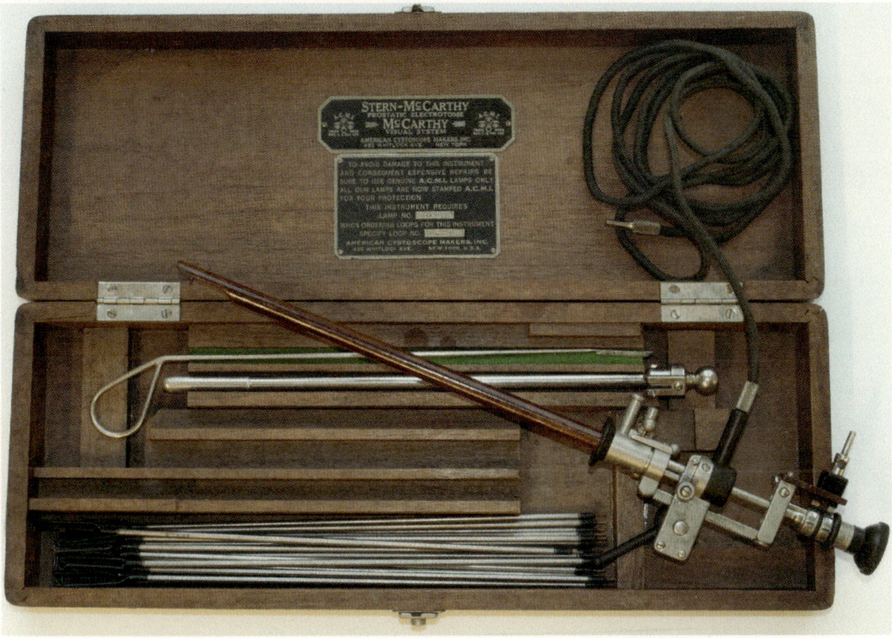

Fig. 5.3 Stern-McCarthy Electrotome (Picture from the William P. Didusch Center for Urologic History, Linthicum, MD)

complications. Bi-polar technology has allowed for resection of larger volume prostates in a shorter period of time with fewer complications, including virtual elimination of the TUR syndrome. Whether a resectoscope uses mono-polar or bi-polar technology, proper insulation is needed to prevent conduction of current along the metal shaft of the sheath. Standard urologic texts written in the last century recommended that TURPs be reserved for small to moderate sized prostates and in fact many recommended that prostates larger than 60 g should be treated with open surgery. Modern bi-polar resectosocpes are routinely capable, in the hands of experienced resectionists, of removing twice that suggested upper volume limit of prostate tissue within the safety margin of 60 min.

Future Challenges

TURP has been often referred to as the gold standard for the surgical management of BPH. It has withstood a number of medical and minimally invasive challenges and continues to maintain its predominance largely due to the adaptability of the technology. TURP came under attack by 3rd party payers concerned about cost containment. Medicare cut reimbursement for TURP when it was the 2nd most common operation in men over age 65, with only cataract surgery being more

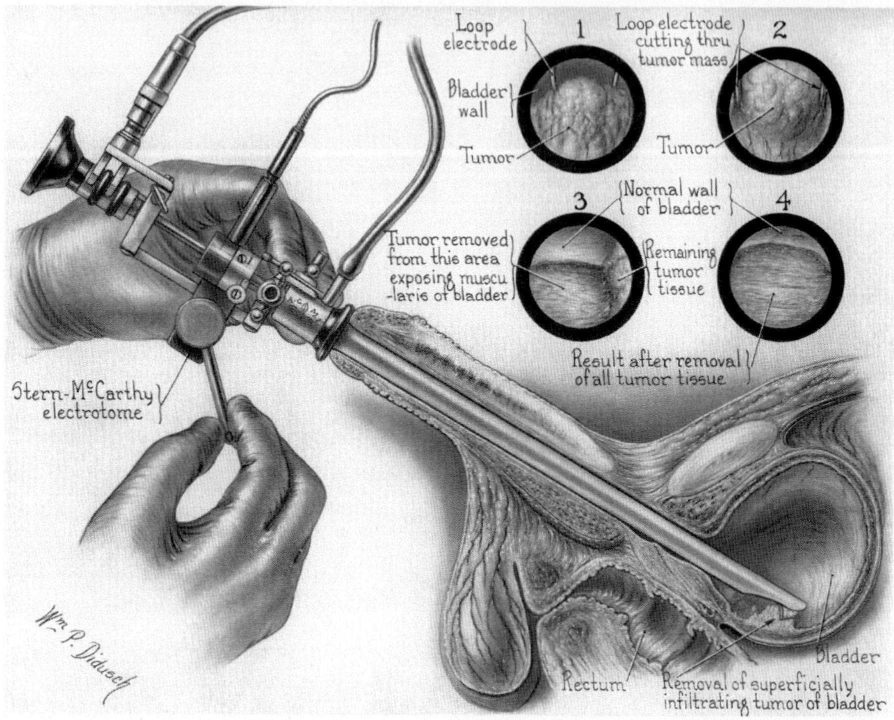

Fig. 5.4 William P. Didusch Illustration on the application of the Stern-McCarthy Resectoscope in the treatment of bladder tumors (Picture from the William P. Didusch Center for Urologic History, Linthicum, MD)

widely performed in this population. The advent of five alpha reductase inhibiters and alpha blockers also were challenges to the position of TURP as the treatment of choice for symptomatic BPH. TURP has largely been relegated to a procedure for symptomatic males who have failed prior attempts at medical management. Nonetheless, TURP has maintained its position of prominence for the surgical management of BPH and has withstood the onslaught of numerous other minimally invasive surgical options.

Transurethral technologies are adaptable to the size of the prostate. The same resectoscope with a Collings knife can adequately treat a small 20–30 cc prostate with a TUIP as efficiently as it can resected 100 g from a large volume prostate with a prominent median lobe. A limitation of the TURP is admittedly in the anti-coagulated patient who cannot transiently come off his anti-coagulant therapy. Many new minimally invasive alternatives are currently undergoing investigation and it is unclear if any of them will have the broad applicability of the TURP. Obviously further studies into genetic, molecular and individualized therapies may in the future discover a means of preventing or retarding the development of symptomatic BPH. Until that time TURP will continue to improve and evolve and maintain a prominent role in the surgical management of BPH.

References

1. Pare A. The workes of that famous Chirugian Ambrose Pare. Translated by T. Johnson. London; 1634.
2. Bottini E. La galvanocaustica nelia practica chirugica. Norvara; 1874.
3. Young HH. A new procedure, punch operation for small prostatic bars and contracture of prostatic orifice. JAMA. 1913;60:253–7.
4. Braasch WF. Median bar excisor. JAMA. 1918;70:758–9.
5. Stern M. Resection of obstructions at the vesical orifice. JAMA. 1926;87:1726–30.
6. Davis TM. Prostatic operation. Prospects of the patient with prostatic disease vs. resection. JAMA. 1931;97:1674–9.
7. McCarthy JF. Suggestion as to procedure in the use of the McCarthy visualized prostatic urethrotome. J Urol. 1932;28:265–71.
8. Oconnor JL, Bloom DA. William T. Bovie and electrosurgery. Surgery. 1996;119(4):390–6.
9. Hopkins HH. Optical principles of the endoscope. In: Berci G, editor. Endoscopy. New York: Appleton-Century-Crofts; 1976. p. 3–26.

Chapter 6
History of Transurethral Resection and Fulguration of Bladder Tumors

Harry Herr

Introduction

Transurethral resection (TURB) is the essential surgical procedure used to diagnose, stage and treat bladder tumors. TURB is an ideal operation—focal, targeted, patient-centered, single-port, minimally invasive through a natural orifice (the urethra), safe, and repeatable. Urologists today are armed with a dazzling array of sophisticated endoscopic instruments. Modern flexible digital cystoscopes and video-assisted resectoscopes combine the essentials—access, superior optics, working elements, and energy—to detect, decipher and destroy tumors growing in the bladder. Current endoscopes provide magnified high-definition views of the bladder interior, permitting visual removal of bladder tumors using panoply of cutting loops, forceps or graspers and their targeted destruction by electrocautery or laser energy. The methods, means and skills we enjoy today began in the nineteenth century and refined in the 20th owing to collective genius and ingenuity of many surgeons, scientists, inventors, and visionary entrepreneurs.

Bladder Tumors from Antiquity to Endoscopic era

Although likely they were recognized in antiquity, bladder tumors were mentioned first by Lacuna in 1551. Despite scattered reports of excision of an occasional tumor found during lithotomy, the first operations targeting bladder tumor were performed in the 16th and 17th centuries. Up to the eighteenth century, surgeons removed

H. Herr, M.D.
Department of Urology, Memorial Sloan-Kettering Cancer Center, Weill Cornell Medical College, New York, NY 10065, USA
e-mail: herrh@mskcc.org

S.R. Patel et al. (eds.), *The History of Technologic Advancements in Urology*,
DOI 10.1007/978-3-319-61691-9_6

bladder tumors blindly through a dilated urethra, or open suprapubic or lateral perineal incision, using ligatures, ecrasement (steel-wire loop), arrachement (tearing out), enucleation, or cauterization.

During the eighteenth century, the so-called *carnosities* of the bladder became more clearly understood in scattered works on the pathologic anatomy of bladder tumors, polyps, ulcerations, and carcinomas. The first landmark in the history of bladder tumors was Chopart's classical work, "Traite des Maladies des Voies Urinaires." He noted essential differences between various kinds of bladder tumors and regarded "fungosities of the bladder" as benign tumors subject to cancerous degeneration. As a result, the nineteenth century witnessed a marked advance in the knowledge of bladder tumor pathology soundly based on histologic structure. For example, Civiale differentiated papillary fungoid type of growths from solid cancerous tumors. Definition of these lesions, now described as low-grade papillary tumors separate from high-grade solid tumors, was highly relevant because the more common papillary growths were the only tumors early endoscopists could treat successfully. Solid tumors were usually invasive and far too advanced for local excision [1].

Early Endoscopic Era

Table 6.1 lists landmark developments in the endoscopic access and improved treatment surgical treatments of bladder tumors [2]. Beginning with Bozzini in 1806, physicians, armed only with speculum, candle and mirror, began to explore body cavities and learn endoscopic anatomy by practical experience. The urinary tract was first explored by inspection through crude specula inserted into the urethral meatus, chiefly in women. Surgeons attempted to seize pedunculated growths transurethrally, tie the pedicle and blindly tear away as much tissue as possible, usually with unsatisfactory results.

In the mid-nineteenth century, Desormeaux introduced his endoscope, and cystoscopy became established as a practical, although difficult, means of clinical investigation. He designed his instrument around a paraffin flamed that burned more brightly by the addition of turpentine. In 1853, Desormeaux was able to perform the first true endoscopic operation when he extracted a papilloma through the urethra using his urethroscope [3]. Trouve made a critical contribution to cystoscopy in 1873 when he moved the light source (a glowing hot platinum wire) to the inner tip of his "Polyscope." In 1876, Rutenberg, attempting to improve vision within the female bladder, designed his "Blasenspiegel" through which he was the first to observe the larger surfaces of the bladder. Later, the dermatologist Grunfeld improved endoscopic surgery in the urethra and bladder. He developed a urethroscope, as well as endoscopic loop threaders, scissors, forceps, and knives, and was the first to operate in the bladder under direct control of the eye when he removed a bladder papilloma through his urethroscope in 1881. In 1885, Grunfeld developed the "Polypenkneipe," the first cystoscope specifically designed to remove tumors from the urethra and bladder [4].

Table 6.1 Landmark innovations leading to modern endoscopic treatment of bladder tumors

Year	Individual	Innovation
1806	P. Bozzini	Lichtleiter
1853	A. J. Desormeaux	First endoscopic operation—extraction of urethral papilloma
1873	G. Trouve	Polyscope—electroendoscopy
1876	D. Rutenberg	Blasenspiegel—air cystoscopy
1877	M. Nitze	Cystoscope
1878	T. Edison	Incandescent light bulb
1881	J. Grunfeld	Polypenkneipe—first removal of bladder papilloma
1894	M. Nitze	Operating cystoscope
1908	R. Wappler	Monopolar high-frequency (Oudin) current—the resonator
1910	E. Beer	Fulguration of bladder tumors
1911	E. Frank	Bipolar electrocoagulation of bladder tumors
1926	M. Stern	First resectoscope
1928	W. T. Bovie	Separate current for coagulation and cutting
1931	J. McCarthy	Improved Stern resectoscope for bladder tumors
1931	T. Davis	Combined cutting current with diathermy, dual-action foot switch
1938	R. Nesbit	One-handed resectoscope
1959	H. Hopkins	Rod-lens fiberoptic system. Led to flexible cystoscopy
1970	W.S Boyle and G. S. Smith	Charge-coupled-device (CCD)—led to digital endoscopy and video-assisted TURB

Max Nitze and the Operating Cystoscope

Maximilian Nitze introduced the first direct-vision cystoscope in 1877, which markedly improved vision inside the bladder but offered limited operating capability [5]. Never satisfied, from 1891 to 1894, Nitze designed and constructed the first practical operating cystoscope (Fig. 6.1). He became the first to coagulate a bladder polyp visualized with Edison's new light bulb and using cold and hot wire loops for galvanocautery. He initiated systematic cystoscopic treatment of bladder tumors and reported removal of tumors from 150 cases with only 1 death and 20 recurrences. Using curette, cutting forceps, cautery, and wire loop, he was able to remove many papillary tumors cleanly [6]. Others followed his lead, and in 1905, Weinrich reported treating 101 cases of bladder tumors by the Nitze method with 71% recoveries without a recurrence. The procedure was mostly excision of pedunculated tumors with a portion of mucosa or else twisting off the pedicle at its base. For most European and American urologists, however, the Nitze cystoscope was cumbersome to manipulate, and galvanic cautery using the wire loop proved to be an unreliable means of tissue destruction. With advent of diathermy in the United States, surgery of bladder tumors using Nitze's operating cystoscope was practically abandoned.

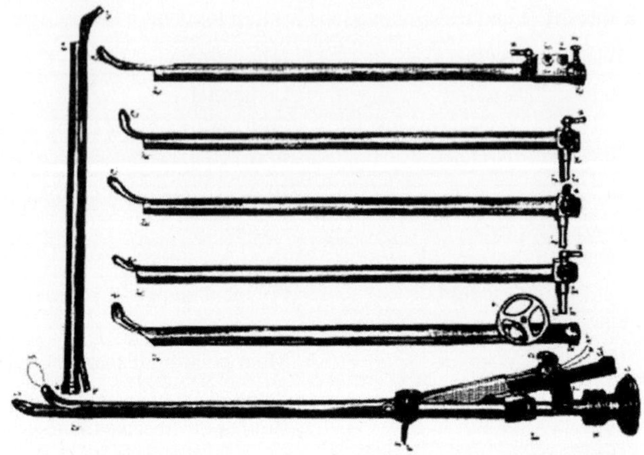

Fig. 6.1 Operating cystoscope, developed by M. Nitze in 1891–1894

Cystofulguration

Nagelschmidt and Doyen in the United States were the first to advocate use of electrically induced heat to treat cancerous growths. Nagelschmidt devised an adequate apparatus for this purpose and is credited with originating the term diathermy. But it was Edwin Beer of New York who really founded electrosurgery of the bladder.

In 1908, Beer, convinced that Nitze's earlier transurethral treatment of bladder tumors was superior to open surgery, conceived the idea of using high-frequency electric current through a catheterizing-cystoscope to coagulate bladder tumors. He used a two-channel Nitze cystoscope (one channel for a 6F copper electrode and the other for irrigation of the bladder) and a monopolar (Oudin) current derived from a resonator made by the American cystoscope maker, Reinhold Wappler. Direct current was applied at various points to papillary growths for 15–30 s at a time, while the bladder was distended with sterile water. Beer treated two women and saw no spark when the full current was thrown on without resistance. Tumor tissue was dessicated at cautery points even under water, and patients experienced no more discomfort than during ordinary cystoscopy. Beer concluded that coagulation was simpler than loop treatment, and in 1910, he reported his successful cases in a landmark article, claiming fulguration to be "proven effective in the cure of bladder papilloma" [7].

For the next 25 years, Beer devoted much of his time to the study of bladder neoplasms and continued to develop and improve his method of treatment, eventually reporting his aggregated experience of cases in 1935. After Beer died in 1938, Reed Nesbit wrote, "Development of this technique by its brilliant discoverer marked one of the greatest advances in the history of urology; it led not only to radical change in the therapeutic management of bladder tumors, but also paved the way for subsequent electroresection methods by proving that high-frequency current could be employed effectively under water" [1]. It did all that and more. Based largely on Beer's pioneering concept, outpatient cystoscopic fulguration of recurrent papillary bladder tumors remains common practice today.

Transurethral Resection

Although cystofulguration was used around the world to destroy benign papillomas and small papillary carcinomas, it was known that not all papillary tumors behaved in an indolent manner. Compounding the problem was that pathologists could not always distinguish between benign, malignant or invasive neoplasms. Even Beer became pessimistic about the efficacy of endoscopic diathermy because it was applicable only to small tumors, did not prevent recurrences, and was ineffective against invasive bladder tumors. Clearly, a more effective means to remove and destroy bladder tumors was needed.

Transurethral resection of bladder tumors could not have developed without the first practical incandescent lamp invented by Thomas Edison in 1879, high frequency electric current devised by Heinrich Hertz in 1888, the vacuum tube permitting continuous current introduced in 1908 by Lee DeForest, application of high-frequency electrical current underwater by Beer in 1910, the fenestrated tube conceived by Hugh Young in 1909, the first practical cutting current by George Wyeth in 1924, and cutting and coagulation current combined into one by Reinhold Wappler in 1931.

In 1926, a urologist in New York named Maximilian Stern introduced a revolutionary new instrument he called a *resectoscope*. Stern's resectoscope consisted of a sheath and working parts assembled in a compact bundle made up of a direct-vision telescope, a light carrier, a water conduit, and a cutting loop or active electrode using a bipolar current. Stern devised a manually controlled gear mechanism to slide a tungsten wire loop back and forth through a fenestra with even movement using the attached control handle (Fig. 6.2). Designed as a punch operation for the prostate, the moveable wire was able to whittle away obstructing prostatic tissue with ease, but the instrument was cumbersome to use in the bladder because it was difficult to engage bladder tissue in the recessed fenestra. However, the cutting loop offered the obvious advantage of removing rather than simply cauterizing bladder tumors [8].

Theodore Davis, who had been an electrical engineer before entering urology, combined the cutting current with a diathermy machine for hemostasis, and in 1931 reported good results. Davis improved the loop by using a larger tungsten wire on Stern's resectoscope, and he provided better insulation (Fig. 6.3). More importantly, working with Bovie, he incorporated cutting and coagulation diathermy, inventing a duel-foot pedal allowing him to switch between either current during surgery.

In 1931, Joseph McCarthy, also of New York, made significant improvements in the resectoscope. McCarthy fashioned a lens system that widened the visual field, used a nonconducting Bakelite sheath, added a rack-and-pinion lever to move an electric-arc cutting loop, incorporated separate currents for coagulation and cutting, and most importantly, moved the wire loop and cutting window to the tip of the instrument. However, the key to success of this instrument was the foroblique telescope developed by Wappler. It provided both a wide-angle view and sufficient magnification allowing precise placement and manipulation of the cutting loop. The chief difference from the Stern instrument, cutting was done toward the bladder

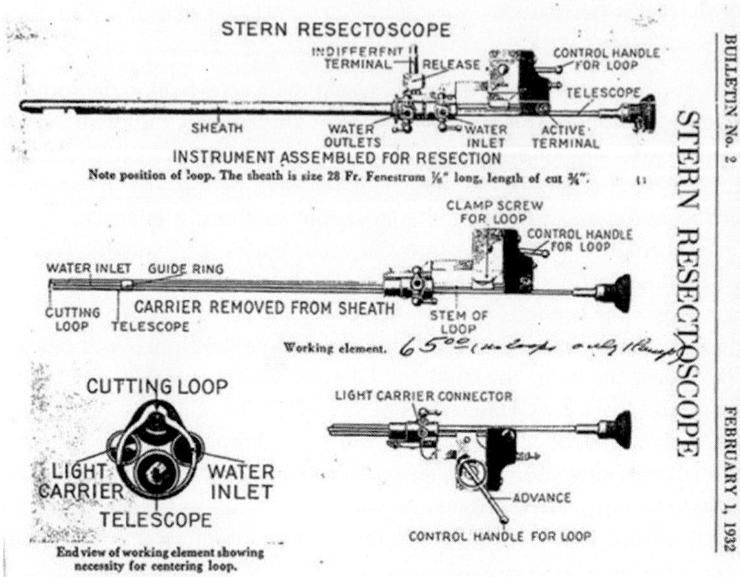

Fig. 6.2 First resectoscope, developed by Maximilian Stern, 1926

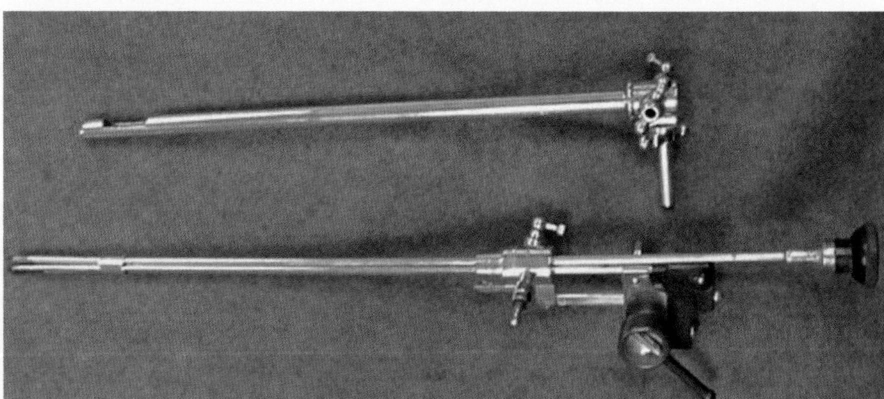

Fig. 6.3 Stern-Davis resectoscope, 1927

(amputating tissue away from the surgeon), while using the McCarthy resectoscope, one cut from within the bladder outward. McCarthy found that his modifications were better adapted to resect vesical neoplasms because with the extended loop, it was easier to engage bladder tumors and to cut slices of tissue back toward the operator under direct visual control [9].

The Stern-McCarthy resectoscope, as it became known, was the first practical cutting-loop resectoscope, and it quickly replaced fulguration to become the dominant method used to diagnose and treat bladder neoplasms for the rest of the twentieth century (Figs. 6.4a, b and 6.5). Numerous modifications of the Stern-McCarthy resectoscope followed, but they were all based on the original design. The most significant of these was a novel one-handed resectoscope devised by Reed Nesbit in 1938 [10]. Nesbit attached a rotating thumb hole and movable carriage with spring for return of the loop, and foreshortened the fenestrum, allowing the loop to extend 1 cm beyond the beak of the sheath to evacuate tissue. Having one hand free allowed the surgeon to elevate the bladder base through the rectum or apply suprapubic pressure to bring tumors within reach of the resectoscope (Fig. 6.6).

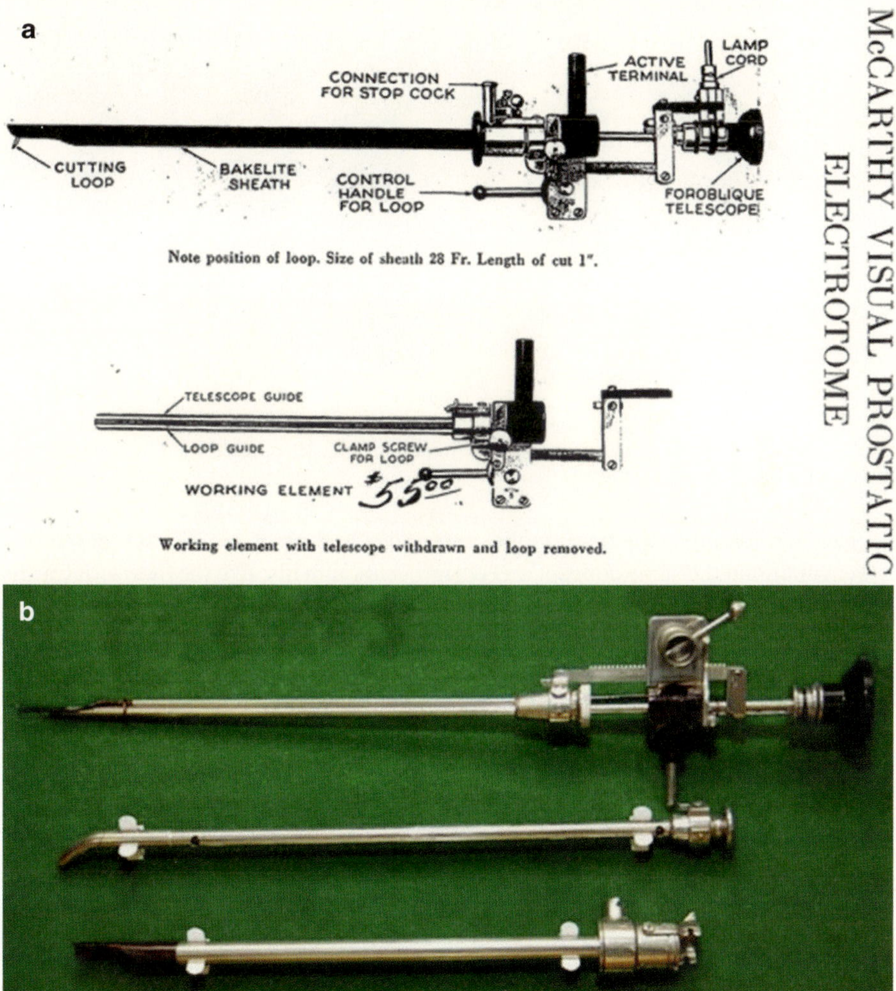

Fig. 6.4 (**a**) Illustration labeling components of Stern-McCarthy resectoscope, 1931. (**b**) Stern-McCarthy resectoscope, 1931

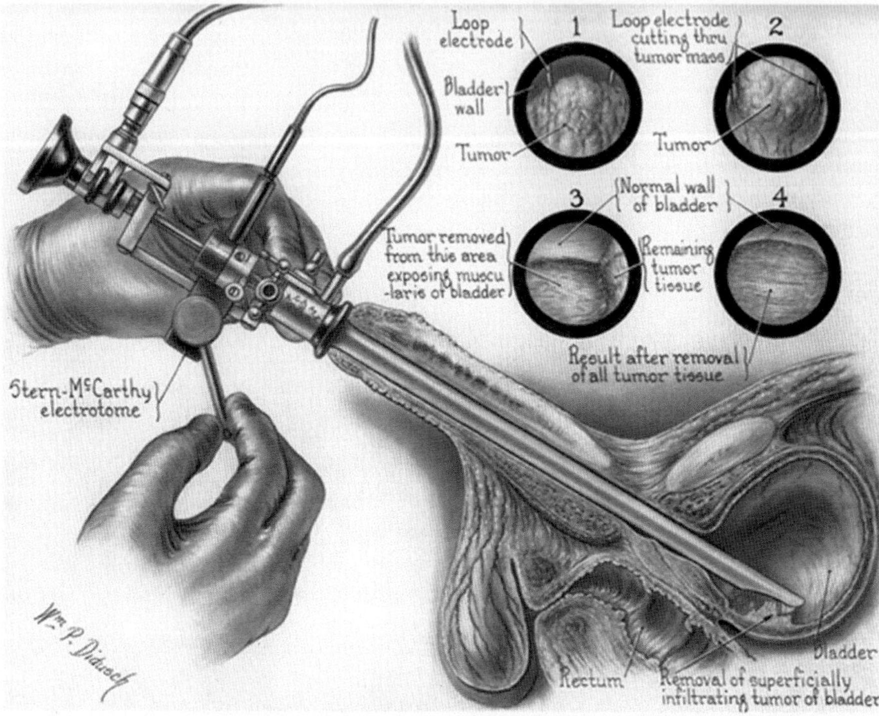

Fig. 6.5 William P Didusch illustration of transurethral resection of bladder tumor using Stern-McCarthy resectoscope (Picture from the William P. Didusch Center for Urologic History, Linthicum, MD)

Nesbit's resectoscope became the forerunner to current modern resectoscopes, which maintain the same concept and design. Although his, like the Stern-McCarthy resectoscope, was developed primarily for transurethral resection of the prostate, TURP has given way to newer methods to relieve prostatic obstruction, whereas TURB remains today a standard operation for bladder tumors. The reasons are obvious: tumors are better removed by resection than destroyed by fulguration, tissue is provided for accurate pathologic evaluation, virtually all superficial and some minimally invasive neoplasms can be cured, and the method can be repeated indefinitely to access the bladder and control recurrent tumors.

Past, Present, and Future

Over the century and a quarter since endoscopy was first conceived in 1806 to the development of the first modern resectoscope in 1931, endoscopic surgery of bladder tumors advanced from an idea to practical reality. Noteworthy individuals and

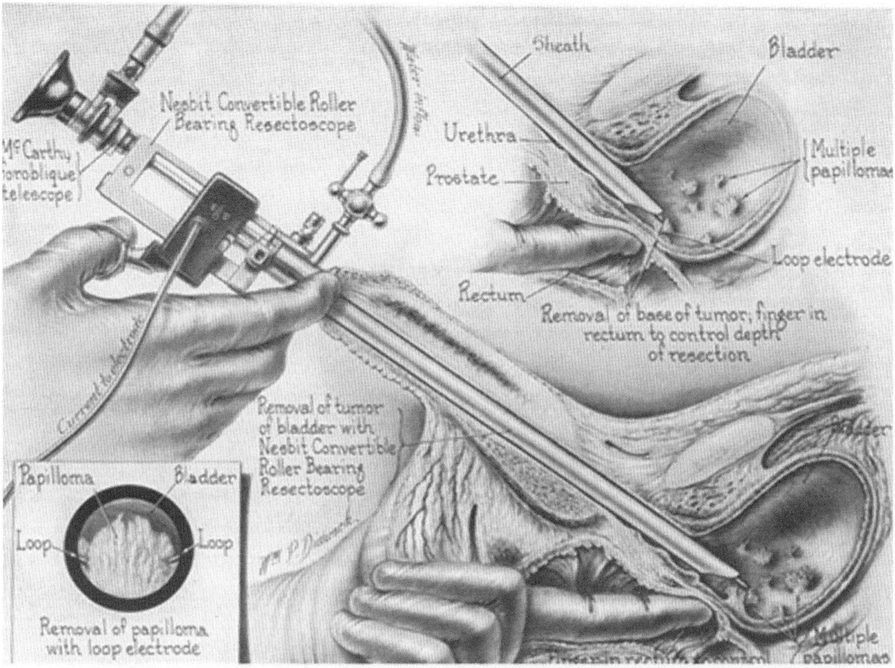

Fig. 6.6 William P Didusch illustration of one-handed Nesbit resectoscope used for transurethral resection of bladder tumor, 1938 (Picture from the William P. Didusch Center for Urologic History, Linthicum, MD)

their innovations each built on discoveries of the past to advance endoscopic treatment of bladder tumors founded on four landmark inventions: a cystoscope, incandescent light bulb, the fenestrated tube, and the application of high-frequency electrical current active in a water environment.

In the second half of the twentieth century, further improvements were created, none more important than introduction of zoom lens and rod-lens system by the physicist Harold Hopkins [11]. Use of glass fibers (fiberoptics), first for illumination and later for flexible optics, was able to carry true video images, and allowed for the creation of flexible endoscopy. Video cameras soon followed, which improved the ergonomics, safety and success rates of tumor resections.

In 1970, Boyle and Smith created the charge-coupled device (CCD)—a semiconductor chip that could record images as a grid of pixels, leading to a move from fiberoptic endoscopy to distal sensor (digital) image-based endoscopy [12]. Digital endoscopes can identify lesions as small as 1 mm at greater distances than was previously possible with fiberoptic technology. Light weight digital cameras were soon attached to the eyepiece of resectoscopes and connected to high definition TV screens to provide superb magnified vision inside the bladder and to facilitate facile transurethral resection. The CCD chip also made possible narrow-band imaging (NBI), a filter that restricts wavelengths of white light to highlight mucosal microvessels, which are enhanced in urothelial tumors in contrast to bland normal mucosa. NBI improves detection and mucosal extent of tumors, facilitating more complete destruction.

Real-time endoscopic histologic tissue and molecular characterization of bladder tumors is on the horizon, with Raman spectroscopy, optical coherence tomography, confocal endomicroscopy, and their disciples projected to become routine in the near future. Enhanced imaging technology represents technical improvements, based on the premise that if one sees better, one resects better, but they are not designed as replacements for the well-established and proven TURB. The basic TURB remains the same as conceived by Stern, Davis, McCarthy and Nesbit nearly a century ago—using a cystoscopic sheath, wide-angle telescope, single-handed working element to guide assortments of loops and coagulating devices into the bladder used to remove and destroy tumors, direct vision light and lens sources within the bladder, saline irrigation (replacing water), separate cutting and coagulation currents and a foot switch to control both. None of this would have happened if not for the genius displayed by countless individuals from multiple disciplines in the twentieth century, who combined their talents to transform Nitze's original concept of an operating cystoscope into today's sophisticated and successful endoscopic treatment of many maladies involving the urinary tract. Arguably, bladder neoplasms are the most significant of these, and suffering patients are the ultimate beneficiaries of their discoveries.

Acknowledgement Assistance and illustrations kindly provided by Tupper Stevens, archivist, William P. Didusch Center for Urologic History, Linthicum, Maryland.

References

1. Zorgniotti A. Bladder cancer in the pre-cystoscopic era. Prog Clin Biol Res. 1984;162A:1–9.
2. Herr HW. Early history of endoscopic treatment of bladder tumors. From Grunfeld's polypenkneipe to Stern-McCarthy resectoscope. J Endourol. 2006;20:85–91.
3. Desormeaux AJ. Del'Endoscope et de ses Applications au Diagnostic et au Traitement des Affections de l'Urethre et de la Vessie. Paris; 1865.
4. Grunfeld J. Polypen der Harnblase, auf endokopischem Wege diagnostiziert und operiert. Wien Med Presse; 1885. p. 89.
5. Herr HW. Max Nitze, the cystoscope and urology. J Urol. 2006;176:1313–6.
6. Nitze M. Ueber intravesicale Operationen von Blasengeschwulsten. Centr Chir. 1895;22:971.
7. Beer E. Removal of neoplasms of the urinary bladder: a new method, employing high frequency (Oudin) currents. JAMA. 1910;54:1768.
8. Stern M. A new cystoscopic instrument employing a cutting current capable of operation in a water medium. Read before the New York Academy of Medicine, January 20, 1926.
9. McCarthy JF. A new apparatus for endoscopic surgery of the prostate, diathermia, and excision of vesical growths. J Urol. 1931;26:695–7.
10. Nesbit RMA. Modification of the Stern-McCarthy resectoscope permitting third dimensional perception during transurethral prostatectomy. J Urol. 1938:646–8.
11. Gow JG. Harold Hopkins and optical systems for urology—an appreciation. Urology. 1998;52:152–7.
12. Boyle WS, Smith GS. Charge coupled semiconductor devices. Bell Syst Tech J. 1970;49:587–93.

Chapter 7
The Birth of Endourology

Arthur D. Smith

Willard Goodwin performed what actually was the first percutaneous nephrostomy in 1955. He and two colleagues had a patient with hydronephrosis and wanted to relieve the pressure, so they inserted a needle [1]. The procedure was considered so extraordinary that their report on it appeared in JAMA. However the technique did not catch on: it was not used again until the 1970s, when it gained popularity because open drainage for bilateral ureteral obstruction was so hazardous. The patients who required the procedure were quite ill, with bleeding tendencies arising from uremia and the underlying problem that caused the obstruction in the first place. Both the ureter and the renal hilum frequently were not accessible because of enlarged lymph nodes; thus the insertion of the needle.

In 1977, a patient who had received radiation therapy for cancer of the prostate presented with ureteral obstruction. He had undergone ureteral reimplantation but postoperatively developed a leak at the anastomotic site. It would have been desirable to insert a stent into the ureter, but this was not possible because the anastomotic site was not accessible with a rigid cystoscope. The only stent that was available at this time was the Gibbon's stent which had a closed upper end. We decided to solve the problem by pulling a stent up the ureter from the kidney. A percutaneous nephrostomy was created, and a 6Fr catheter was guided down the ureter so that the tip could be retrieved cystoscopically [2]. We then attached a filiform dilator and follower, as well as the Gibbons stent and positioned it to allow splinting of the anastomosis and appropriate drainage of the kidney [3] (Fig. 7.1). Subsequently a redesigned retrograde stent made it easier to use [4].

Shortly after we treated this patient, we had another whose kidney was obstructed by a ureteroileal stone. Once again, a nephrostomy was performed and a catheter advanced down the ureter to the ileal loop and retrieved cystoscopically. A stone

A.D. Smith, M.D.
The Arthur Smith Institute of Urology, 450 Lakeville Road, Lake Success, NY 11042, USA
e-mail: asmith1@northwell.edu

S.R. Patel et al. (eds.), *The History of Technologic Advancements in Urology*,
DOI 10.1007/978-3-319-61691-9_7

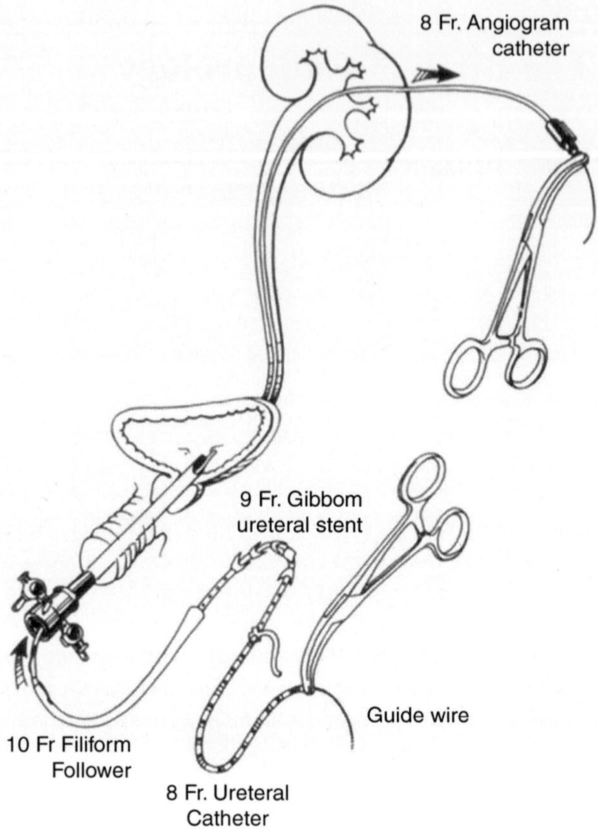

Fig. 7.1 Steps required to pull a Gibbons stent into the ureter

basket was attached to the tip of this catheter, and the stone was captured under fluoroscopic control [5] (Fig. 7.2).

In the days before ureteroscopy, blind stone basketing was the only technique available for endoscopic stone removal. If this extraction failed, or if there was more than one stone, it frequently was difficult to salvage the situation because the ureter resisted second and third passages of a stone basket. The problem was solved by advancing a catheter antegrade down the ureter and attaching a basket that could then be pulled up as often as necessary [6] (Fig. 7.3).

Patients who had repeated resections of bladder tumors sometimes developed ureteral meatal stenosis. Cystoscopic viewing of the ureteral orifice was not possible. If one advanced a catheter down the ureter from a percutaneous nephrostomy to the site of the stricture, one could resect over this site under fluoroscopic control and then stent the ureter if appropriate [7] (Fig. 7.4). In addition, it was possible to perform a meatotomy by attaching an adapted ureteral catheter with an exposed section of stylet to dilate and cut the orifice. A further application of the antegrade catheter was used in patients who developed ureteral strictures after ileal conduit surgery. The stricture could be bypassed, dilated and stented.

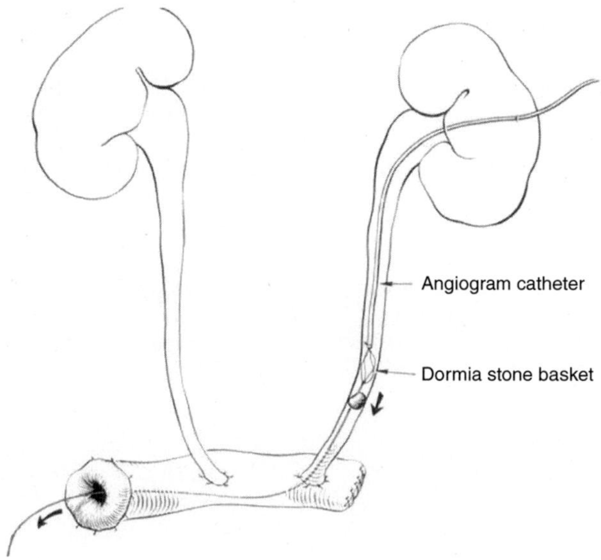

Fig. 7.2 Controlled retrograde extraction of ureteroileal stone. (**a**) Technique, (**b**) Special stone basket that can be opened from either the proximal or the distal end

In the 1960s and early 1970s, ileal conduit diversion was commonly performed for the management of neurogenic bladder in paraplegic and quadriplegic patients. These patients frequently developed kidney stones, which had to be removed surgically. In quadriplegic patients with stone recurrence, a nephrostomy tube frequently was left in place and attempts were made to dissolve the stones with citric acid, magnesium carbonate and glucono-delta-lactone (Renacidin) [8]. This technique was later extended to patients with recurrent struvite stones without initial removal of the bulk of the stone (Fig. 7.5).

Let it be said that the technique worked, but it took more than a month to dissolve a stone. At that time, this was acceptable at the Veterans Administration hospital (as it was then called), but not in the real world. Moreover, Renacidin had many side effects, such as marked mucosal edema and hypermagnesemia. Fortunately, a urology surgery resident, Curtis Sheldon, was standing at the bedside and knew exactly what to do to revive the patient. The technique proved more successful and less dangerous for chemolysis of cystine and uric acid stones [9].

Several patients who had nephrostomy drainage tubes did not want to undergo chemolysis, and they therefore needed frequent changes of their drainage tubes (usually a Foley catheter). Moreover, we routinely injected only 3 mL of liquid into the balloon of the foley catheter, which meant they often fell out. If the catheter had been out of the nephrostomy tract for less than 1 day, it was usually possible to reestablish the tract by inserting a 5Fr catheter at the skin site and instilling a small amount of contrast medium. The tract become partially visible and a guidewire and more contrast medium could be injected to guide catheter insertion. The complete tract could then be dilated and new nephrostomy tube inserted.

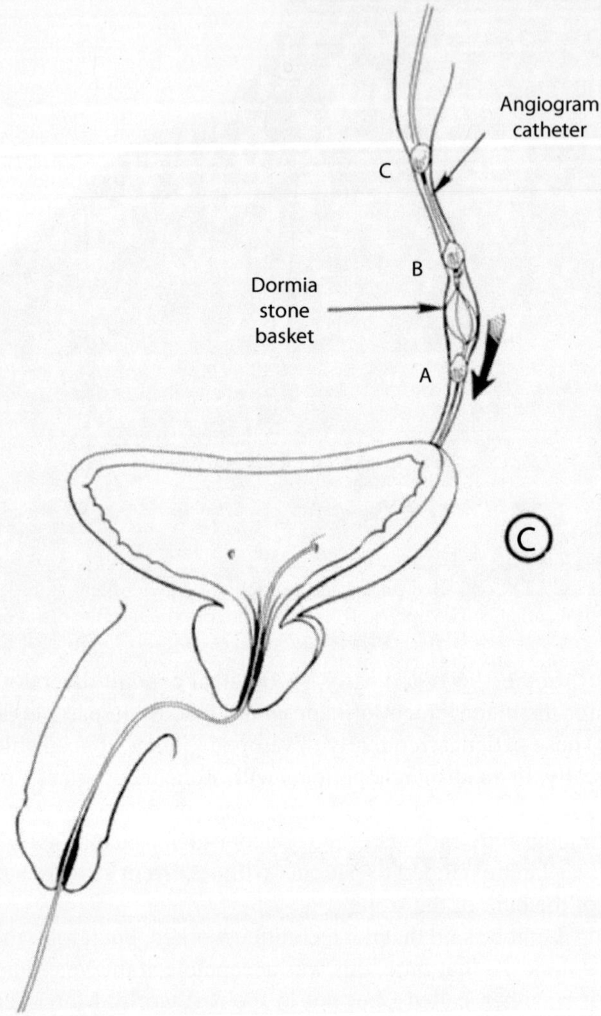

Fig. 7.3 Controlled ureteral stone basketing

It proved difficult to maintain a Foley catheter in the kidney, as the balloon would obstruct one or several calices. The best drainage device available at the time was a circle nephrostomy tube. [10] This tube entered through an upper calix and exited from a lower calix, allowing drainage without obstruction of any part of the kidney. In addition, the tube could be changed easily by attaching a new catheter to the old one and railroading it into position. To convert a nephrostomy tube already in place to a circle tube, the tube was removed and a stone basket inserted into the renal pelvis. A second puncture was then performed, usually into an upper calix and the guidewire it contained was directed toward the open stone basket. When it entered the basket, the basket was closed and the wire was pulled out through the original nephrostomy site. A catheter was then advanced over this captured guidewire, the tract was dilated and a circle tube was inserted. This technique was also used in patients who developed meatal stenosis after cutaneous ureterostomy.

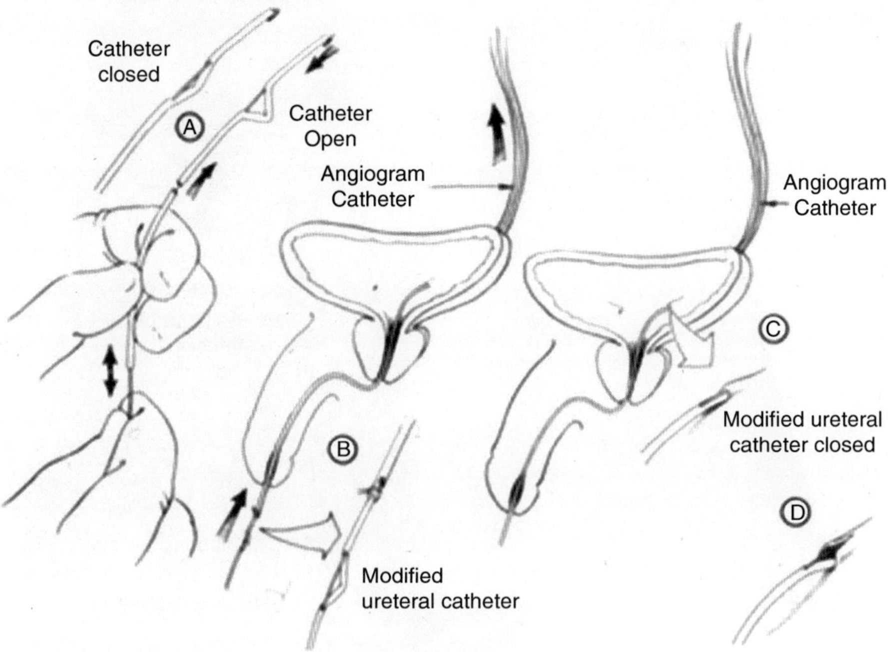

Fig. 7.4 Controlled ureteral meatotomy

All of the techniques were developed with the assistance of Robert Miller, an interventional radiologist at the Veterans Administration (now Veterans Affairs) Hospital in Minneapolis. Subsequently, I moved to the University of Minnesota campus and began working with Kurt Amplatz and Wilfrido Castaneda-Zuniga. They had a very capable technician who could manufacture any desired device overnight.

It was at this time—in 1979—that we had another development that had nothing to do with equipment. The Chairman of the Department of Urologic Surgery at the University of Minnesota, the late Dr. Erwin E. Fraley, had been pondering what we were doing. He had an intense interest in language, and he thought our new techniques deserved a name of their own. The one he created was "endourology," which was accepted immediately by the profession [6]. We had created a new specialty, which employed the skills of urologists and interventional radiologists.

It soon became clear that if we wanted to remove stones, we needed a stable nephrostomy tube tract so that if an instrument slipped out of the tract, it would be reinserted easily. This required antegrade insertion of a second guidewire down the ureter from the nephrostomy site. We started calling this extra guidewire the "safety guidewire."

If the ureteroplevic junction was not enlarged, it often was difficult to direct this guidewire down the ureter. It often required a shaped catheter that could direct the guidewire in the direction we wanted it to go. This was achieved by heating the tip of a 5Fr catheter over a Bunsen burner until it was very flexible and then bending it into an appropriate configuration and cooling the catheter tip with cold sterile water. This was not convenient, but it worked well.

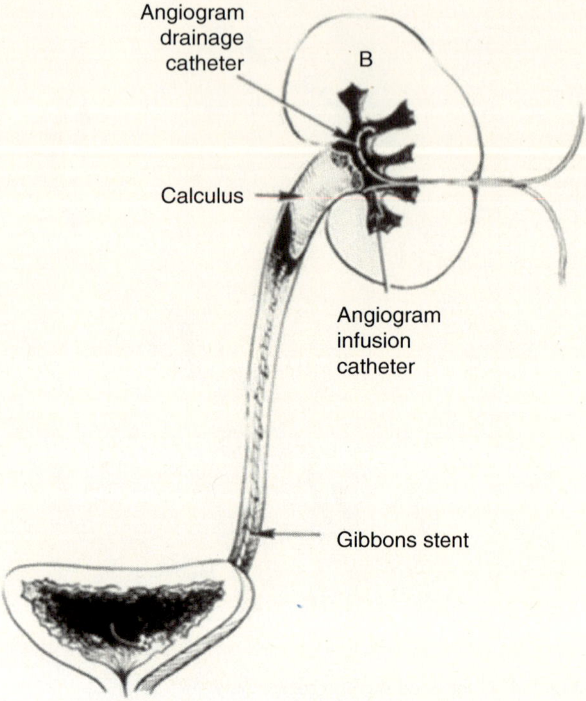

Fig. 7.5 During chemolysis, it is important to ensure good drainage

The next phase was to figure out how to dilate the nephrostomy tract adequately. Initially, we cut the metal tip of a follower off and advanced it over the 5Fr catheter. Then our technician fused these parts into a long tube, which we exchanged for larger tubes in sequence. When using this technique, we could not see when the dilating device was traversing the ureteropelvic junction and worried that we would damage this area. So we inserted a metal ring between the area between the 5Fr catheter and the dilator (Fig. 7.6). Then we could see where all the parts of the device were. Once we could dilate the tract easily, we wanted a sheath through which we could access the kidney. We used a hollow tube that was passed over the final dilator.

We then had to decide how far we could dilate the nephrostomy tract. We decided that the sheath should have an inner diameter of 30Fr, as this would accommodate a 1 cm kidney stone. It also would easily allow passage of a 26Fr nephroscope while allowing egress of water, thereby ensuring no build-up of intrapelvic pressure. This entire assembly was the beginning of the Amplatz dilating system that we still use today.

The access sheath was used in a variety of ways to extract stones (Fig. 7.7). Stone baskets were employed, as well as grasping forceps originally used to remove gall-stones. One patient had multiple small stones and we tried the Ellick evacuator. This did not work: with suction, the renal pelvis collapsed onto the tip of the access

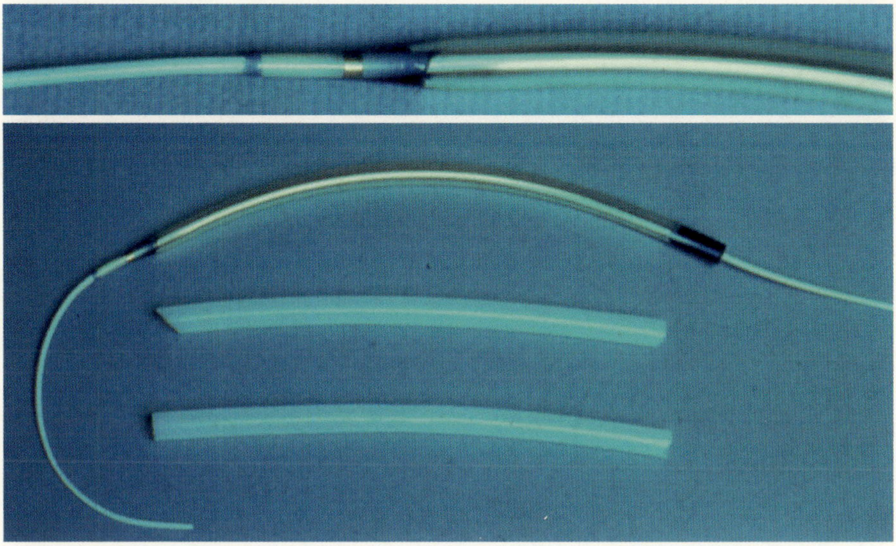

Fig. 7.6 Original Amplatz dilators and sheath. Note the metal radiopaque marker

sheath. When we cut the tip of the sheath at an angle, this did not occur. Access sheaths now have a terminal angle.

We also needed a suitable nephrostomy tube to place at the end of the procedure. We initially though that the Stamey suprapubic catheter was suitable but decided that the introducer was too dangerous to use in the kidney. Our technician cut off the needle tip and replaced the body of the needle with a coiled wire tube that enabled a Malecot tip to be flattened so it could be advanced over a guidewire through a narrow tract.

In 1982, I moved to Long Island Jewish Medical Center and continued to remove stones percutaneously. Over the course of time, we had a need to remove stones from many obese patients, a problem that is becoming increasingly common. The Stamey nephrostomy tube proved inadequate, as it did not splint the ureteropelvic junction; and when obese patients rolled over in bed, the panniculus moved and the nephrostomy tube slipped out. We elected to use the Malecot-type catheter with a tail that extended down the ureter, creating the re-entry nephrostomy tube, which was produced commercially by Boston Scientific and Cook Urological.

Some patients were referred to me after a failed pyeloplasty and clamping of the established nephrostomy tube caused pain and fever. I believed that simple dilation would be inadequate; that the ureteropelvic junction had to be incised. This incision was splinted with a 14Fr catheter at the upper end and a 7Fr catheter at the lower end, which was coiled in the bladder [11, 12]. The tube was positioned so that there were side holes in the renal pelvis but none at the ureteropelvic junction. The change in diameter occurred in the upper third of the ureter (endopyelotomy stent; Cook Urological).

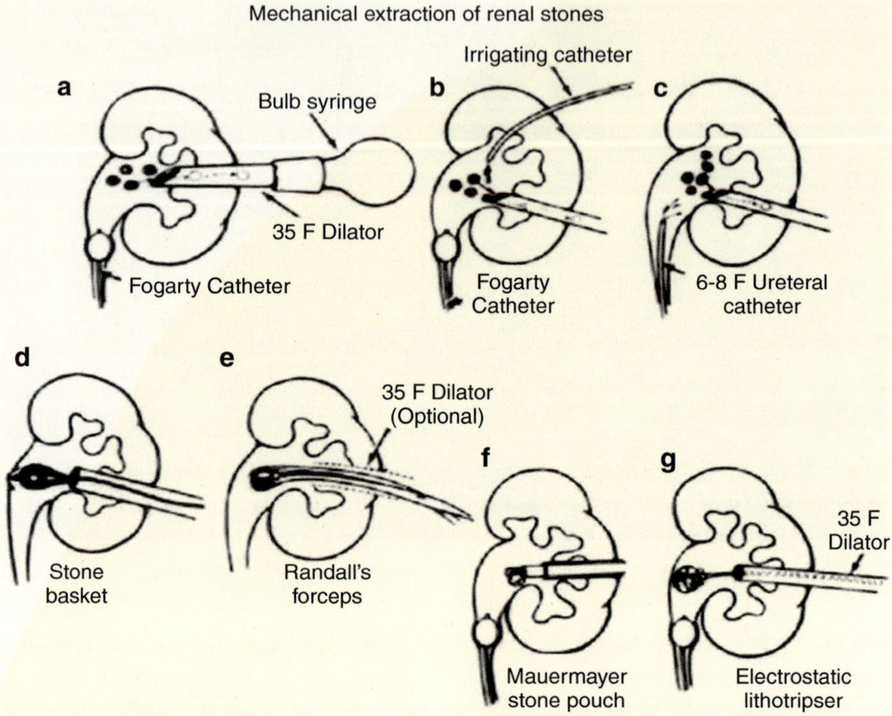

Fig. 7.7 Different irrigations and extraction methods for kidney stones. (**a–c**) Flushing techniques. (**d**, **e**) Grasping techniques. (**f**, **g**) Crushing techniques

Our next endeavor was removal of upper-tract transitional cell carcinoma. Our idea was that if low grade tumors could be resected from the bladder without cystectomy (as was well known), why not do the same thing from the ureter or kidney? Ureteral tumors could be removed ureteroscopically, but larger tumors in the pelvicaliceal system could not be resected adequately. We developed a technique for percutaneous resection with subsequent topical chemotherapy or Nd:YAG laser ablation [13]. A recent review of the long-term outcome of more than 200 cases proved that we were able to spare 83% from nephrectomy.

It has been exciting over the past 35 years to see all the fundamental changes that have occurred in our management of patients by pursuing minimally invasive operations. The list of publications on the subject has become too long to be convenient! We have dramatically reduced morbidity and allowed our patients a far more rapid return to their normal daily activities. These changes came about through the collaboration of physicians in different specialties and working with industry to evolve better and safer equipment. It has been a most satisfying journey.

References

1. Goodwin WE, Casey WC, Woolf VV. Percutaneous trocar (needle) nephrostomy in hydronephrosis. JAMA. 1955;157:891–4.
2. Smith AD, Lange PH, Miller RP, Reinke DB. Introduction of Gibbons ureteral stent facilitated by antecedent percutaneous nephrostomy. J Urol. 1978;120:543–4.
3. Smith AD, Lange PH, Miller RP, Reinke DB. Percutaneous dilation of ureteroileal strictures and insertion of Gibbons ureteral stents. Urology. 1979;13:24–6.
4. Smith AD, Miller RP, Reinke DB, Lange PH, Fraley EE. Insertion of Gibbons ureteral stents using endourologic techniques. Urology. 1979;14:330–6.
5. Smith AD, Lange PH, Reinke DB, Miller RP. Extraction of ureteral calculi from patients with ileal loops: a new technique. J Urol. 1978;120:623–5.
6. Smith AD, Lange PH, Fraley EE. Applications of percutaneous nephrostomy: new challenges and opportunities in endourology. J Urol. 1979;121:382.
7. Smith AD, Lange PH, Miller RP, Reinke DB. Controlled meatotomy. J Urol. 1979;121:587–9.
8. Sheldon CA, Smith AD. Chemolysis of calculi. Urol Clin North Am. 1982;9:121–30.
9. Smith AD, Lange PH, Miller RP, Reinke DB. Dissolution of cystine calculi by irrigation with acetylcysteine through percutaneous nephrostomy. Urology. 1979;13:422–3.
10. Smith AD, Fraley EE, Castandeda-Zuniga WR, Aplatz K. Percutaneous circle tube nephrostomy. J Urol. 1982;127:29–30.
11. Karlin GS, Smith AD. Endopyelotomy. Urol Clin North Am. 1988;15:439–44.
12. Badlani GH, Smith AD. Stent for endopyelotomy. Urol Clin North Am. 1988;15:445–8.
13. Orihuela E, Smith AD. Percutaneous treatment of transitional cell carcinoma of the upper urinary tract. Urol Clin North Am. 1988;15:425–31.

Chapter 8
History of the Development of Guidewires, Access Sheaths, Baskets, and Ureteral Stents

Natalia Hernandez Bustos, Alan Yaghoubian, Sarah Mozafarpour, and Brian Eisner

Guidewires

Guidewires are a mainstay of endourologic procedures, as they provide safe access to the urinary tract and allow the passage of catheters and stents [1]. The development of guidewires in urology began with the application of angiographic tools in urologic endoscopy. Fritzche et al. reported the use of angiographic guidewires in 7 patients with ureteral obstruction in 1981 [2]. The authors noted in this study that their methods allow the "placement of angiographic guide wires and catheters past ureteral obstacles when standard urological retrograde procedures are not feasible technically." The transvesical approach was described as where a 6Fr open-ended polyethylene catheter was placed at the ureterovesical junction and followed by advancing a 0.035 in. diameter guide wire [2]. The authors noted several advantages of the angiographic catheters and wires that allowed their urological application. The smaller diameter floppy tip reduced the risk of ureteral injury. A curve could be applied to the wire to facilitate manipulation and a wide range of shapes and sizes available for angiography allowed the urologist to attach a stone basket to the catheter for multiple passages through the level of obstruction [2]. Advances over subsequent years created specialized categories of guidewires which allowed the urologist to select the most appropriate tool for a given circumstance. These wires include hydrophilic straight and angled guidewires (used for bypassing more difficult obstructions or for the tortuous ureter), the hybrid wires (wires with a hydrophilic distal tip for bypassing obstructing stones and a nitinol core which is kink resistant to be used as a working wire) and stiffer wires such as Amplatz extra stiff (used to straighten ureter or for stabilization when passing dilating catheters and access sheaths) [1, 3]. More recent studies have evaluated the mechanical

N.H. Bustos (✉) • A. Yaghoubian • S. Mozafarpour • B. Eisner
Department of Urology, Massachusetts General Hospital, Harvard Medical School, Boston, MA 02114, USA
e-mail: BEISNER@mgh.harvard.edu

S.R. Patel et al. (eds.), *The History of Technologic Advancements in Urology*,
DOI 10.1007/978-3-319-61691-9_8

characteristics and performance elements of guidewires, including tip bending, resistance, pull force, shaft bending resistance, tip puncture force, shaft stiffness, and lubricity [1, 4]. The authors corroborated that hybrid wires offer the combination of the hydrophilic tip and stiffer shaft than standard wires, while the extra stiff wires may be best-suited for placement of ureteral access sheaths or larger stents. Interestingly they also noted that "brand name" guidewires designed for the same purposes may differ from one manufacturer to the next.

There has been some controversy in the literature regarding the use of safety wires during either semi-rigid or flexible ureteroscopy. The safety wire, positioned alongside the ureteroscope during endoscopic manipulation, maintains ureteral access to the upper tract and facilitates stent placement in the case of ureteral injury or bleeding which obscures the surgeon's field of view. Proponents of the safety wire feel that in extreme cases and unanticipated intraoperative complications, the use safety wire will decrease the rate of nephrostomy tube placement or other complication by allowing allowing for safe placement of a stent. Early ureteroscopy series originating from the mid 1980s consistently advocated for the routine use of safety wire for these reasons [5, 6]. However, more recent studies have called this dogma into question within the last decade. Advocates for the elimination of the safety wire from routine semi-rigid and flexible ureteroscopy argue that with the advent of improved optics, smaller more maneuverable ureteroscopes, and advancements in procedure technique allow the urologist to safely perform the procedure without a the safety wire [7–10]. Although the aforementioned series have demonstrated the feasibility of omitting the safety wire during ureteroscopy, it is still commonly used in practice by many [11].

Ureteral Access Sheaths

During the first successful ureteroscopic evaluations of the upper urinary tract, Takayasu and Aso observed that the major challenge was the insertion of the scope into the ureter. To solve this problem, they introduced the concept of the ureteral access sheath (UAS) in 1974—they reported a guide tube made of Teflon that allowed the passage of the ureteroscope to the upper tract [12]. In a subsequent study which occurred during an 18-month period from 1984–1985, Newman et al. described a novel ureteral access sheath dilator system in 1985 and subsequently described a series of 43 procedures during which a ureteral access sheath set was used [13, 14]. They demonstrated a 51% stone free rate, 92% rate of successful ureteral stricture dilation, and 88% success rate of diagnostic evaluation of upper tract filling defects [13, 14]. Ureteral perforation due to access sheath placement/dilation were observed in 18% of procedures. The "peel-away" introducer sheath was first reported in 1987 by Rich et al.—this was a 60 cm sheath available in sizes ranging from 8 to 18 FR that was placed over a 0.038 in. guidewire. The sheath included two knobs which were used to peel the sheath and adjust to the appropriate length for the procedure. The authors reported use of this sheath for retrograde and antegrade stone basket extraction, flushing stones into the renal pelvis, retrograde stent placement, and catheterization of tortuous ureters [15]. Though early reported complications of ureteral access sheaths limited their widespread adoption, a renewed interest in these devices has occurred with the newer generation of access sheaths. First described by Kourambas et al., in 2001, the latest generation of ureteral access sheaths had an impregnated wire and hydrophilic coating, facilitating safer insertion [11, 16]. In their 2001 study, the authors randomized 59 patients to semi-rigid or flexible ureteroscopy with or without a ureteral access sheath and reported that routine use of ureteral access sheath was associated with decreased operative time and cost without an increase in complication rate. In the ensuing 3 years, additional studies on these devices noted that ureteral access sheaths decreased renal pelvis pressures during ureteroscopy (which may decrease risk of postoperative pain and infection) and also increased the time between repairs of flexible ureteroscopes due to minimizing ureteroscope damage [17–19]. In 2003, Delvecchio et al. reported long-term follow up of patients who had undergone ureteroscopy with UAS with a stricture rate of 1.4% which suggests that the use of UAS does not increase the risk of stricture development compared with ureteroscopy performed without a sheath [20]. Most recently, the CROES Ureteroscopy Global Study, a multicenter study of the use of ureteral access sheath evaluated 2239 patients treated with ureteroscopy (67% of whom had an access sheath used during ureteroscopy)—there were no observed differences in stone free rate or ureteral trauma, but UAS were associated with a 50% reduction in sepsis after ureteroscopy (4.7% sepsis rate in patients in whom UAS was used compared with 9% for no UAS) [21]. A 2014 survey of the Endourological Society with 414 respondents from 44 countries noted that 58% of surgeons routinely use a UAS for every flexible ureteroscopy procedure [22].

Stone Retrieval Devices

The initial description of a stone retrieval device was the Davis Stone extractor, described in 1953 by Thomas A. Davis [23]. This device, developed from a 5Fr ureteral catheter incorporating a monofilament Nylon thread, was used for extraction of distal ureteral stones smaller than 0.5 cm [23–25]. Nearly 15 years later, Constantian reported a success rate of 88% in a 10 year series of procedures which incorporated the Davis Stone Extractor [24]. In 1982 Enrico Dormia reported the use of the Dormia or helical basket in patients with proximal ureteral stones [26]. Under fluoroscopic guidance, a six-crossed or a three-crossed spiral basket (chosen based on stone size) was passed through a cystoscope and into the ureter. The helical design of this basket allowed engaging of the stone with rotational movement of the device after placing the basket in a proximal position. Dormia reported a 94% success rate for stone removal [26, 27]. The ensuing decade saw the development

7. Dickstein RJ, Kreshover JE, Babayan RK, et al. Is a safety wire necessary during routine flexible ureteroscopy? J Endourol. 2010;24:1589.
8. Eandi JA, Hu B, Low RK. Evaluation of the impact and need for use of a safety guidewire during ureteroscopy. J Endourol. 2008;22:1653.
9. Dutta R, Vyas A, Landman J, et al. Death of the safety guidewire. J Endourol. 2016;30:941–4.
10. Patel SR, McLaren ID, Nakada SY. The ureteroscope as a safety wire for ureteronephroscopy. J Endourol. 2012;26:351.
11. Rizkala ER, Monga M. Controversies in ureteroscopy: wire, basket, and sheath. Indian J Urol. 2013;29:244.
12. Takayasu H, Aso Y. Recent development for pyeloureteroscopy: guide tube method for its introduction into the ureter. J Urol. 1974;112:176.
13. Newman R, Hunter PT, Hawkins I, et al. A general ureteral dilator-sheathing system. Urology. 1985;25:287.
14. Newman RC, Hunter PT, Hawkins IF, et al. The ureteral access system: a review of the immediate results in 43 cases. J Urol. 1987;137:380.
15. Rich M, Lee WJ, Smith AD. Applications of the peel-away introducer sheath. J Urol. 1987;137:452.
16. Kourambas J, Byrne RR, Preminger GM. Dose a ureteral access sheath facilitate ureteroscopy? J Urol. 2001;165:789.
17. Auge BK, Pietrow PK, Lallas CD, et al. Ureteral access sheath provides protection against elevated renal pressures during routine flexible ureteroscopic stone manipulation. J Endourol. 2004;18:33.
18. Rehman J, Monga M, Landman J, et al. Characterization of intrapelvic pressure during ureteropyeloscopy with ureteral access sheaths. Urology. 2003;61:713.
19. Pietrow PK, Auge BK, Delvecchio FC, et al. Techniques to maximize flexible ureteroscope longevity. Urology. 2002;60:784.
20. Delvecchio FC, Auge BK, Brizuela RM, et al. Assessment of stricture formation with the ureteral access sheath. Urology. 2003;61:518.
21. Traxer O, Wendt-Nordahl G, Sodha H, et al. Differences in renal stone treatment and outcomes for patients treated either with or without the support of a ureteral access sheath: the clinical research office of the endourological society ureteroscopy global study. World J Urol. 2015;33:2137.
22. Dauw CA, Simeon L, Alruwaily AF, et al. Contemporary practice patterns of flexible ureteroscopy for treating renal stones: results of a worldwide survey. J Endourol. 2015;29:1221.
23. Davis TA. Removal of ureteral calculus by a new catheter type extractor. J Urol. 1954;72:346.
24. Constantian HM. Use of the Davis nylon loop extractor for removal of low ureteral calculi. J Urol. 1967;97:248.
25. Warren JW Jr. The Davis loop stone extractor: results of use. J Urol. 1961;86:684.
26. Dormia E. Dormia basket: standard technique, observations, and general concepts. Urology. 1982;20:437.
27. Conlin MJ, Marberger M, Bagley DH. Ureteroscopy: development and instrumentation. Urol Clin North Am. 1997;24:25.
28. Kavoussi L, Clayman RV, Basler J. Flexible, actively deflectable fiberoptic ureteronephroscopy. J Urol. 1989;142:949.
29. Grasso M, Bagley D. A 7.5/8.2 F actively deflectable, flexible ureteroscope: a new device for both diagnostic and therapeutic upper urinary tract endoscopy. Urology. 1994;43:435.
30. Honey RJD. Assessment of a new tipless nitinol stone basket and comparison with an existing flat-wire basket. J Endourol. 1998;12:529.
31. Dretler SP. Ureteroscopy for proximal ureteral calculi: prevention of stone migration. J Endourol. 2000;14:565.
32. Dretler SP. The stone cone: a new generation of basketry. J Urol. 2001;165:1593.
33. Eisner BH, Dretler SP. Use of the stone cone for prevention of calculus retropulsion during holmium:YAG laser lithotripsy: case series and review of the literature. Urol Int. 2009;82:356.

34. Ding H, Wang Z, Du W, et al. NTrap in prevention of stone migration during ureteroscopic lithotripsy for proximal ureteral stones: a meta-analysis. J Endourol. 2012;26:130.
35. Rane A, Bradoo A, Rao P, et al. The use of a novel reverse thermosensitive polymer to prevent ureteral stone retropulsion during intracorporeal lithotripsy: a randomized, controlled trial. J Urol. 2010;183:1417.
36. JA W, Ngo TC, Hagedorn JC, et al. The accordion antiretropulsive device improves stone-free rates during ureteroscopic laser lithotripsy. J Endourol. 2013;27:438.
37. Herman JR. Urology: a view through the retrospectroscope. New York: HarperCollins Publishers; 1973.
38. Tulloch WS. Restoration of the continuity of the ureter by means of polythene tubing. Br J Urol. 1952;24:42.
39. Zimskind PD, Fetter TR, Wilkerson JL. Clinical use of long-term indwelling silicone rubber ureteral splints inserted cystoscopically. J Urol. 1967;97:840.
40. Gibbons RP, Correa RJ Jr, Cummings KB, et al. Experience with indwelling ureteral stent catheters. J Urol. 1976;115:22.
41. Finney RP. Experience with new double J ureteral catheter stent. J Urol. 1978;120:678.
42. Chew BH, Lange D. Advances in ureteral stent development. Curr Opin Urol. 2016;26:277.

Chapter 9
History of Laser Lithotripsy

Paul Bower and Gyan Pareek

The application of lasers for use in the treatment of kidney stones is among the most important developments in the specialty of urology in the last 50 years. As kidney stone prevalence continues to rise from an estimated 5.2% in 1994 to 8.8% in 2012, the importance of the development and evolution of laser technology cannot be understated [1]. Laser applications in urology have given the ability to treat urinary stones in a minimally invasive manner without requiring an open surgical approach. In this chapter, we report on the origin and evolution of laser technology in the field of urology.

Light Amplification for the Stimulated Emission of Radiation (LASER) was a term first coined in 1957 by Gordon Gould [2]. The LASER was based on the principles of the microwave amplification by the stimulated emission of radiation (MASER) device proposed by Joseph Weber in 1952. The first LASER device was built in 1953 at Columbia University by Charles Townes [3, 4]. MASER and LASER technology are both applications based on the principle of stimulated emission proposed by Albert Einstein in 1917 where photons can be generated in the same phase and direction using an electromagnetic field for orientation.

Ruby Laser

The first laser for lithotripsy, the ruby laser, was built 3 years after Gould coined the phrase LASER. The 694 nm laser was first utilized in 1960 by Maiman [5]. The first success for the destruction of urinary stones was performed by Mulvany and Beck in 1968 using the 694 nm ruby laser excited by a xenon lamp [6]. Stones were

P. Bower, M.D. • G. Pareek, M.D., F.A.C.S. (✉)
Division of Urology, Alpert Medical School of Brown University,
Providence, RI 02903, USA
e-mail: gyan_pareek@brown.edu

S.R. Patel et al. (eds.), *The History of Technologic Advancements in Urology*,
DOI 10.1007/978-3-319-61691-9_9

fragmented with energy delivery levels of 50–300 J per pulse of energy. A key discovery during these initial experiences was that destruction of stones was found to be more efficient when the stones were immersed in fluid and when absorption of light was improved by the application of black or blue dye to the stone prior to lithotripsy. Despite these advancements, the ruby laser was found to be clearly too dangerous for use in the clinical setting due to the large amount of heat production.

As the next generation of lasers were in development, efforts were made to separate the shockwave produced from the laser and the pulse in order to potentially reduce the generated heat [7, 8]. Anderholm and colleagues reported that when the plasma produced by the laser was contained between the stone and a transparent solid, the stress wave could be significantly increased to a level of 34 kb, which was 34 times greater than what is measured at the focal point during contemporary shockwave lithotripsy (SWL). The group was able provide evidence that shockwave generation could be isolated from the thermal effects of the laser.

Q-Switching

Yang then used the concept of Q-switching the ruby laser to create 20 ns laser pulses. Q-switching was reported to be a method of generating a laser pulse by introducing an attenuator to prevent stimulated emission while the laser was being pumped [9]. The latter principle allowed energy to be stored in the gain medium of the laser until the energy reached a maximum level. At this level the attenuator (Q-switch) is switched to a level of low attenuation, allowing the light pulse to be quickly generated as the excess energy in the gain medium is rapidly consumed. The result is a giant pulse with a higher peak power than could otherwise be achieved with continuous output. This method had previously been described in 1962 [10]. Using Q-switching, Yang was able to create laser pulses with resulting stress waves measuring between 1 and 20 kb. Using these pulsed lasers, Fair developed a method of focusing the laser onto an optical fiber with the theory that this would result in an acoustic shock wave able to fragment stones without requiring heat and without thermal destruction of surrounding tissues [11]. These finding were important along with the discovery that shortening the pulse duration of the laser led to greater stress wave pressure.

Nd:YAG Laser

In 1983, Watson applied the technique of a pulsed laser focused on an optical fiber to the neodymium-doped yttrium aluminium garnet (Nd:YAG) laser to fragment urinary calculi [12]. The Nd:YAG has a wavelength of 1064 nm which was considered less desirable at that time due to the decreased absorption by the stone at the longer wavelength when compared with the ruby laser. Through the utilization of a pulsed laser with only 1 Joule per 15 ns pulsation, Watson was able to demonstrate fragmentation of calculi. However, the findings also demonstrated difficulty in transmitting the amount of energy generated from the peak of a Q-switched laser through a flexible fiber. Watson then conducted a series of trials using flashlamp pumped tunable dye lasers to investigate optimal wavelength, fiber size, and pulse duration for conducting in vitro laser lithotripsy [13]. Of note, the minimum pulse duration generated by the flashlamp pumped dye laser was 1 μs as opposed to the Q-switch lasers which could produce much shorter pulse durations. In this study it was found that 445 nm had the lowest energy threshold for stone fragmentation, but concern was raised regarding the absorption by hemoglobin at that wavelength with the potential of tissue injury. From further investigation on wavelength, 504 nm was noted to be the optimal wavelength for lithotripsy. Again, supporting earlier findings, it was found that the shortest pulse duration required the least amount of energy for effective lithotripsy. Additional results of Watson's work demonstrated that the smallest fiber size was the most effective at producing fragmentation. The smallest laser fiber tested was the 100 μm fiber. However, the 100 μm fiber was quickly destroyed as focusing the light on such a small fiber was technically difficult. This led to the development of the 200 μm fiber as the optimal fiber diameter. The mechanism of action of these lasers was further studied using microsecond flash photography as well as piezoelectric and optoacoustic detection of stress waves by Teng et al. [14]. It was confirmed that the mechanism of fragmentation for the flashlamp pumped tunable dye lasers was by acoustic wave generated by plasma. Essentially, the laser was absorbed by the stone surface which in turn generated a cloud of free electrons known as a plasma that created an acoustic wave resulting in fragmentation (Fig. 9.1). It was also shown that immersion in water was necessary for the creation of this wave as the amplitude of the wave was reduced by a factor of ten when lithotripsy was performed in air rather than in water.

Watson and Wickham performed the first in vivo laser lithotripsy of urinary stones [15]. In 1986 they published their results of 32 patients having a total of 37 stones that were treated with laser lithotripsy. Thirty three of the calculi were in the ureter, three were in the renal pelvis, and one was in the bladder. The mean diameter of the calculi was 7.9 mm and the mean length was 9.1 mm. The ureteric calculi had been impacted for a mean of 5.9 months. The laser fiber was passed through a 6 FR catheter which was then passed through the ureteroscope. Saline irrigation was then run continuously around the fiber to improve visibility. All stones reached by ureteroscopy were able to be fragmented. The ureter was unscathed after performance of lithotripsy despite some stones requiring 4000 pulses for fragmentation. A later publication of the same series from the London group reviewing the first 100 cases continued to show promising results [16]. All stones reached by ureteroscopy were fragmented to some degree. An overall success rate of 85% was achieved. Thirteen stones accessed by retrograde means were not able to be treated because they were highly mobile and migrated back to the kidney. Of note, 5% of the patients were chosen at random to have "lasertripsy" delivery performed by fluoroscopic and acoustic guidance with a much lower success rate. A radiopaque catheter was used to pass the laser to the level of the stone and lithotripsy was performed using the

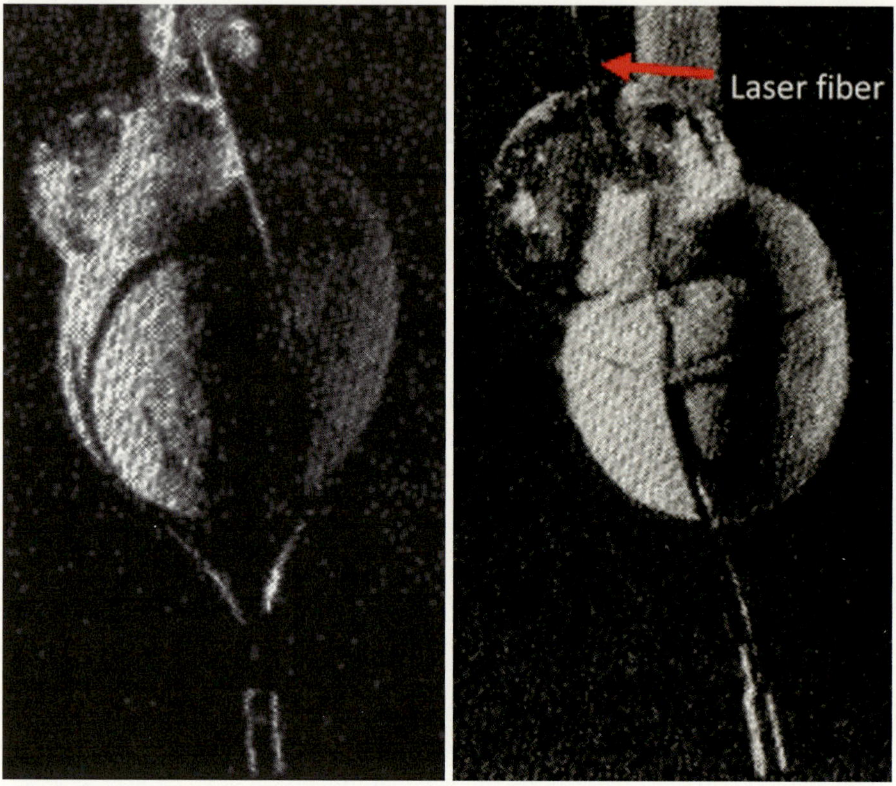

Fig. 9.1 Microsecond flash photography showing plasma and acoustic wave generation by a flash-lamp pumped tunable dye laser at 504 nm [14]

aforementioned acoustic feedback when the fiber was on the stone. No significant ureteral injury was noted with this method. The only noted injury to the ureter from the laser itself were findings of petechiae. Seven ureteral perforations did occur due to endoscopic manipulation out of the 100 cases, and all of these were treated with stenting or percutaneous nephrostomy. The average case length was 1.2 h, but the mean duration of laser use was 30 s. It was noted by Dretler that the laser was significantly more successful at the fragmentation of the reticulated calcium oxalate dihydrate stones rather than the dense calcium oxalate monohydrate stones [8].

Ho:YAG Laser

In 1993 Sayer et al. reported the ex vivo results of the 2100 nm holmium:YAG (Ho:YAG) laser for use in the setting of lithotripsy [17]. Ho:YAG presented as an ideal candidate to perform laser lithotripsy due to the ability of applying laser energy through small, flexible quartz fibers. Interesting experiments were performed on ureter specimens obtained at the time of radical nephrectomy for renal cell carcinoma. The stones were placed in the ureters and laser lithotripsy was performed with ureteroscopic delivery of the laser via a 400 μ fiber monitored by video. Stones of several different compositions were used with the laser set to 5 Hz and 0.5 J/pulse, and the total energy to complete stone fragmentation was recorded (Table 9.1). It was noted that lithotripsy was reasonably effective for all stone compositions tested. The frequency and power settings were then increased in a stepwise manner, and lithotripsy was performed at increasingly higher settings. Ureteric specimens were sent to pathology after completion of lithotripsy, and results were recorded (Table 9.2). Finally, the ureters were intentionally perforated at varying settings, and these pathology results were also recorded as well as the time to ureteral perforation (Table 9.3). It was noted that settings of 5 Hz with 0.5 J/s were safe settings, but ureteric injury occurred at higher power and frequency settings. These injuries many times were not visible on ureteroscopy. Coagulative necrosis was noted at the site of injury although the mechanism for lithotripsy of the holmium:YAG laser was at the time thought to be the same as the pulsed dye lasers, namely throught the generation of acoustic shockwaves (Fig. 9.2). It was later shown that Ho:YAG laser mechanism of fragmentation was through the generation of thermal energy [18]. The Ho:YAG laser has a significantly longer pulse duration than the pulsed coumarin dye laser (250–350 μs vs 1 μs), and that difference along with the observation of the effect of

Table 9.1 Complete stone fragmentation [17]

Stone composition	Size of stone (mm)	Total energy (kJ)
Struvite/ CaApatite	3 × 4 × 3	0.11
Uric acid	5 × 4 × 2	0.04
Amm acid urate	4 × 4 × 5	0.16
Uric acid	4 × 3 × 2	0.01
Amm acid urate	5 × 4 × 3	0.12
Struvite/ CaApatite	6 × 7 × 5	0.26
Struvite	3 × 4 × 5	0.13

Note: All stones fragmented with 0.7 J/pulse at 5 Hz

Table 9.2 Fragmentation with varying power and frequency [17]

J/pulse	Frequency (Hz)	Total energy (kJ)	Pathology
0.5	5	0.13	Denuded mucosa
0.5	10	0.15	Necrosis: submucosa
0.5	15	0.13	Transmural fracture
0.5	20	0.11	Transmural fracture
1.0	5	0.20	Transmural fracture
1.5	5	0.13	Large fracture

Note: Ammonium acid urate stones (3 × 3 × 4 mm)

Table 9.3 Intentional ureteral wall perforation [17]

Power settings	Total energy (kJ)	Time to perforation (s)	Pathology
0.5 J, 5 Hz	0.03	11.4	1 mm fissure
0.5 J, 10 Hz	0.01	4.4	1–2 mm fissure
0.5 J, 15 Hz	0.01	1.4	Prominent fissure
0.5 J, 20 Hz	<0.01	0.3	Large fissure
1.0 J, 5 Hz	0.1	1.2	Large fissure
1.5 J, 5 Hz	0.01	0.8	Large, irregular fissure
2.0 J, 5 Hz	<0.01	0.2	Large, branching fissure

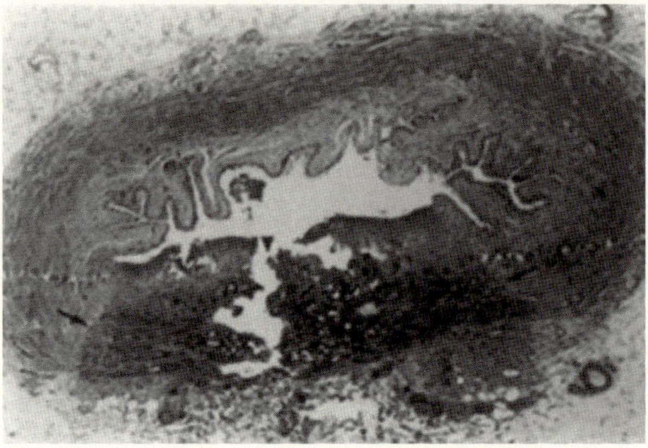

Fig. 9.2 Coagulative necrosis of ureter (*arrows*) with transmural fissure (*arrowhead*)

high temperatures led Vasssar et al. to question the proposed mechanism of laser-induced shockwave lithotripsy (LISL), as had been shown with the flashpump pulsed dye laser (Fig. 9.2). Experiments similar to those conducted in 1987 were performed which demostrated lithotripsy occurring prior to the development of a shockwave from collapse of the vapor bubble, no significant pressure generated from the Ho:YAG laser with a pulse length of 250 μs, and no significant lithotripsy occuring when the incidence angle of the laser was 90° in relation to the stone despite adequate contact with the vapor bubble. In addition, lithotripsy was more effective when stones were dry and carried out in air and when the stone temperature started at 20 °C as opposed to −80 °C. It has thus been theorized that the vapor bubble generated allows fragmentation to take place by conducting the thermal effects of the laser onto the stone. Finally, as further confirmation of the thermal mechanism, breakdown products were found on the surfaces of treated stones that indicated stone surface temperatures >206° at the time of lithotripsy.

With safe settings being established ev vivo by Sayer, Ho:YAG was initially utilized in 1993 in vivo by Denstedt et al. [19]. A preliminary series of 25 patients treated with 27 procedures was reported, including 4 patients who were treated via flexible nephroscopy during percutaneous nephrolithotomy (PCNL). All 4 of the PCNL patients had successful results, but the initial series reported a 65% success rate using Ho:YAG as a sole modality, and an attempt at fluoroscopic rather than visual control of the laser led to a ureteral perforation. However, the completion of same series showed efficacy as a sole modality at a rate at 85% after treatment of 75 patients with 79 procedures [20]. In six cases electrohydraulic lithotripsy was used as an adjunct to fragment ureteral stones either due to attempts at expediting the procedure with large stones (n = 4) or due to difficulty initially applying the laser probe safely (n = 2). The overall stone free rate was reported to be 95% although 81% of the patients had follow up imaging. The authors began lithotripsy using a 400 μ fiber at the minimum available settings (0.5 J for first 31 patients using prototype, 0.2 J for all remaining patients using the then commercially available laser), increasing the power incrementally by 0.1 J until the desired fragmentation had occurred. Flexible ureteroscopy was available for use, and all proximal ureteric stones were approached using a 9.8 FR or 10.5 FR flexible ureteroscope. 6.9 FR, 9.5 FR and 11.5 FR rigid ureteroscopes were available, and balloon dilation of the ureter with a 6 mm × 10 cm balloon was performed for all procedures where use of an instrument greater than 6.9 FR was anticipated. A total of eight laser lithotripsy procedures were performed as an adjunct to the Swiss Lithoclast during PCNL, although 3 of these patients were found to have residual stone at follow up. Similar results were reported by Grasso with success rates of 96% for ureteric stone and 88.5% for renal stones [21]. Grasso had the 200 μ fiber available to maximize deflection in the treatment of difficult to reach stones, such as stones in the lower pole.

Ho:YAG is unique in its versatility as a laser for urologic purposes. In addition to its ability to treat all kinds of stone composition, Ho:YAG is able to perform cutting and coagulation of tissues that other lasers are not able to perform [22]. At a wavelength of 2100 nm Ho:YAG is absorbed in water readily resulting in a thermal injury zone of 0.5–1 mm, which is small enough for precision cutting but large enough for coagulation to occur. This is in contrast to the neodymium:YAG (Nd:YAG) laser which is has a wavelength of 1064 nm and is absorbed over a distance of 4–6 mm. The Nd:YAG laser produces a coagulation effect that can be found deep to what is immediately visible to the surgeon, but does not produce a cutting effect. Also in contrast, the CO_2 laser, which is absorbed over a distance 0.05 mm and produces an exceedingly precise cut, does not produce hemostasis due to the size of small vessels being significantly larger than the distance of absorption. Due to the outstanding lithotripsy results along with the cutting and coagulation properties (tumor ablation and stricture treatment), there has been widespread adoption of the Ho:YAG laser as the workhorse laser for urologic applications.

FREDDY Laser

Although most other laser systems are beyond the purview of this discussion, mention should be made of the Frequency doubled double-pulse Nd:YAG (FREDDY) laser. The FREDDY system utilizes Q-switching and a potassium trihydrogen phosphate (KTP) crystal to pulse the laser and double the frequency of 20% of the laser output, respectively. The resulting 0.3–1.5 μs pulse lengths are significantly shorter than that of Ho:YAG and allow for the photoacoustic mechanism of lithotripsy. The KTP crystal converts 20% of the laser power output from 1064 nm to 532 nm, similar to the wavelength of the previously used coumarin pulsed dye laser. The 532 wavelength output creates the plasma cloud which then absorbs the 1064 nm energy resulting in expansion and contraction of the plasma [23]. This mechanism was meant to combine the safety of the photoacoustic approach with the versatility to treat stones of all compositions. It was also advertised as a low cost system, costing 30% of the common competitor, with a reusable fiber that rarely needed replacement [24]. The FREDDY laser was able to deliver with regards to safety. When directed at rabbit bladders, only minimal edema was noted after 300 pulses of 120 mJ each [24]. In contrast, the Ho:YAG laser has been shown to perforate through the ureter after 2 pulses [25]. Initial clinical experience in 2000 reported a 95% stone free rate for ureteral stones with no reported complications [26]. However, despite providing a 1064 nm pulse to augment the photoacoustic mechanism found in the pulsed dye lasers, concern quickly arose regarding the ability for FREDDY to treat hard stones. Confirming previously published reports of decreased efficacy with the FREDDY system, Yates et al compared the results of FREDDY and the Ho:YAG laser [27]. Thirty patients were treated with each system, with each cohort having a similar distribution of stone location. The FREDDY laser system was noted to have a 76.7% stone free rate at follow up compared with 93.3% in the Ho:YAG group. In addition, costs reported were nearly equivalent. The lack of cost savings, inability to perform cutting or coagulation needed for other procedures, as well as the corroboration of previously reported lower stone free rates led to the FREDDY laser to be largely abandoned in the community and at most academic centers [28].

Conclusion

The development of laser lithotripsy from a ruby laser capable of performing lithotripsy on test bench at 50–300 J to the current Ho:YAG laser capable of rapidly and safely treating greater than 90% of ureteral stones in a minimally invasive manner has transformed urologic stone surgery. Combined with the use of modern flexible ureteroscopes and instruments such as ureteral sheaths to improve drainage and visualization during treatment of large stones, laser lithotripsy with Ho:YAG has become the mainstay procedure for stone treatment for many urologists. Laser lithotripsy is quickly overtaking SWL as the most common procedure performed for treatment of stones, with open stone surgery nearly obsolete [29]. Although a future aim for use of a photoacoustic mechanism causing minimal ureteral trauma in the treatment of all stone compositions may be useful, it will be difficult to justify the economics of purchasing a second laser system alongside the exceedingly effective and versatile Ho:YAG laser.

References

1. Scales CD Jr, Smith AC, Hanley JM, Saigal CS. Urologic diseases in America project. Prevalence of kidney stones in the United States. Eur Urol. 2012;62:160–5.
2. Gould GR. The LASER, light amplification by stimulated emission of radiation. In: Franken PA, Sands RH (Eds). The Ann Arbor Conference on Optical Pumping, the University of Michigan, 15 June through 18 June 1959. p. 128.
3. Weber J. Amplification of microwave radiation by substances not in thermal equilibrium. IEEE Trans Electron Devices. 1953;3:1.
4. Gordon J, Zeiger H, Townes C. The Maser—new type of microwave amplifier, frequency standard, and spectrometer. Phys Rev. 1955;99(4):1264.
5. Maiman TH. Stimulated optical radiation in ruby. Nature. 1960;187:493.
6. Mulvaney WP, Beck CW. The laser bean in urology. J Urol. 1968;99:112–5.
7. Anderholm NC. Laser generated stress waves. Appl Phys Lett. 1970;16:113.
8. Dretler SP. Laser lithotripsy: a review of 20 years of research and clinical applications. Lasers Surg Med. 1988;8:341–56.
9. Yang LC. Stress waves generated in thin metallic fibers by a Q-switched ruby laser. J Appl Phys. 1974;45:2601.
10. McClung FJ, Hellwarth RW. Giant optical pulsations from ruby. J Appl Phys. 1962;33:828.
11. Fair HD. In vitro destruction of urinary calculi by laser-induced stress waves. Med Instrum. 1978;12:100–10.
12. Watson GM, Wickham JEA, Mills TN, Bown SG, Swain P, Salmon PR. Laser fragmentation of renal calculi. Br J Urol. 1983;55:613–61.
13. Watson GM, Murray S, Dretler SP, Parrish JA. The pulsed dye laser for fragmenting urinary calculi. J Urol. 1987;138:195–8.
14. Teng P, Nishioka NS, Anderson RR, et al. Acoustic studies of the role of immersion in plasma mediated laser ablation. IEEE J Quantum Electron. 1987;QE-23(10):1845–52.
15. Watson GM, Wickham JEA. Initial experience with a pulsed dye laser for ureteric calculi. Lancet. 1986;1:1357–8.
16. Coptcoat MJ, Watson GM, Wickham JEA. Lasertripsy for ureteral stones: 100 clinical cases. J Endourol. 1987;1(2):119.
17. Sayer J, Johnson DE, Price RE, et al. Ureteral lithotripsy with the holmium:YAG laser. J Clin Laser Med Surg. 1993;11(2):61.
18. Vassar GJ, Chan KF, Teichman JMH, et al. Holmium:YAG lithortripsy: photothermal mechanism. J Endourol. 1999;13(3):181–90.
19. Denstedt JD, Razvi HA, Sales JL, Eberwein PM. Preliminary experience with holmium:YAG laser lithotripsy. J Endourol. 1995;9(3):255.
20. Razvi HA, Denstedt JD, Chun SS, et al. Intracorporeal lithotripsy with the holmium:YAG laser. J Urol. 1996;156:912–4.
21. Grasso M. Experience with the holmium laser as an endoscopic lithotrite. Urology. 1996;48:199–206.
22. Wollin TA, Denstedt JD. The holmium laser in urology. J Clin Laser Med Surg. 1998;16(1):13.
23. Marks AJ, Teichman JMH. Lasers in clinical urology: state of the art and new horizons. World J Urol. 2007;25:227–33.
24. Zorcher T, Hochberger J, Schrott KM, Kuhn R, Schafhauser W. In vitro study concerning the efficacy of the frequency-doubled double-pulse neodymium:YAG laser (FREDDY) for lithotripsy of calculi in the urinary tract. Lasers Surg Med. 1999;25:38–42.
25. Santa-Cruz RW, Leveillee RJ, Krongrad A. Ex vivo comparison of four lithotripters commonly used in the ureter: what does it take to perforate? J Endourol. 1998;12(5):417–22.
26. Shafhauser W, Zorcher W, et al. Erste klinische erfahrungen mit neuem frequenzverdoppltem doppelpuls neodym:YAG laser in der therapie der urolithiasis. Poster presentation at the DGU, Hamburg, Germany, 2000.

27. Yates J, Zabbo A, Pareek G. A comparison of the FREDDY and holmium lasers during ureteroscopic lithotripsy. Lasers Surg Med. 2007;39:637–40.
28. Dubosq F, Pasqui F, Girard F, Beley S, Lesaux N, Gattegno B, Thibault P, Traxer O. Endoscopic lithotripsy and the FREDDY laser: initial experience. J Endourol. 2006;20(5):296–9.
29. Oberlin DT, Flum AS, Bachrach L, Matulewicz RS, Flury SC. Contemporary surgical trends in the management of upper tract calculi. J Urol. 2015;193:880–4.

Chapter 10
History and Development of Lasers in the Treatment of BPH

Johann P. Ingimarsson and Amy E. Krambeck

Lasers have become a fundamental tool in the modern clinical practice of multiple surgical specialties, with urology having one of the higher utilization rates. The term "laser" is an acronym for Light Amplification by Stimulated Emission of Radiation, thus lasers are devices that generate an intense beam of coherent monochromatic light (or other electromagnetic radiation) by stimulated emission of photons from excited atoms or molecules. Since lasers are capable of precisely focusing intense energy it is not surprising that they have been effectively utilized in clinical scenarios such as: wart removal, stone fracturing, and treatment of benign prostatic hyperplasia (BPH). This chapter focuses on the history of laser development and the various different lasers used in the treatment of benign prostatic hyperplasia.

Early Work

The theoretical work behind laser reaches back to the early work of physicists Max Planck and Albert Einstein. Plank, in 1900, deduced the relationship between energy and frequency of radiation and that energy would be absorbed or emitted in discrete packets or quanta, later known as quantum theory [1, 2]. Einstein in 1905 proposed that light also delivers it energy in quanta, called photons [3] and in 1917 that electrons could be stimulated to emit light of a particular wavelength, known as simulated emission. This is the fundamental mechanism by which laser works [4]. It took some time to go from theory to practice, but in the 1958, based on prior work by Basov and Prokhorov in Russia, as well as their own, Charles Townes of Columbia University and Arthur Schawlow of Bell Labs published a paper on "optical microwave Amplification by Stimulated Emission of Radiation," thus laying the theoretical groundwork for the laser

J.P. Ingimarsson, M.D. (✉) • A.E. Krambeck, M.D.
Mayo Clinic, Department of Urology, Rochester, MN 55902, USA
e-mail: johanningimars@gmail.com

S.R. Patel et al. (eds.), *The History of Technologic Advancements in Urology*,
DOI 10.1007/978-3-319-61691-9_10

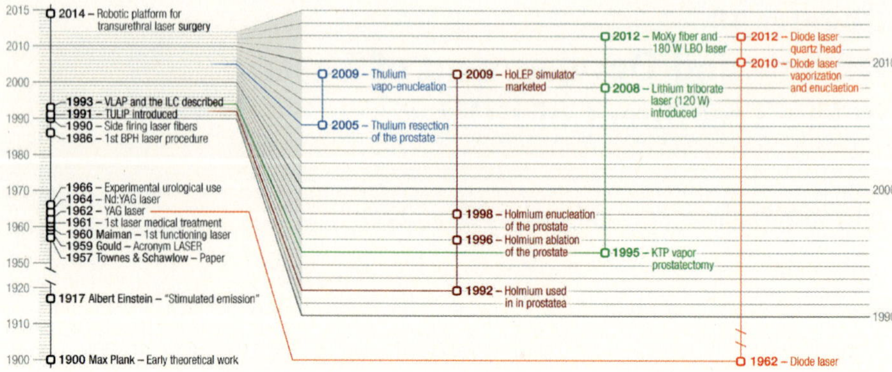

Fig. 10.1 Time line of laser development. Outline of laser conception to current clinical use

construction [5]. Gordon Gould, in November of 1957, an undergraduate student at Columbia had filed for a patent for a "Light Amplification by Stimulated Emission of Radiation," thus coining the acronym L.A.S.E.R. His patent was declined and awarded to Townes and Schawlow, sparking a 30 year court battle over patent rights. Townes, Basov and Prokhorov were awarded the Nobel Prize for their work on lasers in 1964 [6].

Two years after Townes and Schawlow were awarded their patent, Theodore Maiman at Hughes Research Laboratories built the first functional laser using a synthetic ruby and a flash lamp; the year was 1960 [7].

The medical world was quick to adopt the laser technology. In 1961 Dr. Charles Campbell used an optical ruby laser to successfully destroy a retinal tumor [8]. The first recorded urological laser research was performed by Parson et al. in 1966, on the effects of lasers on canine bladders [9]. Little progress was made over the next 20 years until treatment for benign disease was first described in 1986 in a canine model using a laser followed by electrocautery for hemostasis [10]. Two years later the first human studies were published, a report on 6 patients with "direct contact laser vaporization of obstructing median bar" prostatic hyperplasia [11].

Since the first human description, there has been tremendous development in the clinical use of lasers for BPH. Laser development for the treatment of BPH can roughly be divided into: (1) the creation and development of new lasers, (2) the introduction and long term reporting of procedures and operative technique to utilize lasers, as well as the development of fibers and accessories to optimize these procedure, and (3) development of adjuncts, such as training modules and robotic system. These will be detailed below.

Laser Developments

While numerous lasers have been develop since the 1960s, both for clinical and non-clinical use, this text will focus on the development and modification of the two basic laser platforms that have been used to treat BPH, the yttrium aluminum garnet (YAG) based solid lasers and semiconductor diode lasers.

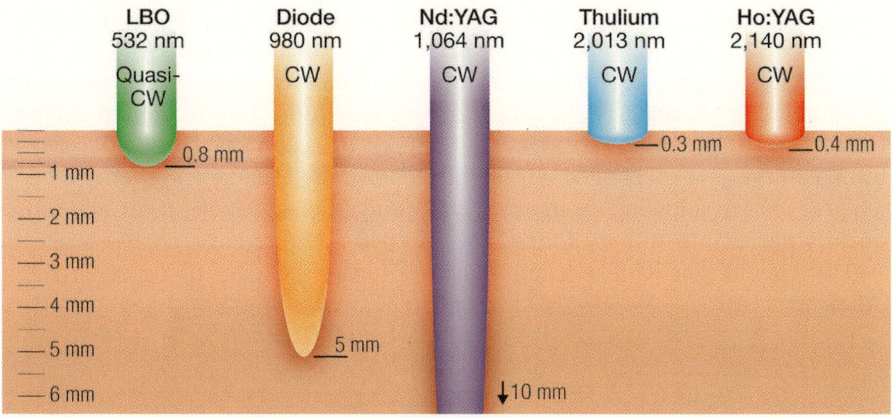

Fig. 10.2 Comparison of different laser wavelenghts and depths of tissue penetration

Yttrium Aluminum Garnet Solid Lasers

The first yttrium aluminum garnet (Y_3 Al_5 O_{12}) laser was developed by Bell Laboratories in 1962 [12]. While other solid phase lasers have been created, for the purposes of BPH laser surgeries, the YAG laser is the base model for all of the subsequent solid phase lasers, because of its efficiency, optical quality, and high thermal conductivity, which permits high rates of repetition.

Nd:YAG Lasers

Inserting, or "doping" a YAG crystal with rare earth mineral was shortly found to be a good way to alter the physical properties of laser and in 1964 Bell Laboratories introduced the neodymium-doped YAG (Nd:YAG) [12]. It's 1064-nm (near infrared) wavelength is outside the absorption peaks of both water and hemoglobin. This translates into deep soft tissue penetration, up to 1 cm. Such deep tissue penetration, adversely affects the accuracy of its cut, with adjacent tissues being affected. The Nd:YAG laser is very hemostatic and can coagulate blood vessels as large as 5 mm in diameter [13]. The first report of Nd:YAG for the treatment of human BPH as in 1988 [11].

532 nm Lasers (Nd;YAG with Potassium-Titinyl-Phosphate or Lithium Triborate)

Passing a Nd;YAG laser through a potassium-titinyl-phosphate (KTP) crystal doubles it frequency and halves it wave length (532 nm), bringing it to the green electromagnetic spectrum. It was introduced to BPH surgery in 1993 because its wavelength is at the absorption peak of hemoglobin [14]. When applied, the KTP laser rapidly heats hemoglobin causing vaporization of surrounding water and tissue. It's depth of penetration is around 0.8 mm, allowing for more accurate utilization then the Nd:YAG. One disadvantage of KTP laser energy is that tissue carbonization can be observed, rather than a true ablative effect [15]. In an attempt to optimize the benefits of the 532 nm wave length the 120 W lithium triborate (LBO) laser (GreenLight HPS) was introduced in 2006 [16]. In the HPS system the KTP crystal is exchanged out for LBO, offering the same wave length, but at a higher energy, allowing for more effective and efficient vaporization, and subsequently decreasing surgery times [15]. In 2010 a higher energy LBO laser, the 180 W GreenLight XPS was introduced to further increase tissue vaporization efficiency [16].

Holmium:YAG Laser

Doping the YAG crystal with the rare earth element holmium instead of neodymium changes the physical characteristics of the laser and causes a 2100 nm beam to be emitted, near the absorption peak of water. The effect is a laser that superheats water, creating a vaporization bubble at the tip of the delivery fiber. The bubble expands rapidly, destabilizing molecules in the tissue it contacts, tearing the tissue apart in a photomechanical fashion, followed by tissue evaporation. The absorption depth in tissue is 0.4 mm, allowing for a more precise incision than the prior Ng:YAG based lasers. The holmium: YAG laser provides excellent hemostasis, especially if delivered in a pulsed mode [13]. It was first introduced in experimental urology in 1990 and the first human use of the holmium:YAG laser was described in 1992 [17]. With time the holmium:YAG lasers have been offered in sequentially more powerful versions, originally in 20 W, now available from 50 to 120 W.

Thulium:YAG Laser

The thulium laser was developed with the intent to more precisely match the water absorption peak in soft tissue. When the YAG crystal is doped with thulium it emits around 2000 nm wavelength laser, with a 0.25 mm depth of penetration. The result is a laser with similar hemostasis as the holmium laser, with minimal collateral tissue damage. It is administered at a higher energy setting and a continuous rather than a pulsed mode, arguing for more efficient tissue vaporization [13]. The first reported use of the thulium: YAG laser in human prostates was in 2005 [18]. Similar to the other lasers, subsequent higher energy thulium lasers have been introduced, now available in up to 150 W.

Semiconductor Diode Lasers

Distinctly mechanically different from the YAG based solid lasers are the semiconductor diode lasers. Laser light is produced using light-emitting diodes (LEDs) between reflecting mirrors in a resonator tube. They are smaller, more energy efficient, and less expensive than most other lasers now in use. The semiconductor laser wavelength can be tuned by various modifications. In general, their depth of penetration (0.5–5 mm) is more than of the 532 nm, holmium and thulium lasers, although the exact penetration depth is dependent on the wave length [13]. In 1996, interstitial laser coagulation of the prostate was performed using an 830 nm diode laser [19]. In 2007 a 980 nm diode laser was used for BPH [20]. Initially offered in 120 W, the diode laser became available in 200 W in 2009. In 2013 a 1318 nm diode lasers (Eraser) was eventually introduced for BPH [21].

Technique

The various lasers mentioned above have been used to treat BPH by different techniques with different results. These can roughly be divided into interstitial coagulation necrosis, transurethral ablation or vaporization, resection, enucleation and combined techniques with or without electrocautery.

Interstitial Coagulation

Interstitial laser coagulation with Nd:YAG laser was an early development in the treatment of BPH. First described in 1993, the main feature of this method was preservation of the prostatic urethra and its urothelium [22]. The procedure is performed by placing laser-diffusing fibers directly into the prostatic adenoma, either via the transurethral cystoscopic approach, or the perineal approach. Laser energy then produces coagulation necrosis within the adenoma, which subsequently undergoes atrophy [23]. This method is safe in anticoagulated patients, but substantial tissue edema occurs with this method resulting in prolonged (7–21 days) postoperative catheterization. Retreatment rates were as high as 20% at 2 years, and 50% at 5 years. Due to the recognized limitations of the interstitial laser coagulation technique several authors have concluded that this modality should probably be restricted to selected, high-risk patients [24]. Ablations and vaporizations.

While the actual physiological mechanism differs, based on the physical properties by which the laser cause tissues injury as described above, the core idea with ablative and vaporizing techniques is the same. With ablation or vaporization dissolution of the tissue from the urethra and the adenoma occurs, thus shrinking the prostatic volume. Initially described in the 1980s, only a handful of ablative/vaporizing cases were reported until the invention of the side firing laser fiber in 1990 after which its use increased exponentially [25].

One of the first ablative techniques to take advantage of the side firing laser was the transurethral ultrasound-guided laser-induced prostatectomy (TULIP), described in 1991 [26] with first clinical results reported in 1993 [27–29]. With the TULIP technique, ultrasound was used to guide a side firing fiber with a Nd:YAG laser. By lasing the prostatic adenoma transurethrally an area of heat-induced coagulative necrosis is created, which extends approximately 1 cm into the tissue. To unobstruct the prostate, TULIP relies on coagulation necrosis of the BPH with subsequent tissue sloughing. While it had reasonable outcomes, TULIP was eventually abandoned as it was and both costly and cumbersome to execute.

Another early technique, was visual laser ablation of the prostate (VLAP) using Ng:YAG laser, first described in 1993 by Norris et al. Long term results were reported in 1995 [30]. Unlike TULIP, which utilized ultrasound guidance, in VLAP the laser was visually guided through a transurethral scope, but otherwise both VLAP and TULIP utilized the same tissue and treatment principles. Furthermore, VLAP was easier to learn and perform than TULIP, but it was limited to prostates 40 g and smaller. Delayed sloughing and edema of the tissue caused by the VLAP procedure lead to irritative lower urinary tract syndrome (LUTS) and urinary retention requiring catheterization in up to 30% of cases, extending in some patients to 3 months [30]. Thus, despite the benefits and ease of use, VLAP fell out of clinical utilization.

The KTP laser was initially introduced in BPH as an adjunct to VLAP, where it was used to make a bladder neck incision at the end of the case [31]. The first pure KTP vaporization procedure, also known as photoselective vaporization of the prostate (PVP), using a 60 W laser and a side firing laser fiber was described in 1998, [32], with the same authors reporting 2 year outcomes in 2000. An 80 W laser was described in 2003 with 2 year results in 2005 [33]. A year later the LBO 532 nm laser (GreenLight HPS) was introduced and the 2 year data was presented in 2010 [34]. In 2011, a case was described using the most recent version, the 180 W LBO laser (Green Light XPS). With the 180 W LBO laser, a new design of a side firing laser fiber (MoXy) was introduced. It included inbuilt saline circulation for cooling and laser fiber preservation, increasing fiber longevity. The combination of the 180 W LBO laser with the fiber was reported to vaporize tissue at twice the speed that could be achieved with the 120 W laser. The GOLIATH study, comparing the 180 W LBO laser vaporization to TURP at 2 years in a randomized trial, was published in 2016, exhibiting efficacy and safety outcomes to be similar between the two procedures [35].

The holmium:YAG laser entered the BPH world in the same fashion as the KTP, as an adjunct to Ng:YAG VLAP. The next step was prostate vaporization in the same 'painting' fashion as the Nd:YAG and KTP lasers, reported in 1996. Although the procedure (called HoLAP, holmium laser ablation of the prostate) which utilizes straight rather than a side firing fiber was easy to learn and effective, it was too time consuming when dealing with larger prostates [36]. For glands smaller than 60 mL it has been shown to have similar long term outcomes compared to PVP [37]. Of note, no new data has been published on HoLAP since 2013.

Thulium lasers have been more utilized in resection and enucleation and limited reports exist on thulium abalation/vaporization.

Diode laser vaporization of the prostate (DiVAP), has been reported with surgical techniques comparable to other vaporization procedures [20]. Although tissue incision is feasible with diode lasers, given the lasers depth of penetration, avoiding deep coagulation can be challenging. Unfortunately, the available evidence on diode lasers is mostly based on low-quality studies with small patient cohorts, making comparison to other laser ablative techniques difficult [38]. However, in a prospective comparison with 120 W GreenLight PVP it was found have better hemostasis, but higher re-treatment rates and complications [39]. In order to address the limitations of DiVAP, a new straight firing quarts coated fiber (Twister fiber) was introduced that does not project a laser beam, but concentrates the energy at the fibers tip. A randomized trial showed that the quartz tipped head used for DiVAP showed similar efficacy as the old fiber, with decreased over-all complications, dysuria and tissue sloughing [40]. Long term outcomes are currently pending.

Resections

Prior to the introduction of the more powerful lasers, ablations and vaporizations were frustratingly slow and inefficient. Therefor this led to the development of prostate laser resections, most notably HoLRP (holmium laser resection of the prostate) which basically simulates traditional TURP [41]. Thulium laser skipped the ablation technique and was first presented in BPH as the thulium laser resection of the prostate tangerine technique [18], followed by simultaneous resection of TURP-like chips and vaporization of tissue, which was proven to be safe and effective [42]. While these technique have acceptable long term outcomes, they have been compared to and found to have inferior results to enucleations with the same lasers [43].

Enucleations

Morbidity aside, simple open prostatectomy has superior long term outcomes when it comes to BPH, especially with large prostate glands. Laser enucleation essentially follows the anatomic principal of a simple prostatectomy via a transurethral approach and without a cystotomy or skin incision. Fraundorfer and Gilling developed the first of these procedures, the Holmium Laser Enucleation of the Prostate (HoLEP) in 1998 [44]. Long term follow up of up to 10 years is available with durable decrease in International Prostate Symptom Score, flow rates and post void residuals. Long term risk of a bladder neck contracture or urethral stricture is 2–7% and retreat rates for adenoma regrowth <1% [45, 46]. Additionally, long term outcomes of a randomized trial comparing HoLEP with TURP demonstrated HoLEP to be at least equivalent to TURP in the with fewer re-operations being necessary [47]. One of the main criticisms of the HoLEP procedure is a long learning curve, limiting its dissemination to the community setting.

Enucleations using similar technique but different lasers have since been described. Enucleation using a thulium laser was described in 2009 [48], 980 nm diode laser in 2010 [49], KPT in 2013 [50] and 1318 nm diode laser in 2013 [51]. Of these, only the thulium vapo enucleation has published 2-year outcomes data, revealing similar data to those reported for HoLEP at that time point [52].

Simulation and Robotics

The development of adjuncts to the existing procedures has already started and may potentially develop further. Simulators instructing laser prostate surgery became available in 2011 for PVP [53], in 2013 for HoLEP and in 2014 for diode lasers (Refs.). All of these simulators have since been validated as teaching tools for these procedures.

Robotic assistance to the laser procedures has recently been introduced. In 2015 a flexible transurethral robot with three working ports was reported to be able to remove bladder lesions en bloc in an experimental model [54]. That same year a robotic platform through a rigid endoscope with a steerable laser fiber was described [55]. Earlier this year a report on a holmium laser robotic template was published. This report describes a robot with two steerable arms or tubes coming out of a rigid endoscope, one for laser fiber and the other for exposure. The authors were able to perform a HoLEP on a simulator and a left lobe enucleation on a human cadaver [56]. Due to the expected additional cost of the robotic systems, it remains to be seen to what extent robotic assistance will be utilized for BPH laser treatments.

This year marks the 30th anniversary of the first described case of laser use in BPH. As listed above, tremendous progress has occurred in the last three decades. With the results of ablative, vaporizing and enucleating procedures being on par with or exceeding the old gold standards of open prostatectomy and TURP, an obvious expectation is that further long term results be reported, especially among the more recent applications. Rigorous detailed studies will enable patients and urologists to contrast the various lasers and procedures when determining the appropriate intervention for BPH.

References

1. Planck M. Über das Gesetz der Energieverteilung im Normalspektrum. Ann Phys. 1901;306:69–122.
2. Planck M. Vorlesungen über die Theorie der Wärmestrahlung. Leipzig: J.A. Barth; 1906.

3. Einstein A. Über einen die Erzeugung und Verwandlung des Lichtes betreffenden heuristischen Gesichtspunkt. Ann Phys. 1905;17:132–48.
4. Einstein A. Quantentheorie der Strahlung. Physikalische Zeitschrift. 1917;18:121–8.
5. Schawlow AL, Towens CH. Infrared and optical masers. Phys Rev. 1958;112:1940.
6. The Official site of the Nobel Prize [web site] 2016 [cited 2016 April 22nd]; Available from: https://www.nobelprize.org/nobel_prizes/physics/laureates/.
7. Maiman TH. Stimulated optical radiation in ruby. Nature. 1960;187:493–4.
8. Campbell CJ, Koester CJ, Curtice V, Noyori KS, Rittler MC. Clinical studies in laser photocoagulation. Arch Ophthalmol. 1965;74:57–65.
9. Parsons RL, Campbell JL, Thomley MW, Butt CG, Gordon TE Jr. The effect of the laser of dog bladders: a preliminary report. J Urol. 1966;95:716–7.
10. Finkelstein LH, Frantz B, Longendorfer LH, DeBias D, Greene C, Monson F. Electroresection followed by neodymium-YAG laser photocoagulation of the dog prostate for establishment of safety parameters. Lasers Surg Med. 1985;5:529–33.
11. Bloiso G, Warner R, Cohen M. Treatment of urethral diseases with neodymium:YAG laser. Urology. 1988;32:106–10.
12. Geusic JE, Marcos HM, Van Uitert LG. Laser oscillations in Nd-doped yttrium aluminum, yttrium gallium and gadolinium garnets. Appl Phys Lett. 1964;4:–182.
13. Bach T, Muschter R, Sroka R, Gravas S, Skolarikos A, Herrmann TR, Bayer T, Knoll T, Abbou CC, Janetschek G, Bachmann A, Rassweiler JJ. Laser treatment of benign prostatic obstruction: basics and physical differences. Eur Urol. 2012;61:317–25.
14. Anson KM, Watson GM, Shah TK, Barnes DG. Laser prostatectomy: our initial experience of a technique in evolution. J Endourol. 1993;7:333–6.
15. Gravas S, Bachmann A, Reich O, Roehrborn CG, Gilling PJ, De La Rosette J. Critical review of lasers in benign prostatic hyperplasia (BPH). BJU Int. 2011;107:1030–43.
16. Zorn KC, Liberman D. GreenLight 180 W XPS photovaporization of the prostate: how I do it. Can J Urol. 2011;18:5918–26.
17. Johnson DE, Cromeens DM, Price RE. Use of the holmium:YAG laser in urology. Lasers Surg Med. 1992;12:353–63.
18. Xia SJ, Zhang YN, Lu J, Sun XW, Zhang J, Zhu YY, et al. Thulium laser resection of prostate—tangerine technique in treatment of benign prostatic hyperplasia. Zhonghua Yi Xue Za Zhi. 2005;85:3225–8.
19. Muschter R, De La Rosette JJ, Whitfield H, Pellerin JP, Madersbacher S, Gillatt D. Initial human clinical experience with diode laser interstitial treatment of benign prostatic hyperplasia. Urology. 1996;48:223–8.
20. Wendt-Nordahl G, Huckele S, Honeck P, Alken P, Knoll T, Michel MS, Häcker A. 980-nm diode laser: a novel laser technology for vaporization of the prostate. Eur Urol. 2007;52:1723–8.
21. Lusuardi L, Myatt A, Sieberer M, Jeschke S, Zimmermann R, Janetschek G. Safety and efficacy of Eraser laser enucleation of the prostate: preliminary report. J Urol. 2011;186:1967–71.
22. Hofstetter A, Alvarez AHA. Treatment of prostatic tumors with interstitial thermocoagulation with neodymium-YAG (a new treatment in minimally invasive surgery). Arch Esp Urol. 1993;46:317–9.
23. Perlmutter AP, Muschter R. Interstitial laser prostatectomy. Mayo Clin Proc. 1998;73:903–7.
24. Daehlin L, Frugård J. Interstitial laser coagulation in the management of lower urinary tract symptoms suggestive of bladder outlet obstruction from benign prostatic hyperplasia: long-term follow-up. BJU Int. 2007;100:89–93.
25. Zarrabi A, Gross AJ. The evolution of lasers in urology. Ther Adv Urol. 2011;3:81–9.
26. Roth RA, Aretz HT. Transurethral ultrasound-guided laser-induced prostatectomy (TULIP procedure): a canine prostate feasibility study. J Urol. 1991;146:1128–35.
27. Flam T, Spitzenpfeil E, Gout A, Peyret C, Chiche R, Thiounn N, Steg A, Zerbib M, Debré B. TULIP: transurethral ultrasound-guided laser-induced prostatectomy. Clinical results after on year. J Urol (Paris). 1993;99:61–6.
28. Schulze H, Martin W, Engelmann U, Senge T. TULIP--transurethral ultrasound-controlled laser-induced prostatectomy: an alternative to TURP? Urologe A. 1993;32:225–31.

29. McCullough DL, Roth RA, Babayan RK, Gordon JO, Reese JH, Crawford ED, Fuselier HA, Smith JA, Murchison RJ, Kaye KW. Transurethral ultrasound-guided laser-induced prostatectomy: national human cooperative study results. J Urol. 1993;150:1607–11.
30. Cowles RS 3rd, Kabalin J, Childs S, Lepor H, Dixon C, Stein B, Zabbo A. A prospective randomized comparison of transurethral resection to visual laser ablation of the prostate for the treatment of benign prostatic hyperplasia. Urology. 1995;46(2):155–60.
31. Farsi HMA. Visual laser ablation of the prostate for patients with acute urinary retention. Br J Urol. 1996;78:90–2.
32. Malek RS, Barrett DM, Kuntzman RS. High-power potassium-titanyl-phosphate (KTP/532) laser vaporization prostatectomy: 24 hours later. Urology. 1993;51:254–6.
33. Sarica K, Alkan E, Lüleci H, Taşci AI. Photoselective vaporization of the enlarged prostate with KTP laser: long-term results in 240 patients. J Endourol. 2005;19:1199–202.
34. Ruszat R, Seitz M, Wyler SF, Abe C, Rieken M, Reich O, Gasser TC, Bachmann A. GreenLight laser vaporization of the prostate: single-center experience and long-term results after 500 procedures. Eur Urol. 2008;54:893–901.
35. Thomas JA, Tubaro A, Barber N, d'Ancona F, Muir G, Witzsch U, Grimm MO, Benejam J, Stolzenburg JU, Riddick A, Pahernik S, Roelink H, Ameye F, Saussine C, Bruyère F, Loidl W, Larner T, Gogoi NK, Hindley R, Muschter R, Thorpe A, Shrotri N, Graham S, Hamann M, Miller K, Schostak M, Capitán C, Knispel H, Bachmann A. A multicenter randomized noninferiority trial comparing GreenLight-XPS laser vaporization of the prostate and transurethral resection of the prostate for the treatment of benign prostatic obstruction: two-yr. outcomes of the GOLIATH study. Eur Urol. 2016;69:94–102.
36. Gilling PJ, Cass CB, Cresswell MD, Malcolm AR, Fraundorfer MR. The use of the holmium laser in the treatment of benign prostatic hyperplasia. J Endourol. 1996;10:459–61.
37. Elshal AM, Elmansy HM, Elhilali MM. Two laser ablation techniques for a prostate less than 60 mL: lessons learned 70 months after a randomized controlled trial. Urology. 2013;82:416–22.
38. Tholomier C, Valdivieso R, Hueber PA, Zorn KC. Photoselective laser ablation of the prostate: a review of the current 2015 tissue ablation options. Can J Urol. 2015;22:s45–52.
39. Ruszat R, Seitz M, Wyler SF, et al. Prospective single-center comparison of 120-W diode-pumped solid state high-intensity system laser vaporization of the prostate for treating benign prostatic hyperplasia. BJU Int. 2009;104:820–5.
40. Shaker HS, Shoeb MS, Yassin MM, Shaker SH. Quartz head contact laser fiber: a novel fiber for laser ablation of the prostate using the 980 nm high power diode laser. J Urol. 2012;187:575–9.
41. Gilling PJ, Cass C, Malcolm A, Cresswell M, Fraundorfer MR, Kabalin JN. Holmium laser resection of the prostate versus neodymium:yttrium-aluminum-garnet visual laser ablation of the prostate: a randomized prospective comparison of two techniques for laser prostatectomy. Urology. 1998;51:573–7.
42. Szlauer R, Götschl R, Razmaria A, Paras L, Schmeller NT. Endoscopic vaporesection of the prostate using the continuous-wave 2-microm thulium laser: outcome and demonstration of the surgical technique. Eur Urol. 2009;55:368–75.
43. Chung JS, Kang PM, Seo WI, CK O, Kim SC, Park SH, Choi JH, Yoon JH, Kang DI, Chung JI. Thulium laser (RevoLix) vaporesection versus vapoenucleation with morcellator (piranha) for the treatment of benign prostatic obstruction: a propensity-matched multicenter analysis. Int J Urol. 2014;21:1156–61.
44. Fraundorfer MR, Gilling PJ. Holmium:YAG laser enucleation of the prostate combined with mechanical morcellation: preliminary results. Eur Urol. 1998;33:69–72.
45. Elmansy HM, Kotb A, Elhilali MM. Holmium laser enucleation of the prostate: long-term durability of clinical outcomes and complication rates during 10 years of followup. J Urol. 2011;186:1972–6.
46. Krambeck AE, Handa SE, Lingeman JE. Experience with more than 1000 holmium laser prostate enucleations for benign prostatic hyperplasia. J Urol. 2013;189:S141–5.

47. Gilling PJ, Wilson LC, King CJ, Westenberg AM, Frampton CM, Fraundorfer MR. Long-term results of a randomized trial comparing holmium laser enucleation of the prostate and transurethral resection of the prostate: results at 7 years. BJU Int. 2012;109:408–11.
48. Bach T, Wendt-Nordahl G, Michel MS, Herrmann TR, Gross AJ. Feasibility and efficacy of thulium:YAG laser enucleation (VapoEnucleation) of the prostate. World J Urol. 2009;27:541–5.
49. Buisan O, Saladie JM, Ruiz JM, Bernal S, Bayona S, Ibarz L. Diode laser enucleation of the prostate (Dilep): technique and initial results. Actas Urol Esp. 2011;35:37–41.
50. Elterman DS, Chughtai B, Lee R, Kurlander L, Yip-Bannicq M, Kaplan SA, Te AE. Comparison of techniques for transurethral laser prostatectomy: standard photoselective vaporization of the prostate versus transurethral laser enucleation of the prostate. J Endourol. 2013;27:751–5.
51. Hruby S, Sieberer M, Schätz T, Jones N, Zimmermann R, Janetschek G, Lusuardi L. Eraser laser enucleation of the prostate: technique and results. Eur Urol. 2013;63:341–6.
52. Netsch C, Engbert A, Bach T, Gross AJ. Long-term outcome following thulium VapoEnucleation of the prostate. World J Urol. 2014;32:1551–8.
53. Shen Y, Konchada V, Zhang N, Jain S, Zhou X, Burke D, Wong C, Carson C, Roehrborn C, Sweet R. Laser surgery simulation platform: toward full-procedure training and rehearsal for benign prostatic hyperplasia (BPH) therapy. Stud Health Technol Inform. 2011;163:574–80.
54. Pickens RB, Bajo A, Simaan N, Herrell D. A pilot ex vivo evaluation of a telerobotic system for transurethral intervention and surveillance. J Endourol. 2015;29:231–4.
55. Russo S, Dario P, Menciassi A. A novel robotic platform for laser-assisted transurethral surgery of the prostate. IEEE Trans Biomed Eng. 2015;62:489–500.
56. Mitchell CR, Hendrick RJ, Webster RJ III, Herrell D. Towards improving transurethral prostate surgery: development and initial experiments with a prototype concentric tube robotic platform. J Endourol. 2016;30(6):692–6.

Chapter 11
The History of Shockwave Lithotripsy

Christian G. Chaussy

The Beginning

In aviation, hypersonic flight in rain presented a considerable challenge for the resilience of the airplane structure. The rain drops created a shockwave which not only destroyed the material at the point of impact, but also caused damage on the interior of the material. Further research under laboratory conditions to try and explain the phenomena was conducted.

To research this collision, high velocity projectiles were fired from a light-gas gun onto a target thereby creating shockwaves (Fig. 11.1a and b). The impact of shockwaves on living tissue was of equal interest to the military. At the end of the 1960s research was conducted at Dornier in collaboration with the Institute of Applied Physics and Electrical Engineering of the University Saarbrücken to, amongst others, determine the reciprocity of shockwaves on organic tissue. In the course of this research it was discovered that shockwaves caused no visible injury when passing through muscle tissue, fat tissue or fascia. Exceptions were bordering areas with high acoustic impendences. It was this project that gave rise to the idea to destroy kidney stones inside the body using shockwaves.

In 1971 at the symposium of the German Physical Society, the first results were presented in which shockwaves, created using high velocity water drops and using a water filled, closed tube as waveguide, were able to destroy kidney stones [1].

The idea was further pursued using a light-gas gun and projectiles were fired with a velocity of up to 5 km/s on a metal target, which was connected to an open water recipient. The shockwaves produced in the target entered the water recipient,

C.G. Chaussy
University of Munich, Munich, Germany

University of Regensburg, Regensburg, Germany

Keck School of Medicine, USC, Los Angeles, CA, USA
e-mail: cgchaussy@gmail.com

S.R. Patel et al. (eds.), *The History of Technologic Advancements in Urology*,
DOI 10.1007/978-3-319-61691-9_11

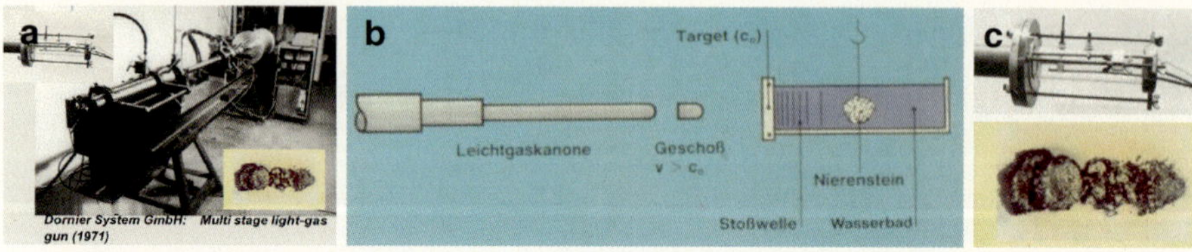

Fig. 11.1 (**a**) Light gas gun. (**b**) Scheme of lithotripsy. (**c**) Target and destructed kidney stone

in which a stone had been placed. Depending on the form of the target, a straight or focused shockwave hit the stone. With a straight wave only small cracks were produced, however with the focused wave substantial fragmentation of the stone was achieved (Fig. 11.1c).

It had thus far been unknown to use shockwaves for therapeutic purposes. Substantial experimental and theoretical studies conducted by an interdisciplinary workgroup, consisting of members of the Department of Urology at the University Munich, the Institute of Surgical Research and Dornier, were therefore required prior clinical application. These studies started in January 1974 [2–8]. The substantial funding for this project, at the time considered as extremely high risk, came from the German Ministry of Research and Technology. Today a similar project would probably not receive public funding, thus such innovation would be impossible.

The costly physical trials could only be justified if there was a likelihood that the shockwave would not damage organs. For this reason the laboratory apparatus in the starting phase of the project was constructed for tests on vital structures (Figs. 11.2 and 11.3). The medical trials conducted were structured in two segments, in-vitro and in-vivo trials. The in-vitro experiments were aimed at determining if the delicate erythrocytes would be destroyed and if the process of erythrocyte proliferation were to be effected. The impact of the shockwave on abdominal and thoracal organs in a small animal were tested during the in-vivo experiments.

In a free standing water bath, probes with a standardized volume of 10 ml dog blood were adjusted into the focal point and the impact of the exposition to up to four shockwaves at 20 kV was studied. Increasing with the number of shockwaves was the concentration of serum haemoglobin to a level of 400 mg/100 ml. The increase seemed not to be relevant in comparison to the total blood volume of the animal. Later in a dog, despite a twentyfold shockwave exposure, no increase in the concentration of serum hemoglobin could be found.

The impact of the shockwave on the proliferative processes in a mixed lymphocyte model was compared to untreated cell cultures in the same way. The reactivity of the exposed lymphocytes did not differ to that of the untreated control group. A change in the stimulation capacity was not found.

For the in-vivo trials the test facility had to be modified. Instead of the water bath a bench was used, with which the shockwave could directly be coupled with the trial animal using a membrane. Using spacers the distance between the membrane and focal point was altered and allowed for the shockwave to act at a certain depth from the skin's surface.

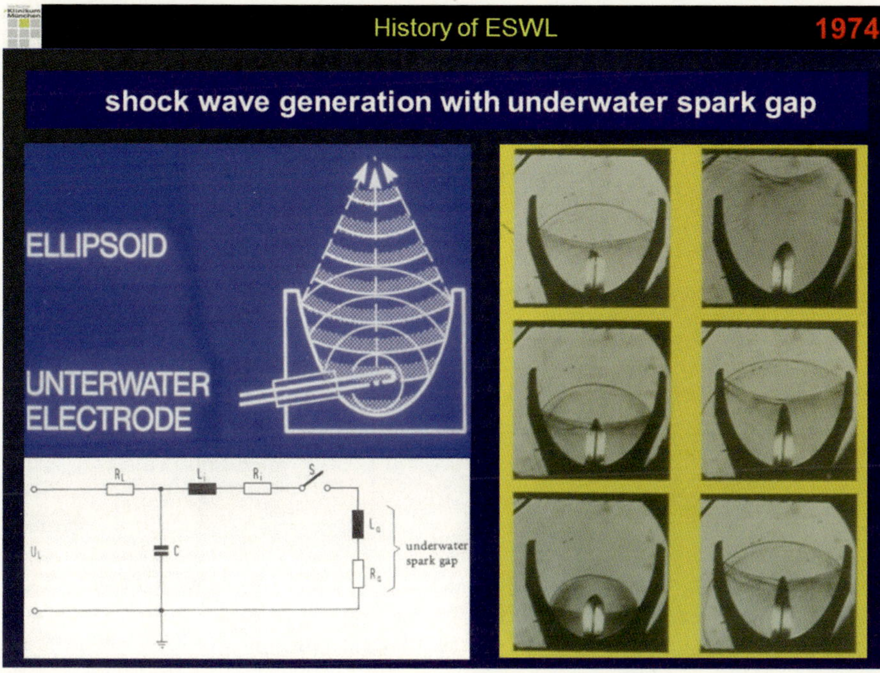

Fig. 11.2 Design of Ellipsoid and Shockwave source and propulsion of pressure waves after underwater spark discharge

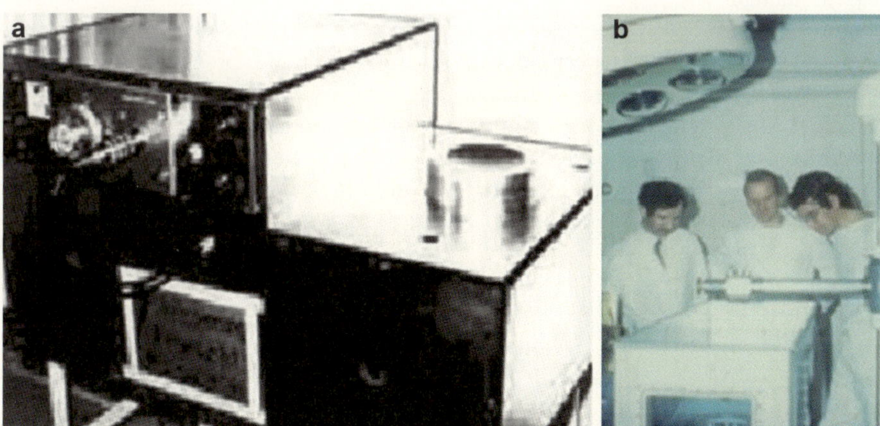

Fig. 11.3 (**a**) First experimental device for in-vitro and in-vivo studies. (**b**) Inspection of an experimental device for larger animals (C. Chaussy, F Eisenberger und B. Forssmann—right to left)

Narcotized rats were fixed to the bench and the thoracic and abdominal area randomly treated with ultrasound at 20 kV. Single shockwave exposure in the thoracic region caused massive lung trauma resulting in the deaths of the animals.

Table 11.1 Results of untargeted shockwave exposition, rat studies (+) in individual cases of petechial bleeding, (+++) massive cell lesions, Ø no bleeding [9]

Exposure 10×	Clinical results	Pathological changes (24 h after experiments)		Pathological changes (14 days after experiment)	
		Macroscopic	Microscopic	Macroscopic	Microscopic
Thorax (n = 20)	Massive hemoptysis	+++	+++	–	–
With sheet of Styrofoam (n = 20)	No result	Ø	Ø	Ø	Ø
Abdominal cavity (n = 20)	No result	Ø	Ø	Ø	Ø
Liver (n = 20)	No result	+	+	Ø	Ø
Colon	No result	+	+	Ø	Ø

This had not been entirely unexpected as the lung possesses other acoustic impedances as muscle or fat. These injuries were prevented by insulating the lung with air-filled materials which stopped the shockwave entering this part of the body. The animals survived ultrasound treatment of the abdominal area with ten shockwaves without any clinical side effects. Histological tests conducted 24 h and 14 days after the treatment showed neither macroscopic nor microscopic pathological changes [9].

Further trials focused specifically on the influence of shockwave exposure on the liver and intestine. The respective organs were eventerated, brought into focus and after successful exposure repositioned. After two exposures the intestine showed petechial bleeding. Massive haemorrhages or lesions of the intestinal wall never occurred. The liver also showed petechial bleeding. After 14 days no pathological alterations could be found on either organ (Table 11.1).

Localization and Stone Model

While the concretions during in-vitro testing in the water bath could be placed into the object's focal point by sight, an accurate and reliable tracing for inside the animal had to be found. The idea of using ultrasound for the positioning was fascinating. The expansion of ultrasound and shockwaves adhere to the same physical laws (Fig. 11.4a and b).

During in- vivo experiments an unambiguous localization only succeeded in exceptions, if the concretion could be located close to the skin surface. A reproducible localization for specific experimental trials or a clinical application did not appear useful.

The emerging ultrasound diagnostic with compound scanners in the B-Scan mode seemed promising for additional information and to reliably locate the stone. Therefore, a B-Scan was integrated, where the pictures were recorded using a fluoroscope. However this method, combined with the A-Scan, did not provide a reliable localization due to the many artifacts. A change of the apparatus to a system of greyscales did not significantly improve the stone identification as the stone shadow, essential to identifying the stone, was generally superimposed by artefacts (Fig. 11.4c).

It proved difficult to find a test subject for the extracorporeal destruction of kidney stones with symptoms comparable to those of a human patient, especially as kidney stones only seldom occur in animals. All attempts using special long term-diets as well as the implantation of exogenous materials, which showed no similarities to a human kidney stone, delivered only unsatisfactory results. Nevertheless, in order to research the treatment of human lithiasis it was completely indispensable to have a simple, reproducible model for large animals.

Initially the idea of injecting liquid resin into the renal calix, which would harden under the influence of body temperature and uric liquid, was pursued. Using acryl acetate the lining of kidney duct system with a renal pelvis calculus was successful (Fig. 11.5a). As these artificial stones did not possess the physical characteristics of a natural kidney stone the destruction into small fragments was not possible.

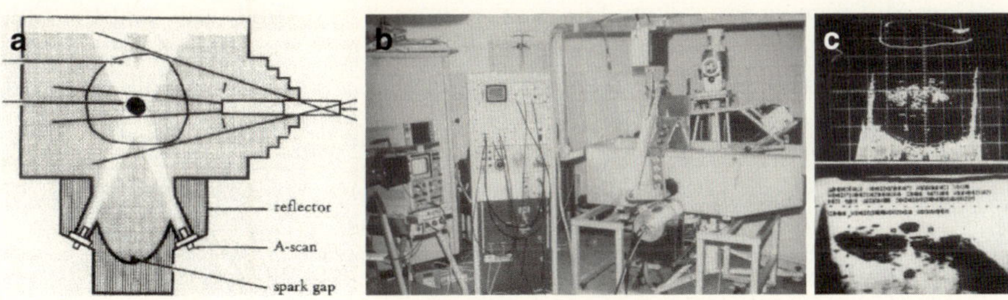

Fig. 11.4 (**a**) Integration of ultrasound scanners. (**b**) Experimental lithotripter with integrated ultrasound scanners. (**c**) Transverse sonogram after stone implantation

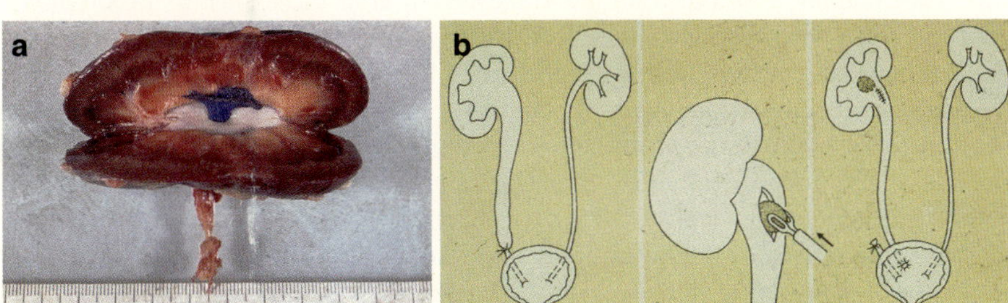

Fig. 11.5 (**a**) Implanted artificial acrylacetate stone. (**b**) Experimental procedure for the implantation of human kidney stones in dogs

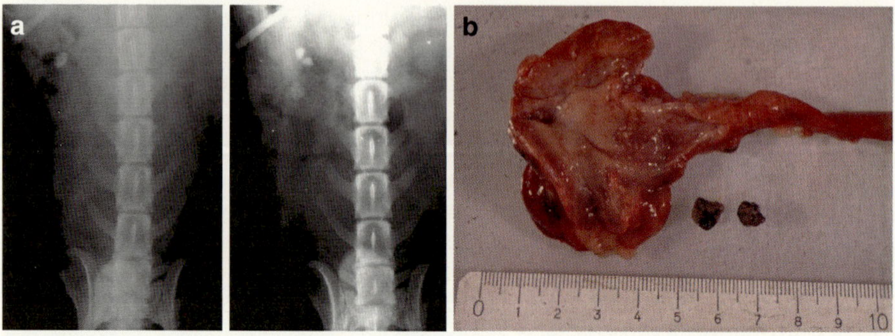

Fig. 11.6 First in-vivo stone destruction (**a**) (a1) X-ray pre and (a2) post shockwave exposure. (**b**) Section specimen

It was therefore decided to implant freshly obtained human kidney stones in the kidney duct system of a dog. Primarily due to size discrepancies between the renal pelvis and the kidney stone, intra-operational technical difficulties in connection with complications in the post-operational course, the initial attempts of implanting sufficiently large kidney stones did not yield the expected results.

A solution to these problems could be achieved by the following procedure:

Dogs did receive an abdominal section under sterile conditions and the right ureter was ligated prevesically. The research animals did later receive a fine median abdominal section and were implanted with a contrast giving human kidney stone with a diameter of between 1 and 2 cm. Afterwards the ureter was re-implanted into the bladder. Following surgery the discharge of urine and the position of the stones was checked in intervals of 8 days using IVP. The intervention did not cause changes in the kidney duct system. The medical requirements for systematic testing of the method in a reproducible animal model were found [10, 11] (Fig. 11.5b).

Despite the ongoing problems of reliable ultrasound tracing the animal testing commenced. In the first step the effects of shockwave exposure on the right kidney were tested in a series of 20 non-stone carrying dogs. Up to ten high energy shockwaves were applied in a grid on the kidney. 48 h after the exposure a section was conducted and tissue samples taken from kidney, liver, spleen, pancreas, duodenum, colon, lungs, ribs and spinal column and tested for shockwaves induced side effects. No macroscopic alterations were found in any of the exposed organs. In some cases slight bleeding was recorded in the lower right pulmonary lobe, but none of these cases induced a haematothorax. Histological studies of these organs showed no pathological changes.

Due to the difficulties in locating the stones using ultrasound, the destruction was only possible in isolated cases (Fig. 11.6). Nevertheless, these were of major importance for the continuation of the project, as the project sponsor had intended to discontinue the subsidies. It proved that extracorporeal shock wave lithotripsy is generally possible and with the first stone destruction the project sponsor could be convinced to authorize further grants.

Localization with X-Rays

To circumvent the deficiencies of ultrasound tracing, the possibility of integrating x-rays into a shockwave apparatus, as a technique to obtain images was considered. An image intensifier and two conventional tubes of X-ray C-arches were integrated in a shockwave apparatus in a way that the central beams would cut the shockwave focal point at an angle of 40° with regards to the ellipsoid axis (Fig. 11.7). Both systems could be rotated around the focal point vertically to the central beams. This should enable one to move the stone shadow out of a bone cover for better identification. X-ray tube and image intensifier could be moved along the central beams to find the best distance for an optimal image.

Further in-vitro tests with low pressure amplitudes of approximately 30 MPa were conducted to define a threshold for the destruction of stones. The capacity of the surge generator was reduced from 2 KF to 20 nF, 40 nF and 60 nF. Using these generators and 50–300 shockwaves in 1 s intervals, the stones could be decomposed into finer particles as had so far been possible with one, strong shockwave (Fig. 11.8).

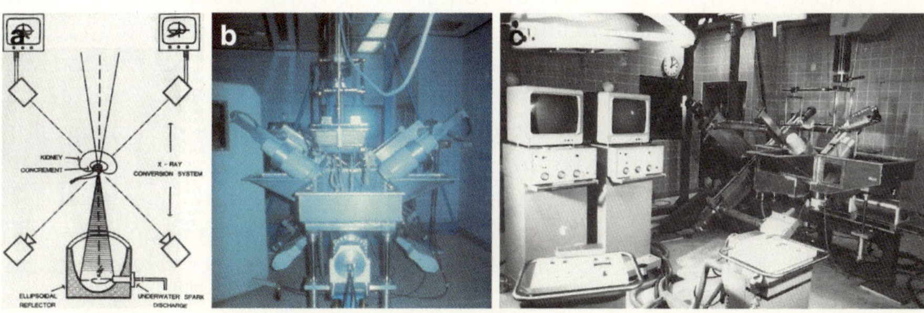

Fig. 11.7 Lithotripter for animal experiments. (**a** and **b**) Principle of X-ray localisation. (**c**) Total view of the experimental setup

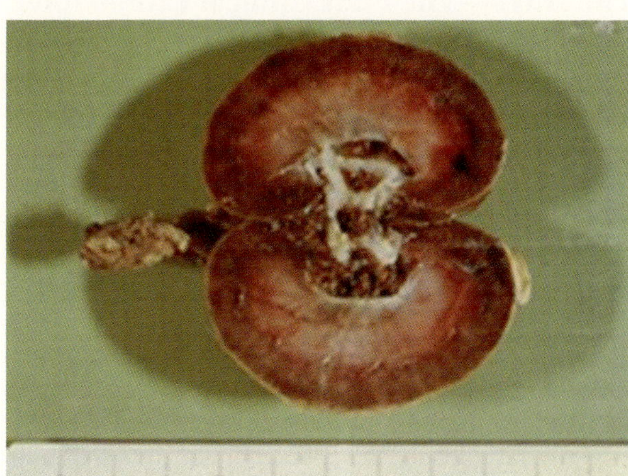

Fig. 11.8 Prepared dissection of a stone bearing dog kidney immediately after shockwave exposure

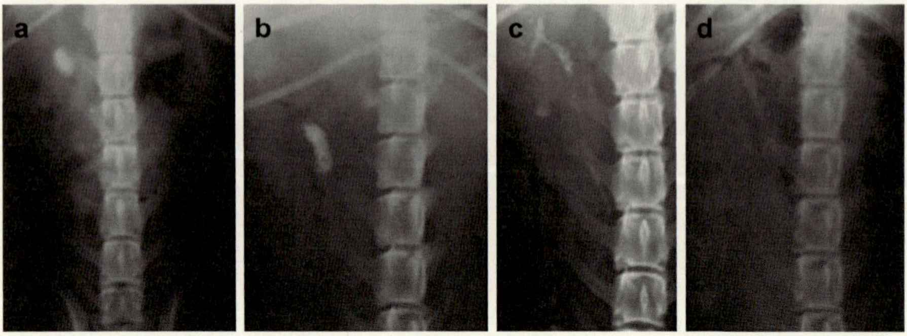

Fig. 11.9 Monitoring of an experimental shockwave exposure (dog) (**a**) before, (**b**) immediately after, (**c**) 1 day after and (**d**) 2 weeks after lithotripsy

A total of 17 dogs implanted with kidney stones were included in the trial series. During and after the trials, no impairments caused by shockwave exposure were found. Thirteen of the animals were stone-free after spontaneously passing the particles. In 11 of these animals, this was achieved after a single shockwave exposure. The remaining three animals received additional treatment 14 days later to further crush larger particles still remaining in the renal pelvis. Following the repeated shockwave exposure two further animals were stone-free after 14 days. In four animals complete stone passage could not be achieved (Fig. 11.9).

Blood samples for laboratory testing were taken from each of the animals prior to and after the shockwave exposure as well as 1 and 2 weeks later. None of the tested parameters showed any significant divergence from the initial values. To assess the possible shockwave effects on the kidney functions split isotope studies on six of the animals, prior to, 4 and 14 days after shockwave exposure were performed with ^{99m}Tc- DMSA [12–14].

The HM1—The First Clinical Lithotripter

The results obtained from the animal experiments justified a transfer of the method into clinical use. The design of the pre-clinical prototype was adapted in size in relation to the patient. In a type of "training program," tracking tests were conducted with volunteers, using the apparatus known as HM1 which was installed in the Institute for Surgical Research in October 1979, to determine the positioning and to practice the treatment process (Fig. 11.10). This initiated some necessary changes on the device; due to the buoyancy during the lowering into the water bath and the adjusting of the stone into focus with an anaesthetised patient a firm fixation was not given. Once the patient stretcher had been equipped with a harness system and changes had been made to the motion axis a reliable localization became possible.

The first, and the following patients were chosen following a strict selection process. Based on the experience gained from the animal testing, it was decided that the stone in the renal pelvis should be no larger than a cherry. Unobstructed

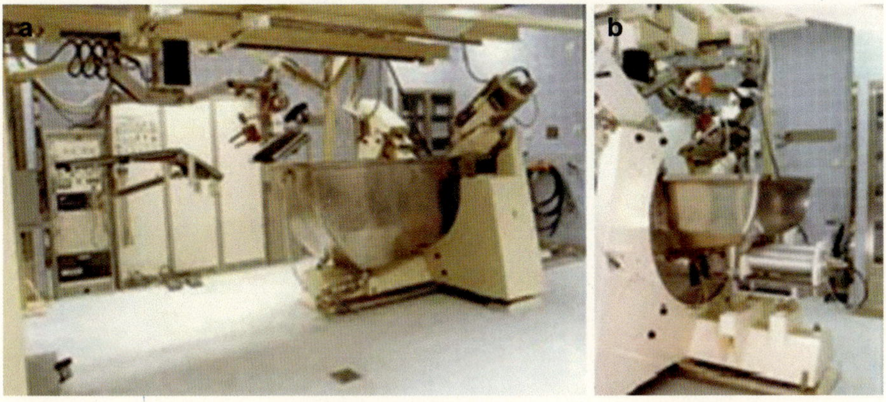

Fig. 11.10 (**a**) Total view of shockwave lithotripter (HM 1). (**b**) Detailed view of the shockwave generator underneath the bathtub

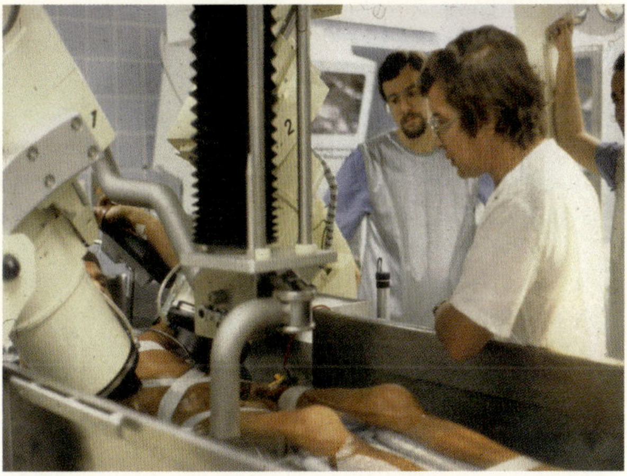

Fig. 11.11 Patient, C. Chaussy and anaesthetist in one of the first treatments

conditions for passages in the urinary tract and the exclusion of an infection in the urinary tract were prerequisites for the passage of the stone particles.

Prerequisite for a fine-grained disintegration was the reliable localization achieved by a high radiographic contrast of the stone. To avoid unexpected complications and to ensure the assessment of possible side effects of a shockwave therapy—though not caused by the shockwave—patients with internal risk factors were not accepted. Based on the requirement parameters for inclusion and exclusion which essentially still apply today were defined.

The first treatment took place on February 7th, 1980. Intubation anaesthesia was used in this and in 13 other cases (Fig. 11.11). However, soon after it was discovered that less strenuous peridural anaesthesia was sufficient for patients. The narcotized patient was harnessed to the stretcher and placed into the water bath using the patient positioning device. The method for tracking and adjusting the stone into the shockwave focal point was identical to the procedure during animal testing (Fig. 11.12).

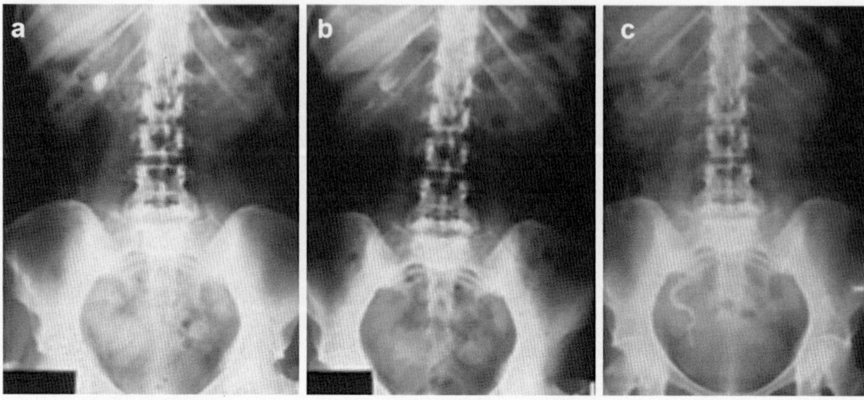

Fig. 11.12 Patient X-ray follow-up (**a**) before (**b**) immediately after shockwave exposure. (**c**) Steinstrasse in distal ureter

To avoid premature breaking of the stone, the shockwave was initially applied with low energy. In intervals of 50–100 shockwave releases the progress of the disintegration was checked. Towards the end of the disintegration process the energy of the shockwave was increased to better shatter larger fragments still remaining. Depending on the size of the stone a total of 500–1500 shockwaves were applied. At the beginning, the time necessary for application was approximately 90 min, caused by repeated changes of the underwater electrode. The treatment time was reduced to 30–45 min after various technical improvements caused an increase in the electrode's life cycle.

In some cases extrasystoles caused by shockwaves could be observed during shockwave exposure, a phenomena which could to this day not fully be explained. By releasing a shockwave triggered by the ECG immediately after the R-Wave this interaction with the conduction system was avoided.

Until May 1982 a total of 221 extracorporeal shockwave lithotripsies, or "ESWL" as it should become known, were conducted on 206 patients. Fifteen patients had to receive a second ESWL to become stone-free and 39% of the patients had already received surgery once or twice on the same kidney before. The majority of the stones (75%) were located in the renal pelvis. Following the first positive experience the method would be extended to renal calyx in 23% of the cases.

Furthermore four high ureteral stones were treated, two of them impacted stones, which nevertheless had to be removed surgically after shockwave exposure. Despite fine fragmentation, the particles could not be passed as they were bound into an organic matrix, comparable to a sack. The particles of the other two stones were passed after just a few days. The stones consisted to 90% of calcium oxalate, 5% magnesium ammonium phosphate and the remaining 5% of different chemical components including uric acid and a cysteine stone.

Further examinations up to 1 year after ESWL showed no anomalies in the laboratory parameters compared to the base line. Also no significant difference in the renal function studies was found. As early as the end of 1980 results from the first 21 patients were published and in 1982 the clinical study was published as well [15–17] (Fig. 11.13) (Table 11.2).

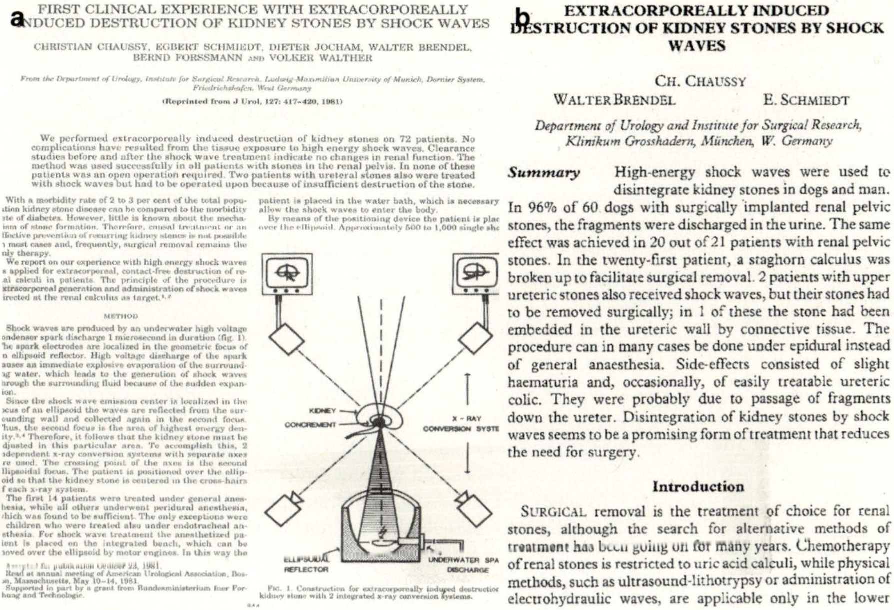

a FIRST CLINICAL EXPERIENCE WITH EXTRACORPOREALLY NDUCED DESTRUCTION OF KIDNEY STONES BY SHOCK WAVES

CHRISTIAN CHAUSSY, EGBERT SCHMIEDT, DIETER JOCHAM, WALTER BRENDEL, BERND FORSSMANN AND VOLKER WALTHER

From the Department of Urology, Institute for Surgical Research, Ludwig-Maximilian University of Munich, Dornier System, Friedrichshafen, West Germany

(Reprinted from J Urol, 127: 417–420, 1981)

We performed extracorporeally induced destruction of kidney stones on 72 patients. No complications have resulted from the tissue exposure to high energy shock waves. Clearance studies before and after the shock wave treatment indicate no changes in renal function. The method was used successfully in all patients with stones in the renal pelvis. In none of these patients was an open operation required. Two patients with ureteral stones also were treated with shock waves but had to be operated upon because of insufficient destruction of the stone.

With a morbidity rate of 2 to 3 per cent of the total popu- ation kidney stone disease can be compared to the morbidity ate of diabetes. However, little is known about the mecha- ism of stone formation. Therefore, causal treatment or an ffective prevention of recurring kidney stones is not possible n most cases and, frequently, surgical removal remains the nly therapy.

We report on our experience with high energy shock waves s applied for extracorporeal, contact-free destruction of re- al calculi in patients. The principle of the procedure is xtracorporeal generation and administration of shock waves irected at the renal calculus as target.[1,2]

METHOD

Shock waves are produced by an underwater high voltage ondenser spark discharge 1 microsecond in duration (fig. 1). 'he spark electrodes are localized in the geometric focus of n ellipsoid reflector. High voltage discharge of the spark auses an immediate explosive evaporation of the surround- ng water, which leads to the generation of shock waves hrough the surrounding fluid because of the sudden expan- ion.

Since the shock wave emission center is localized in the ocus of an ellipsoid the waves are reflected from the sur- ounding wall and collected again in the second focus. 'hus, the second focus is the area of highest energy den- ity.[3,4] Therefore, it follows that the kidney stone must be djusted in this particular area. To accomplish this, 2 ndependent x-ray conversion systems with separate axes re used. The crossing point of the axes is the second llipsoidal focus. The patient is positioned over the ellip- oid so that the kidney stone is centered in the cross-hairs f each x-ray system.

The first 14 patients were treated under general anes- hesia, while all others underwent peridural anesthesia, which was found to be sufficient. The only exceptions were children who were treated also under endotracheal an- sthesia. For shock wave treatment the anesthetized pa- ient is placed on the integrated bench, which can be noved over the ellipsoid by motor engines. In this way the patient is placed in the water bath, which is necessary allow the shock waves to enter the body.

By means of the positioning device the patient is plac over the ellipsoid. Approximately 500 to 1,000 single sho

FIG. 1. Construction for extracorporeally induced destructior kidney stone with 2 integrated x-ray conversion systems.

Accepted for publication October 23, 1981.
Read at annual meeting of American Urological Association, Bos- on, Massachusetts, May 10–14, 1981.
Supported in part by a grant from Bundesministerium fuer For- hung and Technologie.

b **EXTRACORPOREALLY INDUCED DESTRUCTION OF KIDNEY STONES BY SHOCK WAVES**

CH. CHAUSSY
WALTER BRENDEL E. SCHMIEDT

Department of Urology and Institute for Surgical Research, Klinikum Grosshadern, München, W. Germany

Summary High-energy shock waves were used to disintegrate kidney stones in dogs and man. In 96% of 60 dogs with surgically implanted renal pelvic stones, the fragments were discharged in the urine. The same effect was achieved in 20 out of 21 patients with renal pelvic stones. In the twenty-first patient, a staghorn calculus was broken up to facilitate surgical removal. 2 patients with upper ureteric stones also received shock waves, but their stones had to be removed surgically; in 1 of these the stone had been embedded in the ureteric wall by connective tissue. The procedure can in many cases be done under epidural instead of general anaesthesia. Side-effects consisted of slight haematuria and, occasionally, of easily treatable ureteric colic. They were probably due to passage of fragments down the ureter. Disintegration of kidney stones by shock waves seems to be a promising form of treatment that reduces the need for surgery.

Introduction

SURGICAL removal is the treatment of choice for renal stones, although the search for alternative methods of treatment has been going on for many years. Chemotherapy of renal stones is restricted to uric acid calculi, while physical methods, such as ultrasound-lithotrypsy or administration of electrohydraulic waves, are applicable only in the lower

Fig. 11.13 (**a**) Publication of the first clinical results in The Lancet 1980;2: 1265–1268 [15]. (**b**) Publication of first clinical experience in J Urol 1982;127: 417–20 [17]

Table 11.2 Timeline of events in the development of shockwave lithotripsy

Date	Event
1981	The installation of the HM2 in Munich required a space allocation plan. The investment of 2.1 Million DM (in 1981 US $ 855,000) was only possible with the help of the Bavarian insurance companies and the committee for home dialysis (Kuratorium für Heimdialyse = KfH). Without their dedication the project would not have been possible at all [12, 13]
1982	On May 20, 1982 the first lithotripsy center was launched in Munich under the supervision of Ch. Chaussy at the Department of Urology (E. Schmiedt), University of Munich. With this set up fast and further clinical evaluation of the extension of indications was possible. The treatment of staghorn stones by fractionated shockwave exposition in multiple sessions, of infected stones under antibiotic pre-treatment and of multiple stones was possible. Also high risk patients were accepted. Furthermore PCNL, which was initially regarded as competition, was introduced as auxiliary procedure to ESWL. After these successful extensions of indications for ESWL operative indications for stone removal were limited to 10–15% of stone patients [12, 18, 19]
1983	The data and success of ESWL sparked an enormous interest in Germany and worldwide. In 1983 the 2nd lithotripsy center was opened in Stuttgart (F. Eisenberger) [20]
	An FDA study, necessary for approval of ESWL in the USA, was planned at 6 centers. In spite of the great interest displayed by radiologists, it was possible to keep the procedure in the hands of urologists; the main reason was that all principal investigators had to be trained in Munich and the Munich urologists refused to train radiologists

(continued)

Table 11.2 (continued)

Date	Event
1984	The first device in the US was installed in February in Indianapolis (D. Newman, J. Lingeman); another 5 clinics followed. The US FDA study was monitored by G. Drach
	Due to the method's success, the PMA was already granted for general marketing in December. This fast decision was mainly due to the acceptance of the data from the clinical study conducted by the Munich urology clinic which played a significant role because the results of the USA study were not published until 2 years later [21]

References

1. Haeusler E, Kiefer W. Anregung von Stoßwellen in Flüssigkeiten durch Hochgeschwindigkeitswassertropfen. Verhandl. DPG (VI) 1971;6: K 36.
2. Chaussy C, Eisenberger F, Wanner K, Forssmann B, Hepp W, Schmiedt E, Brendel W. The use of shock wave for the destruction of renal calculi without direct contact. Urol Res. 1976;4:175.
3. Chaussy C, Eisenberger F, Wanner K, Forssmann B. Extrakorporale Anwendung von hochenergetischen Stoßwellen - Ein neuer Aspekt in der Behandlung des Harnsteinleidens. Teil II Akt Urol. 1978;9:95–101.
4. Chaussy C, Schmiedt E, Forssmann B, Brendel W. Contact free renal stone destruction by means of shock waves. Eur Surg Res. 1979;11:36.
5. Eisenberger F, Chaussy C, Wanner K. Extrakorporale Anwendung von hochenergetischen Stoßwellen- Ein neuer Aspekt in der Behandlung des Harnsteinleidens. Akt Urol. 1977;8:3–15.
6. Eisenberger F, Chaussy C. Contact-free renal stone fragmentation with shock waves. Urol Res. 1978;6:111.
7. Forssmann B, Hepp W, Chaussy C, Eisenberger F, Wanner KA. Method for no-contact destruction of kidney stones by means of shock waves. Biomed Tech. 1977;22:164–8.
8. Forssmann B, Hepp W, Chaussy C, Eisenberger F, Wanner K. Stoßwellen - eine neue Methode für die Nierensteinbehandlung? Verhandl. DPG (VI) 1977;12: K 47.
9. Chaussy C, Schmiedt E, Jocham D, Walther V, Brendel W, Forssmann B, Hepp W. In: Chaussy C, editor. Extracorporeal shock wave lithotripsy - new aspects in the treatment of kidney stone disease. Basel; Munich; Paris: Karger; 1982.
10. Chaussy C, Eisenberger F, Wanner K. The implantation of human kidney stones - a simple experimental model. Urologe A. 1977;16:35–8.
11. Chaussy C, Wieland W, Jocham D, Eisenberger F, Forssmann B. Röntgenologische Steinlokalisation im Modell der berührungsfreien Steinzertrümmerung - Experimentelle Studie. Verh. Ber. Ges. Urol, 30Tagung, 1978: 333–334.
12. Chaussy C, Eisenberger F, Forssmann B. Extracorporeal shockwave lithotripsy (ESWL): a chronology. J Endourol. 2007;21(11):1249–53.
13. Chaussy C, Schmiedt E, Jocham D, Fuchs G, Brendel W. In: Chaussy C, editor. Extracorporeal shock wave lithotripsy. Technical concept, experimental research, and clinical application. Basel; München; Paris: Karger; 1986.
14. Forssmann B, Hepp W, Chaussy C, Jocham D, Schmiedt E, Brendel W. Prototyp für die klinische Anwendung der berührungsfreien Nierensteinzertrümmerung durch Stoßwellen. Biomed Tech. 1980;25(Suppl):414–6.
15. Chaussy C, Brendel W, Schmiedt E. Extracorporeally induced destruction of kidney stones by shock waves. Lancet. 1980;2:1265–8.
16. Chaussy C, Schmiedt E, Jocham D, Brendel W, Forssmann B, Moser E. Berührungsfreie Nierensteinzertrümmerung durch Stoßwellen - erste klinische Erfahrungen. Deutsches Ärzteblatt. 1981;18:881–6.

17. Chaussy C, Schmiedt E, Jocham D, Brendel W, Forssmann B, Walther W. First clinical experience with extracorporeally induced destruction of kidney stones by shock waves. J Urol. 1982;127:417–20.
18. Chaussy C, Schmiedt E, Jocham D, Walther V, Brendel W. Stoßwellentherapie zur Behandlung von Nierensteinen. MMW Munch Med Wochenschr. 1983;125:151–5.
19. Chaussy C, Schmiedt E, Jocham D, Schüller J, Brandl H. Extrakorporale Stoßwellenlithotripsie - Beginn einer Umstrukturierung in der Behandlung des Harnsteinleidens? Urologe A. 1984;23:25–9.
20. Miller K, Fuchs G, Rassweiler J, Eisenberger F. Extracorporeal shock wave lithotripsy: one year experience with the Dornier lithotripter. Eur Urol. 1985;11:145–9.
21. Drach GW, Dretler S, Fair W, Finlayson B, Gillenwater J, Griffith D, Lingeman J, Newman D. Report of the United States cooperative study of extracorporeal shock wave lithotripsy. J Urol. 1986;135:1127–33.

Chapter 12
The History and Development of Percutaneous Nephrolithotomy

Sutchin R. Patel and Stephen Y. Nakada

The standard treatment for patients with renal calculi prior to the mid 1950s was open stone surgery. The existence of a relatively avascular plane 5 mm posterior to the midline of the kidney was establish through the work of Joseph Hyrtl in 1882 and Max Brödel in 1902 [1, 2]. However, Howard Kelly, found that the landmarks were reliable in only two thirds of kidneys and thus advocated for pyelotomy as he described it as a safer operation [2]. It was not until 1941, that Rupel and Brown would perform the first nephroscopy by placing a rigid cystoscope through a nephrostomy tract so that stones could be removed during open surgery [3]. The early instruments used to explore the renal pelvis during open surgery had hard right angles so that they could reach the calyces. This was much different from the offset nephroscopes with a straight working channel that would be developed in the future for percutaneous nephrolithotomy [4].

Percutaneous Nephrostomy

Thomas Hillier, a pediatric urologist from Great Ormond Street Hospital for Sick Children described a case report in 1865 entitled "Hydronephrosis in a boy 4 years old repeatedly tapped; recovery" where he repeatedly percutaneously drained a hydronephrotic kidney in a child eventually found to have a ureteropelvic junction obstruction [5]. Willard Goodwin, the first Chair of the Department of Urology at UCLA, was the first to place a percutaneous nephrostomy tube. In 1955, while trying to perform a renal arteriogram, Dr. Goodwin placed a needle into the collecting system of a hydronephrotic kidney. He injected radiopaque contrast, thus

S.R. Patel, M.D., F.A.C.S. (✉) • S.Y. Nakada, M.D., F.A.C.S.
Department of Urology, University of Wisconsin School of Medicine and Public Health, Madison, WI 53726, USA
e-mail: sutchin_patel@yahoo.com

S.R. Patel et al. (eds.), *The History of Technologic Advancements in Urology*,
DOI 10.1007/978-3-319-61691-9_12

performing the first antegrade nephrostogram. He then left a tube to drain the kidney, thereby placing the first modern day nephrostomy tube. In his paper he illustrates the optimal site of puncture as "five fingerbreadths lateral to the midline and at a level where a 13th rib would be if it were to exist" [6, 7]. Dr. Goodwin's percutaneous approach would lead to the realization that a percutaneous tract could be used to access the kidney.

By 1976, Fernström and Johansson were the first to describe a technique for extracting renal calculi through a percutaneous nephrostomy under radiological control [8]. In a later paper they would illustrate the use of polythene dilators for tract dilation [9]. Instruments used to extract renal calculi under radiologic control included the Dormia basket, which was placed through a selecter device used to help aim and manipulate the basket once it was in the renal pelvis, as well as the Randall's forceps, used under fluoroscopy for stone extraction.

Endourology and the Dissemination of PCNL

Dr. Arthur Smith, in 1978, would describe the first antegrade stent placement when he introduced a Gibbons stent through a percutaneous nephrostomy in a patient with a reimplanted ureter with a urine leak to allow the urinary leak to seal [10]. He would coin the term "endourology" to describe a closed, controlled manipulation of the genitourinary tract. Once his residents read this title, they, along with some of the radiologists, immediately changed it to the "end of urology" [11]. Dr. Smith's early experiments would usher in the new field of endourology and forever change how we approach the treatment of renal and ureteral calculi (Fig. 12.1). One of his early papers with Drs Zuniga, Clayman and Amplatz describes a series of 63 calculi extracted from 25 patients with a high success rate [12]. The main failures occurred in stones that could not be reached due to narrow infundibula or with stones embedded in swollen mucosa. A firsthand account of the birth of endourology can be found in Chap. 7 of this text.

Dr. Smith's collaboration with Kurt Amplatz, an interventional radiologist and medical inventor, would lead to numerous innovations which would further advance PCNL. Many wires and dilators still bear Dr. Amplatz's name today [11] (Fig. 12.2). A number of adjunctive instruments and various stone baskets which had been developed during the era of blind-stone basketing would find immediate application in the removal of stone fragments during PCNL. In 1926, W.A. Council developed a multiple wire cage for the extraction of calculi [13]. A number of modifications to earlier extraction instruments would be made eventually leading to Dormia's flexible extractor (1958) with a wire cage with significant tensile strength but flexible enough to cause little trauma [14].

When trying to dilate a nephrostomy tract, filiform followers on the end of angiographic catheters were originally used. Dr. Smith wrote, *"However this proved to be difficult to manipulate over a guidewire, so we designed dilators to fit over the*

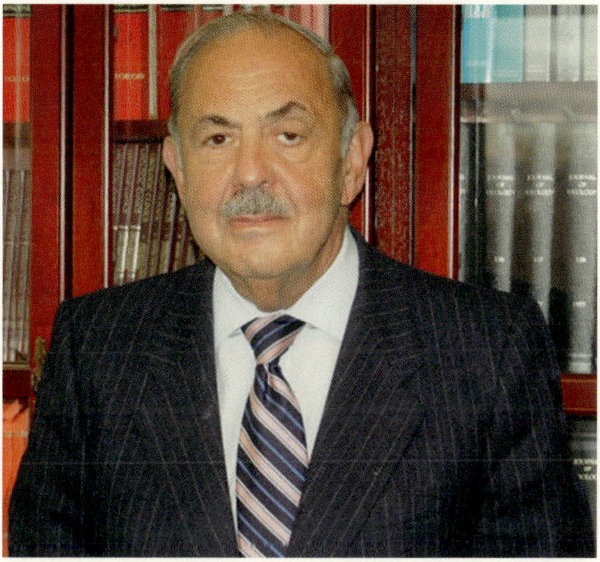

Fig. 12.1 Dr. Arthur Smith, the Father of Endourology

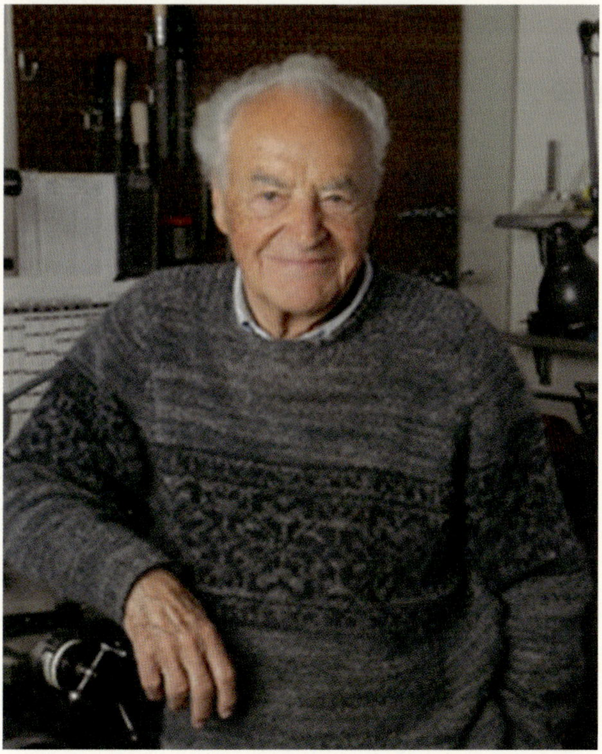

Fig. 12.2 Dr. Kurt Amplatz, radiologist and medical device inventor

angiographic catheter. We then found that we were dilating the ureteropelvic junction and causing extravasations so we placed a metal band at the tip of the dilator to differentiate the parts of the system" [11]. Much of the equipment we use today for PCNL was developed in this era. The fascial and balloon dilators that Dr. Amplatz developed are still used today and the coaxial sequential telescoping metal dilators developed by Dr. Alken were also used during this era.

Dr. Wickham describes the initial procedure as being performed over several days. After placement of a small caliber nephrostomy tube, the tract was serially dilated over several days to 22Fr to 26Fr prior to removal of the nephrostomy tube and insertion of a standard rigid 21Fr cystoscope used to access the caliceal system [12]. As the technique became more successful it was advanced to a one stage procedure.

Despite the development of PCNL, the dissemination of the technique would be largely due to the creation of the Endourological Society as well as the use of courses using the porcine model to teach the technique to practicing urologists. In 1984 at the 2nd World Congress on Percutaneous Renal Surgery in Mainz, West Germany, more than 3000 cases of PCNL were presented with a success rate exceeding 90%. It was during this time period that PCNL was deemed to be a preferable alternative to open surgery [15]. The Endourological Society was formed prior to the 3rd WCE in New York and the society and its members, under the leadership of Dr. Arthur Smith, were largely responsible for many of the innovations that would lead to the evolution of PCNL. Dr. Ralph Clayman was instrumental in helping to disseminate the technique by creating a model with the porcine kidney as a central part of teaching courses in endourology to allow the practicing urologist to adapt the procedure throughout the United States [11].

It was thus in the 1980s that PCNL underwent a rapid evolution as you saw a paradigm shift of stone treatment towards a more minimally invasive approach. The technique of PCNL gained popularity in Europe through the pioneering achievements of Alken and colleagues in Germany, Marberger in Austria and Drs Wickham and Kellet in the United Kingdom. In the United States, the technique gained acceptance following further development by Dr. Segura's group at the Mayo Clinic and with Dr. Smith and Dr. Clayman at the University of Minnesota. Initially PCNL was reserved only for patients who were poor candidates for open surgery but with rapid development in equipment and ancillary tools, PCNL would soon become the treatment of choice for large stones [4, 16].

Optics

The history of rigid optical urologic endoscopes is well documented and is covered in this text in Chap. 3 [16]. Philipp Bozzini developed his lichtleiter, or "light conductor" in 1806 for viewing orifices in the human body [17]. Antonin Desormeaux (who has been called "the father of endoscopy") would develop an open tube endoscope to examine the bladder in 1867, using his device to perform the first endoscopic surgery [16]. Maximilian Nitze and Joseph Leiter, in 1879, are credited with developing the first modern cystoscope [18]. In the late 1950s, Harold Hopkins invented the rod-lens system, which reduced the air space in between lenses with long rods of glass thereby improving the clarity and resolution of the image [19, 20]. The advances in optics led to better cystoscopes which were in turn used as the early nephroscopes. In the 1980s the rigid cystoscope would be replaced by offset nephroscopes with a large straight working channel allowing the use of numerous adjunctive instruments from triradiate graspers to electrohydraulic lithotripters [4].

Advances in illumination would play a significant role in improving the cystoscope as it evolved from indirect illumination to heated platinum wires followed by the incandescent lightbulb [16, 21]. The first fiber-optic endoscope was developed by Basil Hirschowitz in 1957 for use in gastroenterology [22]. Victor Fray Marshall would perform the first antegrade nephroscopy and ureteroscopy using a fiberscope during an open exploration to visualize the pelvis and distal ureter in 1960 [23]. Modern fiberoptics, introduced in the 1960s, coincided with the development of flexible endoscopy/nephroscopy, and aided in less invasive stone clearance. Improvements in imaging culminated with the development of the charged couple device (CCD) by George Smith and Willard Boyle in 1969 for electronic video recording [16].

Lithotripsy

Man has been breaking stone since the beginning of time. With improvements in technology, we have become increasingly efficient and safer in our ability to pulverize larger and harder stones. Thus the modern development of various lithotripsy devices and the introduction of the holmium laser have improved the efficiency of stone fragmentation and clearance [9]. In the early 1970s the ultrasonic lithotrite was developed. Karl Kurth in 1977 provided a means for removing large stones through a nephrostomy tract when he described the use of an ultrasonic lithotrite, previously developed for bladder stones, during PCNL to fragment a staghorn calculus [24]. In 1913 Reinhold Wappler would make the observation that "when a spark is brought into contact with both the hard and soft species of bladder calculi, it causes them to disintegrate" [9]. However it would not be until 1950 that LA Yutkin would obtain a patent for the application of electrohydraulic shock waves. He called his discovery the "electro-hydraulic effect," to describe the submerged powerful high-voltage arc discharge in a liquid [25]. Pneumatic lithotripsy was introduced in the early 1990s with the development of the Swiss Lithoclast (Boston Scientific) [26]. Combined devices utilizing both ultrasonic and pneumatic lithotripsy would be developed to help facilitate stone fragmentation. The CyberWand lithotripter, a dual ultrasonic driller/corer was developed via a joint venture between Jet Propulsion Laboratories and Cybersonics, Inc. It was created in 2000 to acquire samples from planets, asteroids and comets using low power and a low axial load to drill a 0.5 in. hole in hard rocks such as basalt. It relied on a novel mechanism using piezoelectric wafers to produce high frequency vibrations which were converted to a hammering action at low frequency. The drill was used successfully to obtain core samples from locations varying from Antarctica to Mars (via the Curiosity rover). It has since been modified and revised to its current dual ultrasonic probe design to be used for PCNL [27].

Light amplification by stimulated emission of radiation (LASER) was originally described by Albert Einstein in 1917. It was not until 1954 that J.P. Gordon and C.H. Townes at Bell Laboratories generated the first stimulated emissions of microwave radiation (MASER). Medical lasers first appeared in the early 1960s [9]. The Nd:YAG, a solid state laser was developed in 1961. Mulvaney and Beck in 1968 carried out the first attempt at calculus destruction using a ruby laser [28, 29]. The introduction of the Holmium:YAG laser represented a major advance in laser lithotripsy devices as it has been shown to effectively fragment all types of urinary calculi. With the combination of flexible nephroscopy and holmium laser lithotripsy, urologists could access and fragment stones in other calyces independent of the initial renal access.

Radiology

Radiological advances would play a significant role in the development of PCNL [30]. In 2002, Dr. Segura would write:

"...it was the wide spread availablility of fluoroscopy that was the key to the popularity the percutaneous nephrostomy tube placement enjoys today. I believe that had there existed something like an "endourology table" in those days, we and not radiology, would be putting these tubes in today" [31].

In 1895 Wilhelm Röentgen observed that a high electric voltage passing through a covered vacuum tube in a dark room caused a platinocyanide covered screen to emit fluorescent light which he termed "x-rays." Röentgen's work would serve as the foundation for the field of radiology and he would be awarded the first Nobel Prize in Physics in 1902 [32]. The development of fluoroscopes, machines which consisted of a cone with an eyepiece at one end and a screen at the other end that could convert x-rays to light, in 1896, allowed one to observe an object without having to process a film or x-ray plate. The development of the image intensifier tube by J.W. Coltman from Westinghouse in the 1948, allowed an image to be intensified nearly 500 times, thus allowing the image on the screen to be visible during normal lighting [32]. Improvements in fluoroscopy would lead to the development of today's C-arms that would further aid in renal access for PCNL.

Knowledge of renal anatomy is paramount to safe access into the collecting system. In the 1990s, Francisco Sampaio's casts of the renal collecting system and vascular anatomy in human cadavers would further aid urologists by helping establish the paradigm that access to the collecting system should be obtained via direct puncture into the fornix of a calyx and not the infundibulum in order to minimizing the risk of bleeding. It would allow better characterization of the renal collecting system in comparison to the vasculature in a 3-dimensional model [33]. Besides the radiologic innovations leading to safer and more accurate renal access, the development of computed tomography by an engineer, Sir Godfrey Hounsfield (who would win the Nobel Prize in Physiology and Medicine in 1979) and a neuroradiologist, Dr. James Ambrose, would over time lead to improvements in pre-surgical planning as well as evaluation of stone free status post-operatively [34, 35].

Further Advances and Characterization of PCNL

A number of advances in technique and technology would continue to challenge how to better treat renal calculi. Dr. John Wickham reported the first tubeless PCNL in 1984 but it didn't gain acceptance until 1987 and the studies by Bellman [36, 37]. A percutaneous renal access robot (PAKY) was developed by Dr. Louis Kavoussi at Johns Hopkins for robotic needle puncture into the collecting system [38]. Supine PCNL was first described by Gabriel Valdivia in 1987 [39].

The increased clinical experience and utilization of PCNL would lead to larger studies such as the Lower Pole I study, the development of AUA guidelines for Staghorn calculi and the large scale international research projects of CROES (Clinical Research Office of the Endourological Society) on PCNL, thus leading to the characterization of stone free rates and complications for the procedure [40–42]. The use of preoperative stone scoring systems (S.T.O.N.E., Guy's and CROES Nephrolithometry scoring systems) are being used to help predict PCNL outcomes including stone free rates, length of hospital stay and complication rates [43]. As we continue to innovate, we will continue to strive to make PCNL more minimally invasive with higher success rates and a lower risk of complications.

Conclusion

An amalgam of many different technologies contributed to the development of PCNL: from the serendipity and foresight that lead to Dr. Willard Goodwin's first nephrostomy tube, the creation of the field of endourology, the advancements in optics, the development of fluoroscopy for intraoperative navigation and computed tomography for pre-operative planning, and the improvements in devices for lithotripsy (Table 12.1). These innovations culminated in the modern day PCNL and allowed us to fulfill the Hippocratic obligation that "I will not cut for stone."

Table 12.1 Timeline of Innovations in the Development of the Modern PCNL (modified from [30])

Year	Innovation [Reference]
1941	Rupel & Brown 1st Nephroscopy [3]
1950s	Development of Modern Fluoroscopy [32]
1950	LA Yutkin patent for electrohydraulic shock wave application [28]
1955	Willard Goodwin performs 1st Percutaneous Nephrostomy Tube Placement [6]
1960	1st Antegrade Nephroscopy and Ureteroscopy by Victor Fray Marshall [23]
1961	Development of Nd:YAG solid state laser [9]
1968	Mulvaney & Beck use Ruby laser for calculus fragmentation [28]
1969	Smith & Boyle develop the Charged Couple Device (CCD) [16]
1970s	Ultrasonic lithotrite developed [9]
1971	1st Computed Tomography Machine Developed by Hounsfield and Ambrose [32]
1976	Fernstrom & Johansson perform 1st stone extraction through nephrostomy [8]
1977	Karl Kurth uses ultrasonic lithotrite for PCNL of staghorn calculus [24]
1978	Arthur Smith places 1st antegrade ureteral stent [10]
1982	Ralph Clayman creates porcine model for nephroscopy and PCNL to help disseminate the technique [11]
1982	1st World Congress of Endourology, London, England
1984	Founding of the Endourological Society
1984	1st Tubeless PCNL performed by Wickham [36]
1987	1st Supine PCNL performed by Valdivia [39]
1992	Pneumatic lithotripsy developed [26]

References

1. Schultheiss D, Engel RM, Crosby RW, et al. Max Brodel (1870-1941) and medical illustration in urology. J Urol. 2000;164:1137–42.
2. Murphy LJ. The history of urology. Springfield: Charles C Thomas Publisher; 1972. p. 226.
3. Rupel E, Brown R. Nephroscopy with removal of stone following nephrostomy for obstructive calculus anuria. J Urol. 1941;46:177–82.
4. Yuhico MP, Ko R. The current status of percutaneous nephrolithotomy in the management of kidney stones. Minerva Urol Nefrol. 2008;60:159–75.
5. Bloom DA, Morgan RJ, Scardino PL. Thomas Hillier and percutaneous nephrostomy. Urology. 1989;33:347–50.
6. Palapattu GS, Bloom DA, Smith RB, Boxer RJ, Willard E. Goodwin: educator, innovator and pioneer. J Urol. 2004;172:40–4.
7. Goodwin WE, Casey WC, Woolf W. Percutaneous trocar (needle) nephrostomy in hydronephrosis. JAMA. 1955;157:891.
8. Fernstrom I, Johannsson B. Percutaneous pyelolithotomy. A new extraction technique. Scand J Urol Nephrol. 1976;10:257–9.
9. Shah J, Whitfield HN. Urolithiasis through the ages. BJU Int. 2002;89:801–10.
10. Smith AD, Lange PH, Miller RP, Reinke DB. Introduction of the Gibbons ureteral stent facilitated by antecedent percutaneous nephrostomy. J Urol. 1978;120:543–4.
11. Smith AD. A personal perspective on the origins of endourology and the endourological society. J Endourol. 2002;16:705–8.
12. Castaneda-Zuniga WR, Clayman R, Smith A, Rusnak B, Herrera M, Amplatz K. Nephrostolithotomy: percutaneous techniques for urinary calculus removal. J Urol. 2002;167:849–53.

13. Council WA. A new ureteral stone extractor and dilator. JAMA. 1926;86:1907–8.
14. Dormia E. Due nuovi apparecchi per la rimozione dei calculi dall'uretere. Urologia. 1958;25:225–33.
15. Dasgupta P, Rose FK, Wickham JE. Percutaneous renal surgery: a pioneering perspective. J Endourol. 2006;20:167–9.
16. Moran ME. History of ureteroscopy. In: Monga M, editor. Ureteroscopy: indications & technique. New York: Springer Science &Business Media; 2013. p. 3–12.
17. Engel RM. Philipp Bozzini—the father of endoscopy. J Endourol. 2003;17:859–62.
18. Herr HW. Max Nitze, the cystoscope and urology. J Urol. 2006;176:1313–6.
19. Samplaski MK, Jones JS. Two centuries of cystoscopy: the development of imaging, instrumentation and synergistic technologies. BJU Int. 2009;103:154–8.
20. Hopkins HH, Kapany NS. A flexible fiberscope, using static scanning. Nature. 1954;173:39–41.
21. Moran ME. The light bulb, cystoscopy and Thomas Alva Edison. J Endourol. 2010;24:1395–7.
22. Hirschowitz BI. A personal history of the fiberscope. Gastroenterology. 1970;36:864–7.
23. Marshall VF. Fiber optics in urology. J Urol. 1964;91:110–4.
24. Kurth KH, Hohenfellner R, Altwein JE. Ultrasound litholopaxy of a staghorn calculus. J Urol. 1977;117:242–3.
25. Denstedt JD, Clayman RV. Electrohydraulic lithotripsy of renal and ureteral calculi. J Urol. 1990;143:13–7.
26. Denstedt JD, Eberwein PM, Singh RR. The Swiss Lithoclast: a new device for intracorporeal lithotripsy. J Urol. 1992;148:1088–90.
27. Patel R, Faiena I, Elsamra S. From moon rocks to kidney stones: a look at the evolution of the cyberwand. J Urol. 2016;195(4S, supplement):e524.
28. Gross AJ, Herrmann TR. History of lasers. World J Urol. 2007;25:217–20.
29. Mulvaney WP, Beck CW. The laser beam in urology. J Urol. 1968;99:112–5.
30. Patel SR, Nakada SY. The modern history and evolution of percutaneous nephrolithotomy. J Endourol. 2015;29:153–7.
31. Segura JW. Percutaneous trocar (needle) nephrostomy in hydronephrosis. Editorial Comment. J Urol. 2001;167:829.
32. Kotecha R, Toledo-Pereyra LH. Beyond the radiograph: radiological advances in surgery. J Invest Surg. 2011;24:195–8.
33. Sampaio FJ, Zanier JF, Aragao AH, Favorito LA. Intrarenal access: 3-dimensional anatomical study. J Urol. 1992;148:1769–73.
34. Thiruchelvan N, Mostafid H, Ubhayakar G. Planning percutaneous nephrolithotomy usirn multidetector computed tomography urography, multiplanar reconstruction and three-dimensional reformatting. BJU Int. 2005;95:1280–4.
35. Park J, Hong B, Park T, Park HK. Effectiveness of noncontrast computed tomography in evaluation of residual stones after percutaneous nephrolithotomy. J Endourol. 2007;21:684–7.
36. Wickham JE, Miller RA, Kellet MJ, et al. Percutaneous nephrolithotomy: one stage or two? Br J Urol. 1984;56:582–5.
37. Bellman GC, Davidoff R. Candela et al. Tubeless percutaneous renal surgery. J Urol. 1997;157:1578–82.
38. Caddeddu JA, Stoianovici D, Kavoussi LR. Robotic surgery in urology. Urol Clin North Am. 1998;25:75–85.
39. Valdivia-Uria JG, Lanchares E, Villarroya S, Taberner J, Abril G, Aranda JM. Nefrolitectomia percutanea: Tecnica simplificada (nota previa). [Percutaneous nephrolithotomy: simplified technique (preliminary report)]. Arch Esp Urol. 1987;40:177–80.
40. Albala DM, Assimos DG, clayman RV, Denstedt JD, Grasso M, Gutierrez-Aceves J, Kahn RI, Leveillee RJ, Lingeman JE, Macaluso JN Jr, Munch LC, Nakada SY, Newman RC, Pearle MS, Preminger GM, Teichman J, Woods JR. Lower Pole I: a prospective randomized trial of extracorporeal shock wave lithotripsy and percutaneous nephrostolithotomy for lower pole nephrolithiasis-initial results. J Urol. 2001;166:2072–80.

41. Preminger GM, Assimos DG, Lingeman JE, Nakada SY, Pearle MS, Wolf JS Jr., AUA Nephrolithiasis Guideline Panel. Chapter 1: AUA guideline on management of staghorn calculi: diagnosis and treatment recommendations. J Urol. 2005;173:1991–2000.
42. Tefeki A, van Rees Vellinga S, de la Rosetter J. The CROES percutaneous nephrolithotomy global study: final report. J Endourol. 2012;26:1536–9.
43. Labadie K, Okhunov Z, Akhavein A, Moreira DM, Moreno-Palacios J, Del Junco M, Okeke Z, Bird V, Smith AD, Landman J. Evaluation and comparison of urolithiasis scoring systems used in percutaneous kidney stone surgery. J Urol. 2015;193:154–9.

Chapter 13
A Brief History of Radiological Imaging and Its Application in Urology

Lori Mankowski Gettle and Perry J. Pickhardt

Introduction

Imaging of the genitourinary system in its infancy was largely nonspecific and often required surgery to verify the findings. Soon after X-rays were discovered by Wilhelm Roentgen in 1895, abdominal plain films were used to evaluate the kidneys, ureters and bladder, hence the acronym KUB. The radiograph was excellent at visualizing large uroliths, but overlying bowel often obscured soft tissue detail. Eventually, contrast was used to further delineate structures and pathology. Initial contrast materials were instilled in a retrograde fashion and included metal stylets, bismuth or silver compounds and sodium iodide [1]. These methods elucidated information about the ureters and collecting system but still provided little detail about the renal parenchyma. In the 1920's, uroradiology progressed to excretory urography where both anatomic and physiologic information was revealed [1]. Contrast media and cross sectional imaging techniques were refined and genitourinary imaging became more specific and integral in planning surgery and avoiding unnecessary interventions.

Before these advanced techniques, invasive procedures were often required to confirm the suspected diagnosis, as imaging findings often relied on secondary signs. Now there is a wide selection of imaging modalities and protocols that are optimized for detection of specific urologic conditions, ranging from diagnosing adrenal myelolipomas to staging testicular cancer. Imaging techniques have progressed to include both anatomic and functional imaging, such as positron emission tomography-computed tomography (PET-CT) as well as imaging biomarkers, which can predict a patient's response to treatment. Uroradiology crosses all imaging modalities including radiography, ultrasound, computed tomography (CT),

L.M. Gettle, M.D., M.B.A. • P.J. Pickhardt, M.D. (✉)
Abdominal Imaging and Intervention Section, University of Wisconsin School of Medicine and Public Health, Madison, WI 53726, USA
e-mail: ppickhardt2@uwhealth.org

S.R. Patel et al. (eds.), *The History of Technologic Advancements in Urology*,
DOI 10.1007/978-3-319-61691-9_13

magnetic resonance imaging (MRI) and nuclear medicine. Given the broad range of conditions and modalities, this chapter will focus on the brief history of uroradiology with regards to three common urologic conditions: renal cell carcinoma (RCC), urolithiasis, and urothelial carcinoma.

History of Renal Cell Carcinoma Imaging

Abdominal radiographs are limited for detection and diagnosis of renal masses. While findings of renal cell carcinoma could be direct such as enlargement of the renal shadow or calcifications within the mass, these findings were nonspecific and often obscured by normal anatomy. Radiographs more easily detected secondary imaging findings of renal cell carcinoma such as metastatic lesions involving the bones or lung masses (Fig. 13.1). Other indirect signs of renal masses could be seen when enteric contrast was given and mass effect of the enlarged kidney was noted displacing the adjacent colon or stomach. The differential diagnosis remained broad with these indirect signs, as any retroperitoneal mass could cause the same pattern of organ displacement and metastatic disease. Injecting oxygen or carbon dioxide into the perinephric fat could be used in conjunction with x-ray, termed pneumoradiography, to evaluate the renal contour. However this procedure was invasive and often low yield.

Retrograde pyelography was first described by Friedrich Voelcker and Alexander Von Lichtenberg in 1906 using a silver colloid solution, collargol, as contrast. In 1925, William Braasch, a urologist, and Russell Carman, a radiologist, described findings of renal tumors in retrograde pyelography. The secondary signs of renal masses included elongation, shortening, obliteration or distortion of the calyces, renal pelvis, or ureteropelvic junction [2]. They described features that could narrow the differential between inflammatory and neoplastic processes, but often the final diagnosis relied on pathology after surgical resection. Retrograde pyelography was invasive with the risk of infection and perforation by instrumentation. There was additional risk of local toxicity from the heavy metal contrast agents available at the time.

Earl Osborne described the potential for excretory urography after intravenous injection of sodium iodide for the treatment of syphilis in 1923. Opacification of the renal parenchyma as well as the collecting system, ureter, and bladder was seen in some patients [3] (Fig. 13.2). This was forward progress on direct visualization

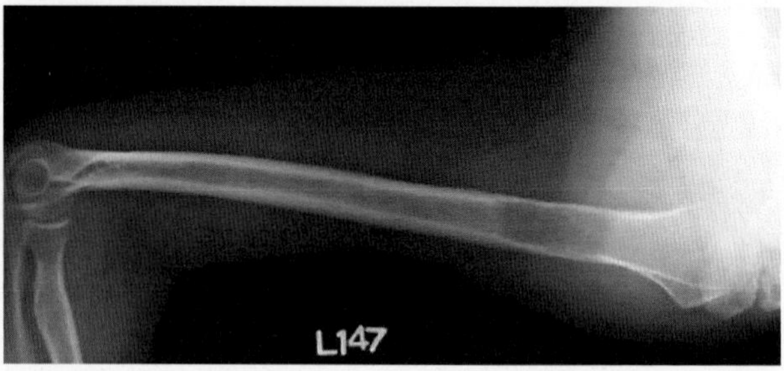

Fig. 13.1 Left humerus radiograph demonstrates a lytic osseous lesion with expansion consistent with a metastatic renal cell carcinoma lesion

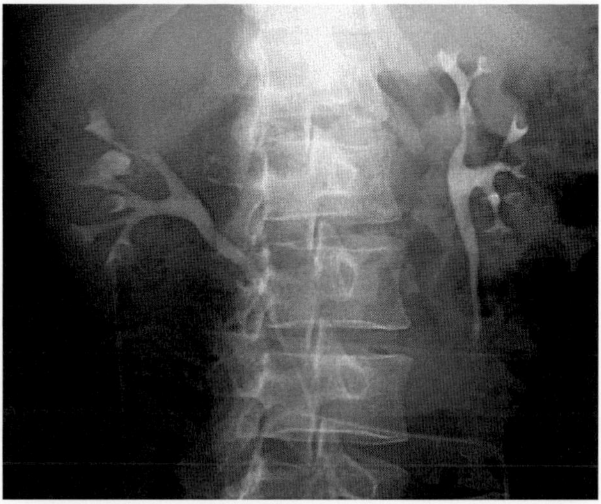

Fig. 13.2 Intravenous urography demonstrates a right upper pole renal cell carcinoma with narrowing of the upper pole major calyx from external compression by the renal mass

of the renal parenchyma, but the contrast agents remained suboptimal and had multiple side effects limiting their use. Experimentation with multiple compounds to find a practical intravenous urographic contrast agent lead Moses Swick to discover Uroselectan in 1929 [1]. Uroselectan had fewer side effects than the previous iodine based contrast agents, was water soluble, and almost entirely excreted in the urine. Intravenous urography eliminated the need for invasive diagnostic instrumentation of the bladder and ureters. The method also provided information regarding renal function, since Uroselectan required functioning nephrons for excretion.

For the next several decades, renal excreted contrast agents were improved. During this period, intravenous excretory urography (also commonly referred to as intravenous pyelography, or IVP) and retrograde pyelography were the mainstays of renal imaging, but serendipitous discovery that injection of these iodinated contrast agents directly into the aorta was generally tolerated opened up the evaluation of kidneys by angiography. In 1957, Arthur Evans reported the angiographic findings of renal cell carcinoma. He describes the procedure using up to an 18-gauge needle to directly puncture the aorta above the celiac axis and inject the same contrast agent used for intravenous urography at that time [4]. With careful technique, angiography was able to differentiate between avascular cysts and vascular masses. The pattern of vasculature seen in renal cell carcinoma was enlarged, disorganized vessels with areas of pooling, but the interpretation could be complicated by necrosis (Fig. 13.3). In his series of 236 cases, Evans reported an accuracy of 95% in detecting malignant renal masses [4]. With the development of the Seldinger technique in 1953, selective angiography became more widely accepted [5]. It was during this period that diagnostic imaging of renal disease moved from the realm of the urologist to the radiologist [1].

Even with the advances in these techniques, aspiration was frequently required to definitively diagnose a cyst versus a solid neoplasm. Cross-sectional imaging removed the dependence on the invasive cyst puncture technique. In 1968, a group from Albert Einstein Medical Center in Philadelphia described the use of amplitude modulation sonography to confidently differentiate between solid and cystic renal masses [6]. The advent of computed tomography (CT) by Godfrey Hounsfield in 1972 rapidly changed the field of uroradiology as CT became the imaging modality of choice for the detection and characterization of renal masses. There was less user variability and multiple post-contrast phases of renal enhancement could be acquired

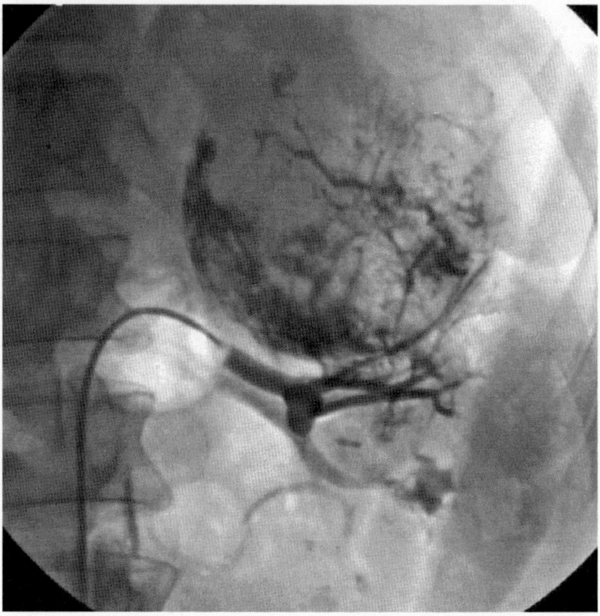

Fig. 13.3 Selective renal artery angiogram using the seldinger technique demonstrates a large left upper pole renal cell carcinoma. There is deformation of the upper pole renal contour along with abnormally enlarged distal vessels and pooling of contrast

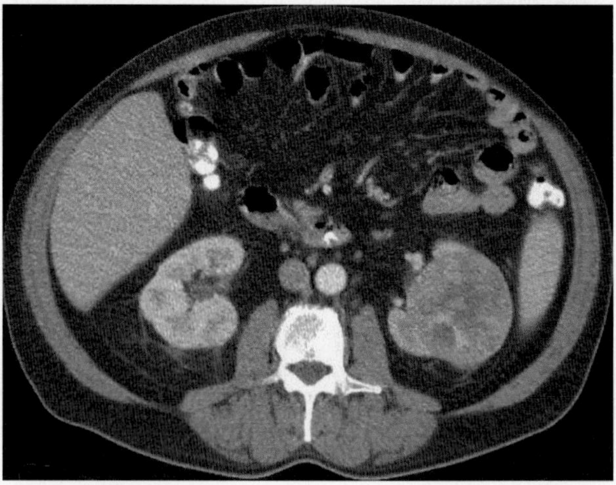

Fig. 13.4 Contrast-enhanced CT demonstrates a heterogenous left interpolar renal cell carcinoma

to more accurately characterize renal masses (Fig. 13.4). In 1986, Morton Bosniak published the well-known renal cyst classification that is still in use today using both CT and US [7] (Figs. 13.5 and 13.6). Now, the Bosniak cyst classification has been optimized for CT with the accumulation of data since that time [8].

Magnetic resonance imaging (MRI) took longer to gain prominence in the field of uroradiology. First developed in the late 1970's, due to its expense and the length of time for an examination, it did not become readily available for imaging of renal masses until almost a decade later [9]. MRI demonstrated usefulness in the evaluation of renal vein and inferior vena cava involvement by renal cell carcinoma [10].

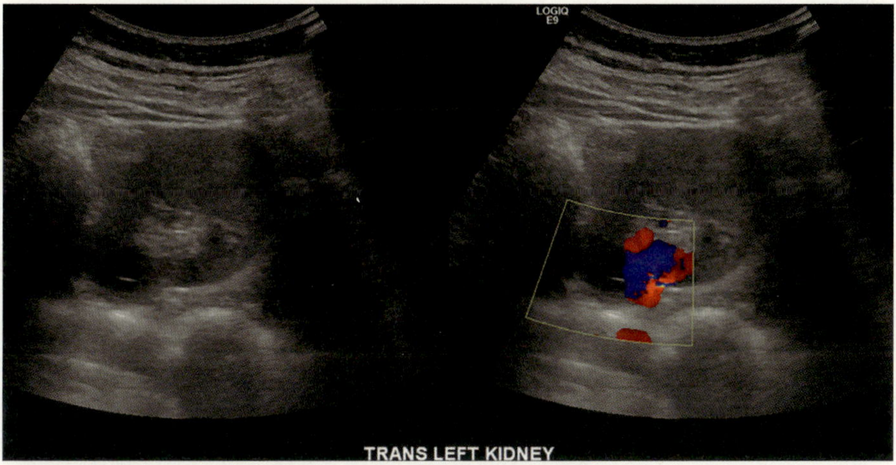

Fig. 13.5 Ultrasound demonstrates a left upper pole Bosniak 2 renal cyst

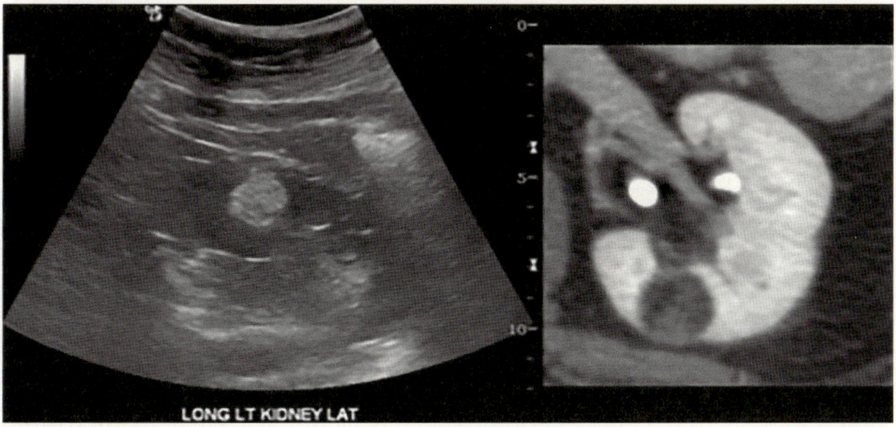

Fig. 13.6 Ultrasound demonstrates a hyperechoic solid left interpolar renal lesion. Contrast-enhanced CT confirms intralesional fat consistent with an angiomyolipoma

MRI is typically used as complementary to CT for renal cell carcinoma diagnosis but is preferred for establishing vascular involvement, and is also indicated if the patient has contraindications for iodinated contrast (Fig. 13.7).

The future of renal cell carcinoma imaging likely includes the addition of contrast enhanced ultrasound (CEUS) in its armamentarium (Fig. 13.8). In the spring of 2016, the United States Food and Drug Administration (FDA) approved an ultrasound contrast agent for the evaluation of liver masses. With the recent FDA approval, the United States will continue to evaluate the diagnosis and characterization of renal lesions using CEUS. The lack of ionizing radiation and the ability to monitor enhancement in real-time, make CEUS an attractive alternative to explore. This technique may also prove useful to guide percutaneous biopsy of renal masses, which is now being performed more commonly.

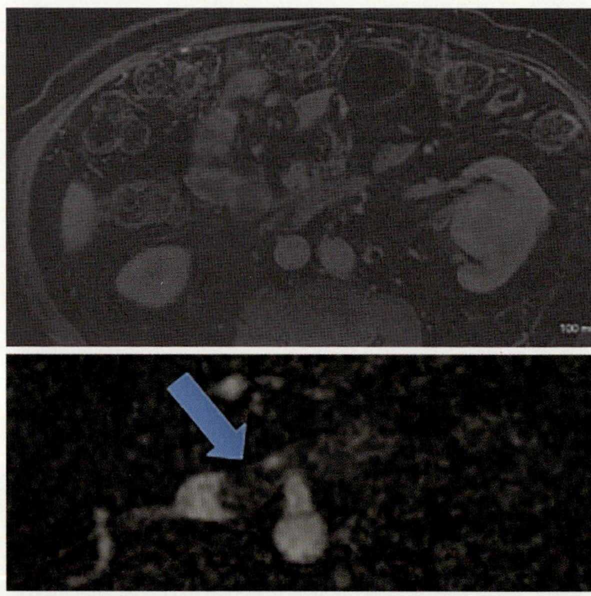

Fig. 13.7 Contrast-enhanced MRI demonstrates heterogenously enhancing left renal cell carcinoma with expansion of the left renal vein and inferior vena cava with tumor thrombus (arrow)

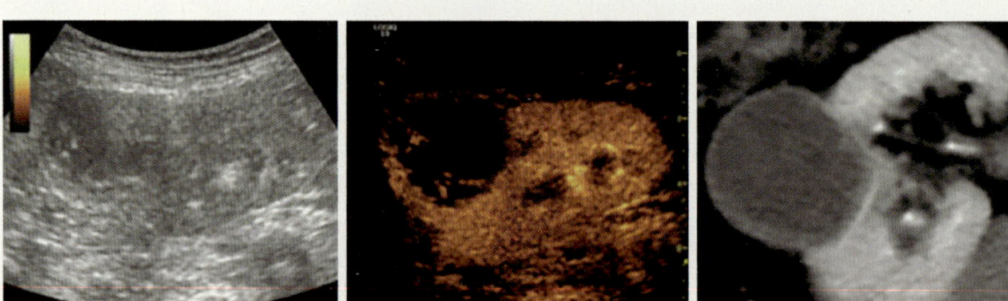

Fig. 13.8 Contrast-enhanced ultrasound (middle image) demonstrates that the thin septations seen on CT are enhancing. This was a clear cell renal cell carcinoma on biopsy

History of Urolithiasis Imaging

Once Wilhelm Roentgen discovered x-rays in 1895, the detection of urolithiasis by radiograph was reported within the following year [1]. This remained the simplest modality for detection of radiopaque stones until CT became readily available. Abdominal radiographs detected 90–95% of stones [11]. Intravenous urography was often used to verify that the stone was within a ureter or causing obstruction. However, if the stone was not radiopaque, the differential remained broad and included hemorrhage and urothelial mass. Ultrasound was highly sensitive for detecting obstruction (98–100%), but much less sensitive for the detecting the cause of the obstructing, usually a ureteral calculus (Figs. 13.9 and 13.10). Faye Laing compared ultrasound and excretory urography in the evaluation of acute flank pain in an emergency department setting in 1985. Gray scale sonography only was performed as opposed to a combination of gray scale and color Doppler ultrasound. Compared to IV urography, only 14% of the obstructing calculi were identified [12].

In 1977, during the early development of CT, stones within renal parenchyma and calyces were described [13]. As CT was more available, the usefulness in discriminating between stones and other filling defects was explored. Michael Federle reported nine cases of urinary calculi seen on CT, with seven of them being occult on radiography [14]. CT offers the ability to rapidly and accurately determine the location of the stone, the degree of obstruction, and differentiate the filling defect from clot or mass (Fig. 13.11). An additional advantage is the ability to detect other causes of flank pain or hematuria. Non-contrast CT remains the imaging study of choice for suspicion of urolithiasis according the most recent American College of Radiology Appropriateness Criteria from 2015 [15].

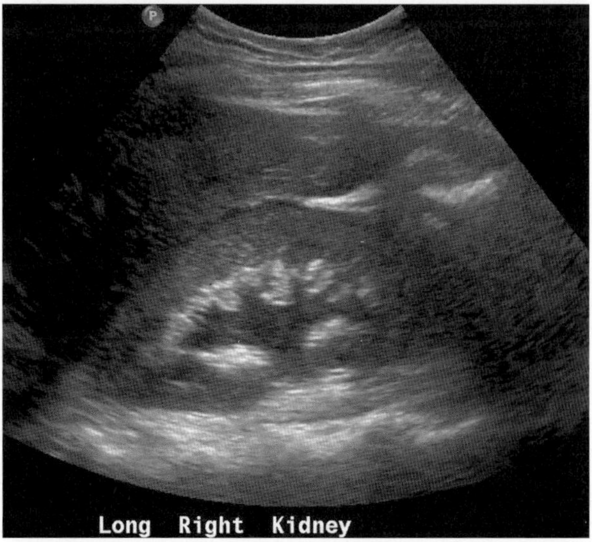

Fig. 13.9 US demonstrates upstream mild right hydronephrosis as a result of obstructing UVJ stone

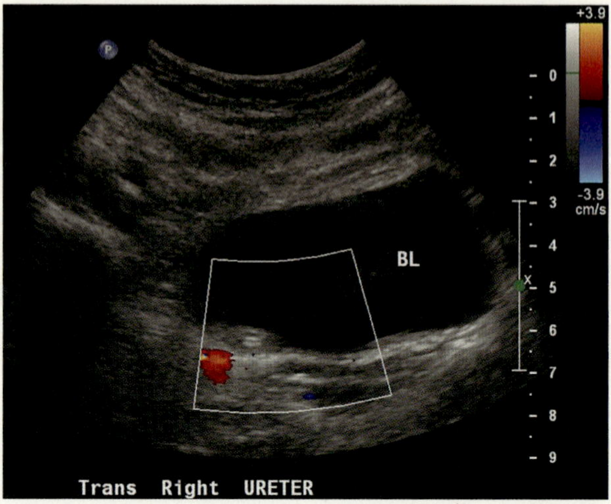

Fig. 13.10 Color Doppler US of the right distal ureter demonstrates an echogenic stone at the ureterovesicle junction

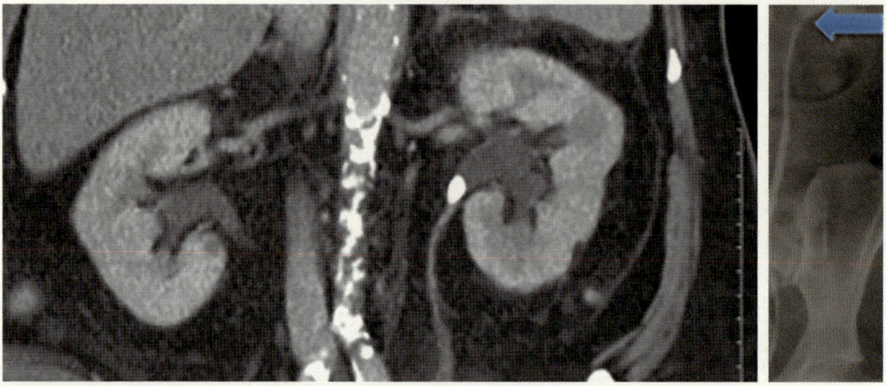

Fig. 13.11 CT demonstrates an obstructing left ureteropelvic junction stone with mild hydronephrosis. Retrograde pyelogram confirms the location of the stone (arrow) before placement of a nephroureteral stent

Dual-energy CT (DECT) improves characterization of urolithiasis composition, which can guide treatment. A study evaluating 213 calculi was 98% sensitive and specific for differentiating uric acid containing stones from non-uric acid containing stones. Dual energy sources did not increase the effective radiation dose compared to an unenhanced CT [16]. As the use of medical imaging has increased, the attention to radiation dose has also gained attention. As urolithiasis is often a recurrent disease, the use of ultrasound in the detection of stone disease has been revitalized. Research was recently published in the New England Journal of Medicine looking at 2759 patients who presented to the emergency department with suspicion of urolithiasis. The conclusion was that the patients imaged with ultrasound as the initial triage received a lower radiation dose while having no difference in overall outcome. The final recommendation by these authors being that ultrasound should be considered as an initial screening modality in the setting of suspected renal calculi [17].

History of Urothelial Carcinoma Imaging

Imaging findings of urothelial carcinoma, previously called transitional cell carcinoma, overlap with renal cell carcinoma and urolithiasis. Urothelial carcinoma may present as an infiltrative renal mass or as a filling defect within the collecting system, ureter, or bladder. Abdominal radiographs have no role in the diagnosis of urothelial cancer. Initially, retrograde pyelography was used for the initial detection of urothelial lesions. A lesion that changed position would suggest a mobile filling defect such as blood clot or radiolucent stone over neoplasm, and dilated, obstructed or eroded calyces could be noted. Limited ability to detect possible parenchymal invasion made retrograde pyelography suboptimal (Fig. 13.12). Intravenous excretory urography was used for detection of urothelial carcinoma for decades, but the radiographic findings were variable and nonspecific, ranging from discrete filling defects to hydronephrosis with an enlarged kidney [18]. The differential diagnosis

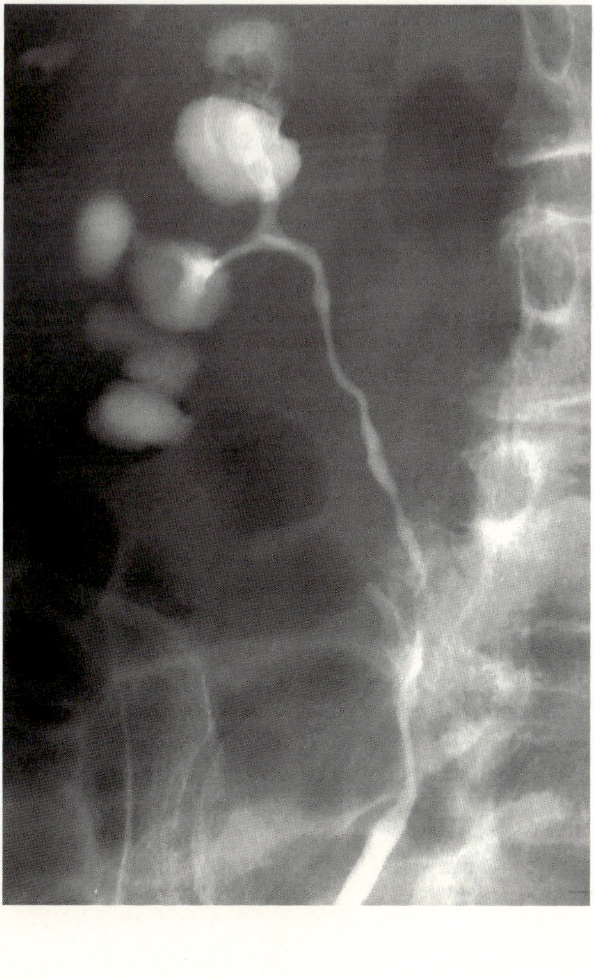

Fig. 13.12 Retrograde pyelography demonstrates irregular long-segment narrowing of the renal pelvis and proximal ureter from an infiltraing urothelial carcinoma. Note marked calieactasis

for these imaging features was broad and included nonradiopaque stones, renal cell carcinoma, and other inflammatory and benign renal lesions.

Sonography was first reported for detection of urothelial carcinoma in 1979, but the imaging appearance overlapped with blood clots [19]. The characteristics on sonography were not sufficiently different from other masses or inflammatory diseases to make a confident diagnosis [18] (Fig. 13.13). CT with and without contrast was evaluated in 13 patients with nonradiopaque collecting system filling defects in 1981, but the results suggested limited utility with the exception of tumor staging [20]. Continued improvement in computed tomography technique led to this modality ultimately surpassing excretory urography as the choice imaging for urothelial carcinoma (Fig. 13.14). In the mid-2000's, excretory urography was compared with CT urography in 128 patients with hematuria who were high risk for urothelial cancer. The overall accuracy for detecting lesions was 94% for

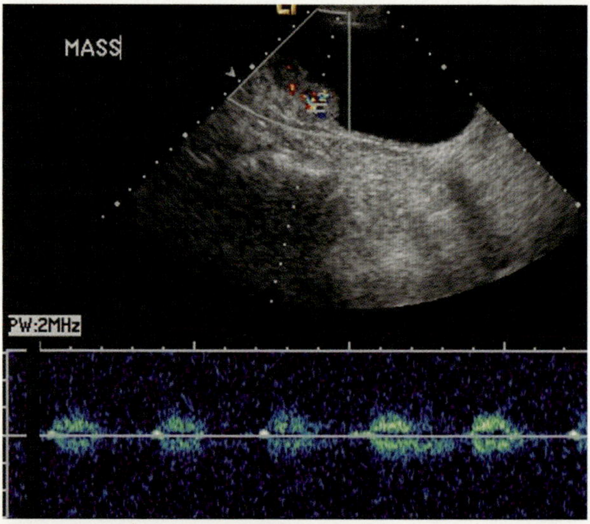

Fig. 13.13 Ultrasound demonstrates a urothelial carcinoma mass near the right ureteral orifice with internal blood flow

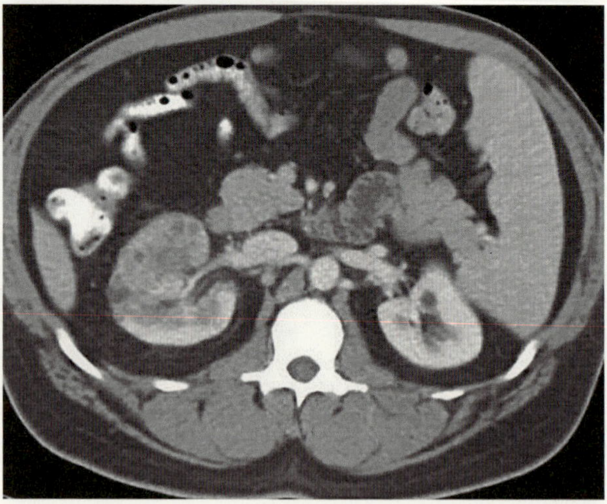

Fig. 13.14 Contrast-enhanced CT demonstrates an infiltrative right urothelial cell carcinoma

CT urography and 81% for excretory urography [21]. The added benefit was that staging could be done at the same time with CT urography (Figs. 13.15 and 13.16).

The current state of practice for suspected urothelial cancer is for CT urography or MR urography to be performed to evaluate the upper urinary tract. As noted before, MR is a longer examination, more expensive, and limited in availability, but lacks ionization radiation and can be used in patients with a contraindication to iodinated contrast. MR urography often fails to detect small lesions secondary to inferior spatial resolution compared to CT [22]. The current recommendation by the American College of Radiology is for CT urography to be performed in the setting of hematuria from presumed urothelial carcinoma [23].

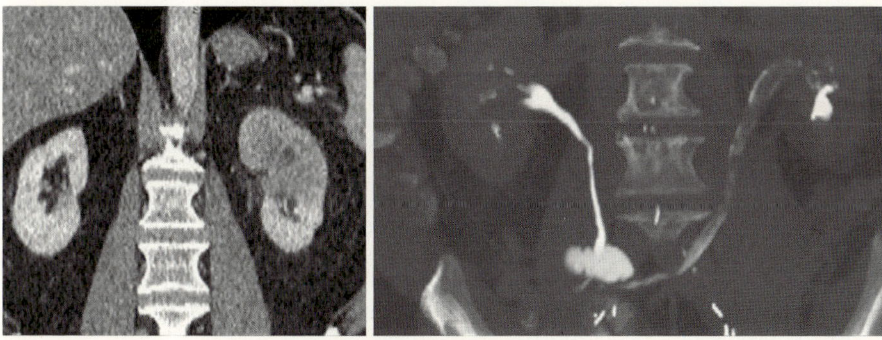

Fig. 13.15 CT urography demonstrating an infiltrative left upper pole urothelial cell carcinoma with multiple lesions in the left ureter after cystectomy

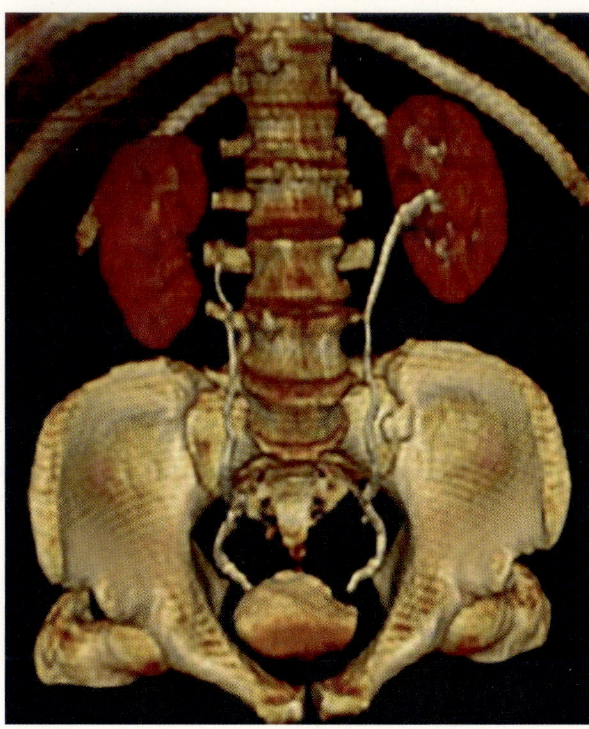

Fig. 13.16 CT urography with 3D reconstructions demonstrates a distal urothelial carcinoma at the left ureterovesicle junction with a mass-like filling defect

Conclusion

Since the discovery of the X-ray in the late Nineteenth century, remarkable advancing in medical imaging have been witnessed over the ensuing 120-plus years. Beyond conventional radiography, the introduction of direct and intravenous contrast techniques allowed for more direct visualization of the kidneys and urinary collecting system. The further development of cross-sectional imaging techniques such as ultrasound, CT, and MR vastly improved the diagnostic capabilities of non-invasive imaging for urologic pathology.

References

1. Elkin M. Stages in the growth of uroradiology. Radiology. 1990;175:297–306.
2. Braasch W, Carman R. The pyelographic and roentgenologic diagnosis of renal tumors. Radiology. 1925;4(6):445–52.
3. Osborne ED, Sutherland CG, Scholl AJ, Rowntree LG. Roentgenography of the urinary tract during excretion of sodium iodide. JAMA. 1923;80(6):368–73.
4. Evans A. Renal cancer: translumbar arteriography for its recognition. Radiology. 1957;69:657–62.
5. Seldinger S. Catheter replacement of the needle in percutaneous arteriography: a new technique. Acta Radiol. 1953;39:368–76.
6. Goldberg BB, Ostrum BJ, Isard JH. Nephrosonography: ultrasound differentiation of renal masses. Radiology. 1968;90:1113–8.
7. Bosniak MA. The current radiological approach to renal cysts. Radiology. 1986;158:1–10.
8. Bosniak MA. The Bosniak renal cyst classification: 25 years later. Radiology. 2012;262(3):781–5.
9. Goldman SM, Sandler CM. Genitourinary imaging: the past 40 years. Radiology. 2000;215:313–24.
10. Choyke PL, Pollack HM. The role of MRI in diseases of the kidney. Radiol Clin North Am. 1988;26(3):617–31.
11. Thornbury JR, Parker TW. Ureteral calculi. Semin Roentgenol. 1982;17:133–9.
12. Laing FC, Jeffrey RB, Wig VW. Ultrasound versus excretory urography in evaluating acute flank pain. Radiology. 1985;154:613–6.
13. Sagel SS, Stanley RJ, Levitt RG, Geisse G. Computed tomography of the kidney. Radiology. 1977;124:359–70.
14. Federle MP, McAninch JW, Kaiser JA, Goodman PC, Roberts J, Mall JC. Computed tomography of renal calculi. Am J Roentgenol. 1981;136:255–8.
15. Moreno CC, Beland MD, Goldfarb S, Harvin HJ, Heilbrun ME, Heller MT, Nikolaidis Preminger GM, Purysko AS, Raman SS, Taffel MT, Vikram R, Want ZJ, Weinfeld RM, Yoo DC, Remer EM, Lockhart ME. Acute Onset Flank Pain – Suspicion of Stone Disease. Available at https://acsearch.acr.org/docs/69362/Narrative/. Accessed 12 Dec 2016.
16. Spek A, Strittmatter F, Graser A, Kufer P, Stief C, Staehler M. Dual energy can accurately differentiate uric acid-containing calculi from calcium stones. World J Urol. 2016;34:1297–302.
17. Smith-Bindman R, Aubin C, Bailitz RN, Bengiamin CA, et al. Ultrasonography versus computed tomography for suspected nephrolithiasis. N Engl J Med. 2014;371:1100–10.
18. Leder RA, Dunnick NR. Transitional cell carcinoma of the pelvicalices and ureter. Am J Roentgenol. 1990;155:713–22.

19. Arger PH, Mulhern CB, Pollack HM, Banner MP, Wein AJ. Ultrasonic evaluation of renal transitional cell carcinoma: preliminary report. Am J Roentgenol. 1979;132:407–11.
20. Pollack HM, Arger PH, Banner MP, Mulhern CB, Coleman BG. Computed tomography of renal pelvic filling defects. Radiology. 1981;138:645–51.
21. Jinzaki M, Matsumoto K, Kikuchi E, Sato K, Horiguchi Y, Nishiwaki Y, Silverman SG. Comparison of CT urography and excretory urography in the detection and localization of urothelial carcinoma of the upper urinary tract. Am J Roentgenol. 2011;196:1102–9.
22. Silverman SG, Leyendecker JR, Amis ES. What is the current role of CT urography and MR urography in the evaluation of the urinary tract. Radiology. 2009;250:309–23.
23. Shen L, Raman SS, Beland MD, et al. Hematuria. Available at https://acsearch.acr.org/docs/69490/Narrative. Accessed 12 Dec 2016.

Chapter 14
Prostate Cancer and Radiation Therapy: A History

Michael E. Moran

Prostate Cancer in History

"*We found the patient complaining of excruciating pains in various parts of the body, which could be compared to nothing except the pains under which persons afflicted with carcinoma occasionally labour. He could not void no urine without the assistance of a catheter. The prostate gland, examined by the rectum was found to be much enlarged and of a stony hardness. I continued to visit him in consultation for nearly a year, at the end of which time he suddenly lost the use of the muscles of his lower limbs and died a fortnight afterwards.*" Sir Benjamin Brodie, 1832 [1].

Prostate cancer is an ancient disease that also affects other species but has a fascinating history which certainly needs a historical introduction prior to proceeding with a history of radiation therapies since they are related by technology [2]. The history of the treatment of prostate cancer is quite complex, given the historical comments of none other than Willet Whitmore, considered by many to be the father of urologic oncology—"*For a patient with prostate cancer, if treatment for cure is necessary, is it possible? If possible is it necessary?*" [3]. Elliot Smith and Warren Dawson noticed among the cemetery burial of the Giza Pyramids (5th Dynasty) that a large osteosarcoma of the femur and two cases of sarcoma of the head of the humerus were described. In 2011 a male mummy was discovered that is estimated to be approximately 2250 years old with metastatic prostate cancer [4]. At about this same time, another report has documented that a Scythian King (Ancient steppes of Russia) who was 2700 BCE also suffered and died of metastatic prostate cancer (Fig. 14.1a). It would be interesting to quote George Johnson on these discoveries. "*In 2001 archeologists excavated a 2700-year-old burial mound in the Russian*

M.E. Moran, M.D.
American Urological Association, William P. Didusch Center for Urologic History, Carolina Urology Associates, Southwest Urology, 1015 Delaware Ave, Suite B, McComb, MS 39648, USA
e-mail: memoran2@juno.com

S.R. Patel et al. (eds.), *The History of Technologic Advancements in Urology*,
DOI 10.1007/978-3-319-61691-9_14

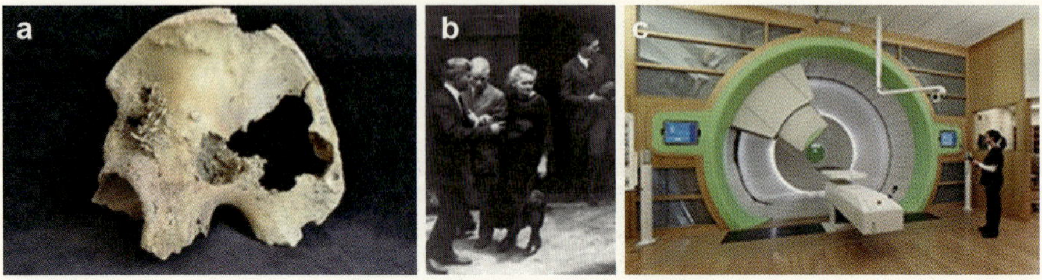

Fig. 14.1 (**a**) Ancient Scythian with metastatic prostate cancer to bone. (**b**) Marie Curie visiting New York City. (**c**) The Proton Accelerator at M.D. Anderson's Cancer Center

republic of Tuva, where nomadic horsemen called the Scythians once thundered across the Eurasian steppes, their leaders dressed in gold. Digging down through two wooden ceilings, the scientist came upon a subterranean chamber. Its floor, covered with a black felt blanket, cushioned two skeletons. Crouched together like lovers, both man and woman wore what remained of their royal vestments. Around the man's neck was a heavy band of twisted gold decorated with a frieze of panthers, ibex, camels, and other beasts. Near his head lay pieces of a headdress: four gold horses and a deer. Golden panthers, more than 2500 of them, bedecked his cape. His riches couldn't save him. When he died—he appeared to have been in his forties—his skeleton was infested with tumors. A pathological analysis, including a close look with a scanning electron microscope, concluded that the nature of the lesions and the pattern of their spread were characteristic of metastatic prostate cancer. Biochemical tests revealed high levels of prostate-specific antigen, or PSA" [5].

Prostate cancer is widely believed to have occurred in ancient humans, though other animals such as rodents and canines also have been discovered to develop prostate cancer [6]. Giovanni Battista Morgagni described both the benign enlargement of the prostate as well as a case he assumes is cancer as well. Matthew Baillie (1761–1823) also had such a case in his classic work, *The Morbid Anatomy of Some of the Most Important Parts of the Human Body* [7]. He even states that "*the most common disease of the prostate gland is scirrhus.*" In Benjamin Brodie's textbook of genitourinary diseases he states, "*I have observed that malignant diseases of the prostate are of rare occurrence*" [2]. It is in his textbook that he described the 60 year old male who would die of metastatic disease with spinal cord compression. He tried to get an autopsy on this gentleman but was unfortunately denied. Now we come to the work of Walter Hayle Walshe (1812–1892), an Irish physician who trained in Edinburgh. He had travelled to Paris and worked with Pierre Charles Alaxandre Louis and Francois L.I. Valleix and became interested in the microscopic investigation of diseased tissues. In 1836 he began to practice in London and was appointed as Professor of Anatomy at the University College of London. He published his most famous work *The Nature and Treatment of Cancer* in 1846 which contained all of the known data about cancer at that time, plus much of his own pathologic findings [8]. The book was organized in two parts—Part One was on the general principles of cancer and had eight chapters; Part Two was on cancers of particular parts and had twelve chapters. It is Chapter V of this section that was titled Cancer of the Urinary Organs that we will pay specific attention to his discussion on prostate cancer, where he essentially had collected the world's data on this malignancy. He began by mentioning that M. Tanchou's tabulated autopsy information on cancer deaths of 8289 fatal cases, only five were from the prostate [8]. He related both of Brodie's cases and noted further cases from M. Mercier the size of an ostrich's egg and two cases from M. Civiale. He noted, "*that cancer affects the prostate as a distinct tumor, or infiltrates the organ more or less extensively. The size of the mass thus produced may, as the descriptions show, be very considerable. All three lobes of the gland appear prone to suffer from the disease; the middle is almost always mentioned as having been specially implicated*" [8]. He then notes the progressive, lethal nature of the disease. "*In all cases on record, except that of Mr. Stafford, cancer of the prostate has proved a disease of advanced life...The duration of life after the outbreak of symptoms in these cases has varied between a few months and several years*" [8]. He went on to recount how the diagnosis is confirmed. "*Examination with the catheter and the finger per rectum, coupled with consideration of symptoms, will commonly render the existence of prostatic tumor matter to certainty*" [8]. Finally he espoused the known therapeutic options. "*The treatment must be purely palliative; and the best palliation is afforded by the carefully managed use of the catheter; especially the elastic-gum kind. In cases of total retention, puncture of the bladder might become necessary; the operation above the pubes is probably the one to be preferred*" [8].

In 1851, John Adams, a surgeon and lecturer on Anatomy at the London Hospital, published his *The Anatomy and Diseases of the Prostate Gland* [9]. He mentions George Langstaff's case of sarcoma of the prostate. He discusses the physical examination as follows, "*A schirrhous prostate conveys to the finger, passed per anum, a sense of gristly hardness, and is usually irregularly nodulated, one lobe being especially affected*" [9]. He also described the sarcoma of the prostate in two cases of children, each about the age of three who rapidly died of their disease. In 1853, Adams also reported on a case of a man age 59 that died of prostate cancer with some histological slides from his prostate and lymph node metastases. In 1860, Henry Thompson wrote his Jacksonian Prize winning treatise, *The Diseases of the Prostate, Their Pathology and Treatment* [10]. To the world's literature, Thompson would add 22 cases, 16 adults and 6 children, tabulating them nicely (Fig. 14.2a). He had very little more to offer, he also recommended the use of opioids when the pain became intolerable and discussed a bit more about the management of hematuria, which he believed was more common than the previous authors. Harrison tried surgery for prostate cancer in 1885 and stated, "*Progressive cancer of the prostate resembling some features of hypertrophy is far more common than is generally believed to be the case*" [11]. Billroth attempted surgical interventions in 1867, Fuller in 1898, Young in 1905. The progressively radical nature of the surgeries and the ultimate demise of the patients resulted in attempts to refine the indications and develop newer strategies for treatment. Harrison lamented, "*...neither castration nor vasectomy is at all likely to be of any avail*"

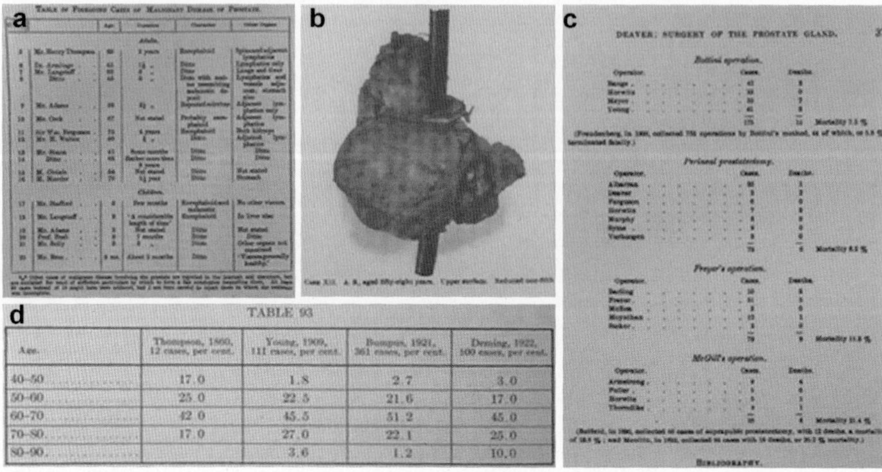

Age.	Thompson, 1860, 12 cases, per cent.	Young, 1909, 111 cases, per cent.	Bumpus, 1921, 361 cases, per cent.	Deming, 1922, 100 cases, per cent.
40–50	17.0	1.8	2.7	3.0
50–60	25.0	22.5	21.6	17.0
60–70	42.0	45.5	51.2	45.0
70–80	17.0	27.0	22.1	25.0
80–90		3.6	1.2	10.0

Fig. 14.2 Early treatment failures. (**a**) Thompson's list of failed therapies. (**b**) Image from Deaver's paper. (**c**) Deaver's listing of failures. (**d**) Hugh Young's list

[11]. But his comments were premature and not associated with the degree of comparison, controlling many factors that would be necessary for this understanding—but it was coming.

In 1891 Friedrich Daniel Von Recklinghausen (1833–1910) was one of Virchow's protégés described the osteoblastic variety of bone metastases that typify prostate cancers [12]. Franck Sasse described a patient presenting with bone pain from metastases in 1894 [13]. The other feature of metastatic prostate cancer was described by Octave Pasteau (1870–1957) when he noted the involvement of the iliac lymph nodes in 87% of cases whereas the inguinal nodes were only involved in 36% of these advanced cases [14]. George Blumer followed this case report and a review of the literature in 1902. He was able to extract from the literature 43 such cases, of which 16 of the total were recorded by Kaufmann. In 22 of these cases, the bones were examined and 70% showed metastatic disease and he states, "*Considering the frequency of prostatic carcinoma it is easily realized that many instances of bone metastases must have been overlooked in the past. If bone metastases occur in such a large proportion of cases of carcinoma of the prostate, it is important to know whether the condition can be recognized clinically*" [15]. He goes on to recount how this might be possible, "*Of the general symptoms emaciation and weakness were most frequently mentioned. Pain of a general character in all the bones, or more local pain in the back and legs was also common. Anemia was noted in some cases, though there are but few records of blood examinations and most of these show merely a secondary anemia*" [15]. He does go on to mention the condition originally described by Sir Benjamin Brodie that began this section of our history, namely metastatic paraplegia. "*Those with more or less marked paraplegia numbered 8 out of the 23 cases. In 4 of these the paraplegia was complete and accompanied by the usual sensory changes, the lack of sphincter control, and the exaggerated reflexes. In the other 4 cases the paralysis was incomplete"* [2].

John Hunter (1728–1793) described the seasonal variations in the size of testicles and compared them to the prostates of various animals. In addition, he surgically removed the testicles and observed the effect upon the prostate [16]. In 1893, W. J. White of Philadelphia reported on the castration of dogs resulting in the atrophy of the glandular mass of the prostate. He advocated castration for the treatment of symptomatic men [17]. Clyde Deming and the group at Yale did studies on primates, also noting atrophy of the prostate in castrated males [18]. Robert Moore and Allister McLellan discovered that female hormones also had activity upon the prostate [19]. In 1936, in was reported that various phosphates were elevated in men with skeletal metastases from prostate cancer. Charles Brenton Huggins (1901–1997) was a Canadian-born physician, attended Harvard's Medical School before going to the University of Michigan for his internship and specialty training in urology. He moved to the University of Chicago where he became interested in the hormonally-induced regression of prostate cancer [20]. In 1940 he published *Quantitative studies of prostatic secretion. 11. The effect of castration and of estro gen injection on the hyperplastic prostate glands of dogs* [21]. He followed this with *The effect of castration on benign hypertrophy in man* [22]. Finally in 1941 his paper, *Studies on prostate cancer: 1. The effects of castration, of estrogen and androgen injection on serum phosphatases in metastatic carcinoma of the prostate* was published [23]. He was given the Nobel Prize in Physiology and Medicine in 1966. "*Prostatic cancer is influenced by androgenic activity in the body. At least with respect to serum phosphatases, disseminated carcinoma of the prostate is inhibited by eliminating androgens, through castration or neutralization of their activity by estrogen injection*" [20]. In that same fateful year, Huggins also presented the case for oral estrogen administration by stilbesterol. In the 1960s the Veterans Administration Cooperative Urologic Research Group (VACURG) noted in one of the largest randomized studies performed, noted the beneficial effects of androgen ablation in men with advanced prostate cancer as well as confirming the significant cardiovascular sequeallae of estrogens [24]. Huggins continued to contribute by noting that the adrenals also contributed androgens and that bilateral adrenalectomy did offer some response. Andrew Schally discovered the structure of the hypothalamic hormone LHRH in 1971 and developed agents to manipulate this system including LHRH agonists and antagonists [25]. He would go on to win the Nobel Prize in 1977 [26]. Anti-androgens were discovered to be synergistic to the effects of hormone suppression with the first agent being aminoglutethimide and the antifungal agent ketoconazole. Steroidal and non-steroidal antiandrogens showed relative poor response to advanced prostate cancer alone, with much better results used in combination with LHRH agents. None of the agents or combinations of agents however cured the patient with metastatic prostate cancer, but improved survival rates only [27].

Early Therapeutic Failures

Surgery for the treatment of prostate cancer was not as dramatic as for other genitourinary cancers, partially because of the deep pelvic location of the prostate, surrounded on all sides *by* anatomical potential disaster—the bladder above, the rectum posteriorly, and large veins and plexuses of veins all around. In 1852 Jean Nicolas Demarquay used the perineal approach common in stone disease to approach the prostate. Küchler in 1866 is given credit for developing the strategies necessary for performing a complete, if not radical perineal prostatectomy in Berlin on cadavers. But it fell to the great Theodor Billroth (1824–1923) who attempted to remove a large tumor "about the size of a duck's egg" from a 30 year old man in 1867 that died of recurrence 14 months after the surgery. He tried again that same year but this patient survived only a few days [28]. Bernhard Rudolph Conrad von Langeneck (1810–1887) also tried to excise cancerous prostate via the perineum in 1876, this was observed by his pupil Heinrich Wilhelm Franz Leisrink who went on to perform a radical perineal prostatectomy in 1883 but the patient died on the 14th postoperative day [29]. The great Austrian surgeon Vincenz Czerny (1842–1916) also tried total prostatectomy twice—both died 12 days to 9 months following the surgery [29]. In 1891, Georg Ferdinand von Kóster (1839–1930) tried a combined total cystectomy along with a perineal prostatectomy with implantation of the ureters into the sigmoid colon, but the patient died 5 days afterwards [29]. In 1904, a new radical perineal approach had been devised by Hugh Hampton Young (1870–1945), and he had his Chief, William Stewart Halsted (1852–1922) assist on his first case and a year later reported upon his first six cases [30]. He stresses the necessity of discovering the cancers early. "*An inverted V cutaneous incision was made in the perineum…By blunt dissection the end of the bulb and central tendon were exposed, and the latter divided, exposing in turn the rectourethralis muscle, the division of which gave free access to the membranous urethra behind the triangular ligament. Urethrotomy upon a grooved staff, was followed by introduction of the prostatic tractor, which was opened out after it reached the bladder…the lateral attachments, which are slight were easily separated by the finger…The posterior surface of the seminal vesicles were then freed by blunt dissection, the now mobile prostate being well out of the wound. In this exposure of the posterior surface of the vesicles I was careful not to break through the fascia of Denonvillier's. The next step was to expose the anterior surface of the bladder, which was easily done by depressing the tractor and making strong traction…it was easily incised at a point in the middle line about one cm. behind the prostatovesicular juncture. By means of scissors the division was continued on each side until the trigone was exposed…the line of incision was carried across the trigone with a scalpel so as to pass about one cm in front of the ureteral orifices…thus exposing the anterior surface of the seminal vesicles and the adjacent vasa deferentia, all of which were carefully freed by blunt dissection with the finger as high up as possible, so as to remove with the vesicles much circumjacent fat and areolar tissues on account of the lymphatics which they contained*" [30]. The first patient did well except for incontinence only to develop stones upon the silk sutures used to perform the anastomosis and undergoing a litholapaxy developed extravasation of urine dying about 4 weeks later. An autopsy revealed that a small focus or cancer was found along the left vas deferens, but no other foci could be identified. In later long-term follow-up studies, Young noted that only about 50% of surgical patients were alive at 5 years in 1937 (Fig. 14.2d). His protégé J. A. C. Colston by 1940 had obtained no better results, except in the degree of incontinence but the same 50% 5-year cancer survival was not very good [31]. Better diagnostic strategies and improved imaging studies were required. Terence John Millin (1900–1979) did develop a retropubic surgical approach in 1947 that seemed to make the surgical approach easier for urologists, as well as sample the pelvic lymphatics in an expanded methodology and this was followed in Philadelphia by Deaver [32]. (Fig. 14.2b and c]. Patrick C. Walsh (1938-) developed the anatomical radical retropubic prostatectomy in 1983 and brought forth the new wave of radical surgeries [33]. For surgery to progress, a tumor marker that isolated the cancers to earlier grades and stages was necessary and the discovery of prostatic specific antigen represented this needed impetus. Next, the complications and side-effects of surgery could be addressed. Finally, the type of surgery could reduce the trauma to the patient and laparoscopic radical prostatectomy begat robotic-assisted radical prostatectomy and the future interventions will come of their own accord [34]. The failure of early historical surgery and the rise of improved technology in radiation therapy represented the next major accomplishments in the management of prostate cancer.

Radiation and History

"*What can be easier than to turn the rays on the lungs of persons afflicted with consumption.*" Thomas Edison, February 1896.

Perhaps given the poor results of surgical intervention in the pre-PSA era, radiation treatments were hoped to add to the patient's survival. Radiation was just discovered by Antoine Henri Becquerel (1852–1908) in 1896. Wilhelm Conrad Röntgen (1845–1923) won the very first Nobel Prize in 1901 for his discovery of X-rays in 1895 and Marie Curie-Sklodowska (1867–1934) with her husband Pierre Curie (1859–1906) discovered radium in 1898 (Fig. 14.1b). The biologic effects of X-rays were described in hand injuries by O. Leppin in 1896. Leopold Freund (1868–1943) used Röntgen rays for treatment of a naevus pilosus with tragic results in 1896. The first skin cancer was treated in 1899 by Thor Stenbeck (1864–1914) and prostate cancer followed in 1904 by Armand Imbert (1850–1922) [35]. Nikola Tesla in 1896 speculated for the New York Times, "*it might be possible to load X-Rays with cancer-fighting drugs or chemicals and project them into the body*" [36]. The beams of the X-rays were not well configured but early reports by E. Loumeau reported favorable responses. The use of radium was introduced by M. Minet and Ernst Desnos by radium catheters in 1908, the Gussenbauer Clinic in Vienna followed in 1902 and Hugh H. Young at Johns Hopkins also adapted applications for use. But no one literally knew how the new X-rays actually worked, though by 1906 Tribondeau and Bergonié stated, "*The effects of irradiation on the cells are more intense the greater their reproductive activity, the longer their mitotic phases, and the less their morphology and functions are established*" [37].

Robert Abbe (1851–1928) was an American surgeon who pioneered the use of radium for cancer therapy in New York City. He became a friend to the Curies, especially Marie Curie and he began to use her newly discovered element, radium for the treatment of malignancies in 1904 [38]. He visited their research laboratory in 1903 that year and returned to the U.S. with a zeal for treating cancer and a supply of radium—at the time there were three known rays emitted from radium designated alpha, beta and gamma (Fig. 14.1b). He was an outspoken opponent of smoking—reporting on 100 cases of smoker's cancers. Abbe was an astute clinician and surgeon; he stated "*No one who ventures to use it [radium] in practice should do so without first testing his particular specimen or specimens on his own skin… He may best choose perhaps the inner side of the calf of his leg for this test*" [39]. Becquerel, Marie and Pierre Curie had already reported skin burns with radium. He was aware of the potential, but blinded to the potential for harm—"*One thing is certain, that the Beta ray, isolated, may be showered for almost indefinite periods upon the skin, with no deleterious effect. Not even erythema ensues after hours of pure Beta therapy, but a sense of comfort follows*" [39]. He studied the effects of ionizing radiation on the growth of tumors, "*Growth composed of overgrown masses of cells returns to orderly growth permanently when given the exact dosage of negative electrons…Growths to which too much is supplied undergo atrophy and, if excessively oversupplied, undergo death*" [39]. He devised methods to directly insert radium rods into tumors, interstitial implantation. It was Abbe who first reported that regular intervals of lower dose treatments worked better than a single large dose, "*If more intensive treatment is necessary, then cumulative or successive attacks are better and an interval of 1 or 2 weeks between treatments works out a better result. Thus, successive blows fall upon the disease, sustaining a long corrective action rather than an intense and destructive one*" [39].

Radiation is a two-headed snake because it is used to treat cancers as well as the cause of others. Radiation is not a new form of carcinogen just recently brought upon humanity since Antoine Henri Becquerel first described this process in February of 1896. Radon has been leaching from the ground since animals and mankind's alluvial beginnings. Uranium was mined by ancient civilizations for the blue-colored pigments it could produce. But no one was aware of the properties of nuclear decay and the subsequent release of particles (alpha, beta, and gamma) until Becquerel discovered radioactivity. Marie and Pierre Curie were both exposed to high doses of ionizing radiation throughout much of their careers. Marie would tell the story of walking around with a vial of radium in her lab pocket because of the glow from the radiation was soothing. She died at the age of 66 from aplastic anemia long thought to be due to her exposure to radium and polonium. Her body was exhumed in 1995 for the honor of being reburied with Pierre in the Panthéon, yet the amount a radiation in her coffin was only 9.7 picocuries (20 times less than the maximum safe limit). The Office de Protection Contre les Rayonnements Ionisants concluded that her terminal cancer was not caused by the radium or polonium, but rather the X-rays she was exposed to from working with her daughter, Iréne Joliot-Curie (who also won a Nobel Prize) performed as medical volunteers in World War I. Iréne would also die from a leukemia when she was aged 58 [40].

The nuclear bombs dropped by the U.S. on Japan in 1945 caused an estimated 150,000 fatalities immediately. The two cities, Hiroshima and Nagasaki were both hit with different types of nuclear weapons—Hiroshima was hit with a uranium-type bomb, whereas Nagasaki was hit with a different uranium-type bomb. One survivor of both nuclear explosions was Tsutomu Yamaguchi who was near enough to the epicenter of the first blast to have skin burns and a blown-out tympanic membrane. But he took the train to his home in Nagasaki just in time for the second bomb. He lived to be 93 years of age, dying in 2010 of cancer of the stomach. The first radioactive experiments were carried out at the University of California Berkeley's cyclotron even before the isolation and purification of plutonium. Lawrence began to publicize the potential benefits of radioactive isotopes to study physiology and potentially treat disease. In fact, a little know sidebar is that Earnest and John Lawrence's mother, Gunda developed cancer and she was transported to Berkeley's Rad Lab where her sons arranged for the first neutron beam therapy from a cyclotron. The University of California, San Francisco took notice and two physicians, Robert Stone and Joseph Hamilton were eager to do research. They had managed to inject two leukemia patients with radioactive sodium but it did not alter the diseases course, nor did it cause side effects. Stone began to use Berkeley's cyclotron to deliver neutron beams to humans. It is estimated that he treated 128 patients from December of 1939 to September of 1941 from his outpatient UCSF tumor clinic. All of the patients were thought to have incurable cancers and nearly ½ of his patients died in 6 months. Hamilton experimented on radioactive iodine which concentrates in the thyroid gland. He would give demonstrations upon himself holding up a Geiger counter to his own thyroid. He eventually developed a fatal leukemia and died in the 1950s [41] (Fig. 14.3).

The earliest organized radiation treatments occurred at centers around the western world such as the Curie Foundation in Paris, the Radiumhemmet in Stockholm, the Christie Hospital and Holt Radium Institute in Manchester, and the Royal Marsden Cancer Hospital in London. Ralston Paterson campaigned to substitute radiotherapy for radical surgery since the surgeries so badly disfigured the patients at the Christie Hospital. Some surgeons, particularly Robert McWhirter and Geoffrey Keynes did less radical surgeries with augmented radiation treatments. But the results were in many ways hampered by poor strategies in patient assignment, the lack of knowledge about radiation physics, the poor methods of focusing the primitive radiation beams, and lack of methods of follow-up as well as quantifying complications [42]. But until these problems could be systematically addressed there would be chaos and incomplete information with no rationale to proceed. This would all be solved by a pioneering group that took the bold step of including a radiation physicist in their midst at the M.D. Anderson Cancer Center in Houston, Texas. From its beginnings under the directorship of the surgeon, R. Lee Clark this center sought to include all aspects of cancer therapies in hopes of improving cure

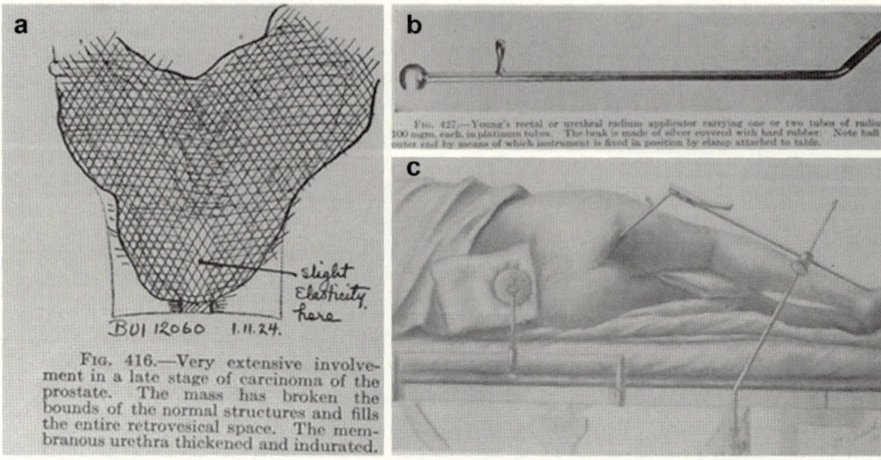

Fig. 14.3 Hugh Young's early radiation therapies. (**a**) First digital rectal examination "map" with extensive local disease (distant metastatic disease could not yet be evaluated). (**b**) His radium delivery catheter. (**c**) Patient positioning for early Johns Hopkin's radiation therapy

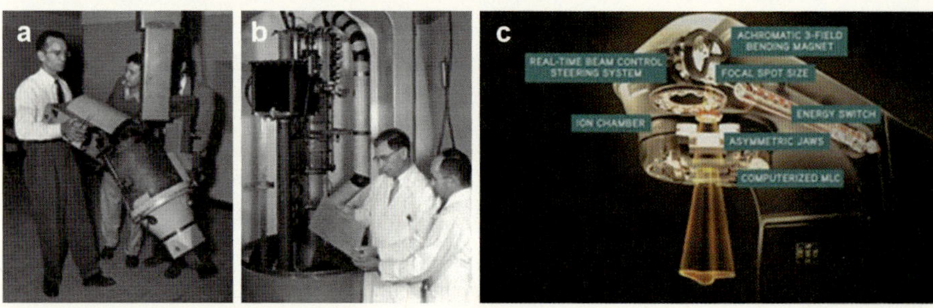

Fig. 14.4 (**a**) The M.D. Anderson Cobolt-60 device called the "Big Gun." (**b**) Stanford's early Linear Accelerator (Megavoltage). (**c**) The technology inside the current modern methods of IMRT and IGRT

rates as did other centers. Clark was unusual for a surgeon because he had done some training at the Radium Institute in Paris and saw first-hand some early reports on brachytherapy and external x-ray beam therapy and stated at the outset—"*I intend to discover the cause of cancer and build the greatest cancer hospital in the world*" [43]. Clark hired Gilbert H. Fletcher to head the new radiation department in October 1947 and promptly brought on board Leonard Grimmett, a physicist from England to the fledgling department. They immediately began to work on a new, safer, cost-effective, high energy delivery unit utilizing Cobalt-59 and then Cobalt-60 (Fig. 14.4a). Utilizing some work and resources of the U.S. Oak Ridge Institute they developed a device that ultimately was produced by General Electric X-Ray Corporation as the prototype for modern X-ray units. Not resting on the laurels of success, they immediately began to plan on upgrades, developing a new

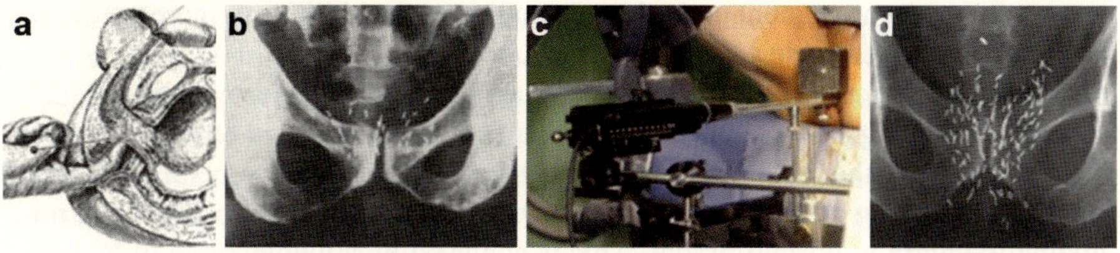

Fig. 14.5 Brachy therapies evolve. (**a**) The first prostate brachytherapies involved digital rectal-guidance. (**b**) X-ray following one of these DRE-guided brachytherapies. (**c**) US-guided transperineal brachytherapy. (**d**) X-ray following this method (many more seeds dispersed regularly)

betatron to harness the electrons and generate megavoltage high-energy beams [43] (Fig. 14.4b). This coupled with sophisticated imaging and ultimately with fiduciary marker placements have allowed for increasingly precise molding and delivery of high energy photons to the prostate to spare surrounding tissues and to minimize long-term side effects. This is the era of IMRT (intensity modulated radiation therapy), IGRT (image guided radiation therapy) and the robotic delivery of ever more precise beams by the CyberKnife® systems [42] (Fig. 14.4c).

Prostate Cancer and Radiation Technologies

Brachytherapy which is the application of radiation sources via a closed system, not via external sources of radiation has several types: surface application, intracavitary, interstitial and intravascular. Almost as soon as Marie and Pierre Curie's discovery of radium in 1898, surface applications to treat skin cancers were reported. In 1911 MacLeod reported on a special catheter to treat prostate cancers and by 1915 Barringer at New York's Memorial Hospital inserted radium needles into the prostate (Fig. 14.5a and b). "*These needles are 4–6 inches long and are inserted through the perineum into the prostate or further into the vesicles. A finger in the rectum is used to guide the needles*" [44]. Rubin Flocks (1906–1975) at the University of Iowa began to use the instillation of colloidal gold (Au198) into the prostate during open prostate surgeries and reported on his initial 20 cases in 1952. He eventually extended his treatments to patients with bulky large, tumors and updated his series of 335 patients with 5-year follow-up with a mere 4.4% local recurrence rate compared to 21–28% noted by others [45]. Willet F. Whitmore, Jr. (1917–1995) was the Chairman of the Urology Service at Memorial Sloan Kettering Cancer Center for 33 years and is considered by many to be the father of urologic oncology introduced brachytherapy with 125I in 1970, though not the first to do so, his trial was the most observed and reported upon, though the method for image-guided implantation of the seeds have improved dose distribution curves and overall improved the outcomes (Fig. 14.5c and d). The high degree of positive biopsy and the relative higher numbers of complications have reduced this therapeutic modalities utility in recent

17. White WJ. The results of double castration in the hypertrophy of the prostate. Ann Surg. 1895;22:1–3.
18. Demming CL, Jenkins RH, Van Wagenen G. Further studies in the endocrinological relationship of prostatic hypertrophy. J Urol. 1935;34:678–85.
19. Moore RA, McClellan AM. Histological study of the effect of the sex hormones on the human prostate. J Urol. 1938;40:641–57.
20. Hansson N, Moll F, Schultheiss D, Krischel M. Remembering Charles B. Huggins' Nobel Prize for hormonal treatment of prostatic cancer at its 50th anniversary. Eur Urol. 2016;69(6):971–2.
21. Huggins CB, Clark PJ. Quantitative studies of prostatic secretion. II. The effect of castration and estrogen injection on the hyperplastic prostate glands of dogs. J Exp Med. 1940;72:747.
22. Huggins CB, Stevens RA. The effect of castration on benign hypertrophy of the prostate in man. J Urol. 1940;43:105.
23. Huggins CB, Hodges CV. Studies on prostate cancer. I. The effects of castration, of estrogen and androgen injection on serum phosphatases in metastatic carcinoma of the prostate. Cancer Res. 1941;1:203.
24. Veterans Administration Cooperative Urological Research Group. Treatment and survival of patients with cancer of the prostate. Surg Gynecol Obstet. 1967;124:1011–7.
25. Schally AV, Kastin AJ, Arimura A. Hypothalamic FSH and LH-regulating hormone. Structure, physiology and clinical studies. Fertil Steril. 1971;22:703–21.
26. Schally AV, Kastin AJ, Coy DHLH. Releasing hormone and its analogues. In J Fertil. 1976;1:1–5.
27. Denmeade SR, Isaacs JT. A history of prostate cancer treatment. Nat Rev Cancer. 2002;2(5):389–96.
28. Billroth T. Chirurgishce Erfahrungen in Zurich 1860-1867. Langenbecks Arch Klin Chir. 1869;10:547–54.
29. Androutsos G. Carcinoma of the prostate. A historical account. J BUON. 2005;10:135–44.
30. Young HH. The early diagnosis and radical cure of carcinoma of the prostate. Bull Johns Hopkins. 1905;16(175):315–21.
31. Colston JAC. Carcinoma of the prostate: a study of the percentage of cases suitable for the radical operation. JAMA. 1943;122(12):781–4.
32. Deaver JB. Surgery of the prostate gland. Am J Med Sci. 1904:1–39.
33. Walsh PC. The discovery of the cavernous nerves and development of nerve sparing radical retropubic prostatectomy. J Urol. 2007;177(5):1632–5.
34. Moran ME. The history of robotic surgery. In: Hemal AK, Menon M, editors. Robotics in genitourinary surgery. New York: Springer; 2011.
35. Dronsfield A, Ellis P. Radium-a key element in early cancer treatment. Educ Chem. 2011;3:56–9.
36. Tesla N. An interesting feature of X-ray radiations. Elect Rev N Y. 1896;29(2):13–4.
37. Bergonié J, Tribondeau L. Interpretation de quelques resultants de la radiothérapie et essai de fixation d'unde technique rationelle. Compt Red Acad Sci. 1906;143:983–5.
38. Silverstone SM. Robert Abbe: founder of radium therapy in America. Bull N Y Acad Med. 1956;32(2):157–67.
39. Abbe R. On what lines is the treatment of malignant disease advancing? Med Rec. 1904;66:1041–3.
40. Goldsmith B. Obsessive genius: the inner world of Marie Curie. New York: W.W. Norton; 2005.
41. Welsome E. The plutonium files: America's secret medical experiments in the cold war. New York: The Dial Press; 1999.
42. Slater JM. From X-rays to ion beams: a short history of radiation therapy. In: Linz U, editor. Ion beam therapy, biological and medical physics, biomedical engineering. New York: Springer; 2012.
43. Oslson JS. Making of cancer history: disease & discovery at the University of Texas M.D. Anderson Cancer Center. Baltimore: Johns Hopkins University Press; 2009.

44. Barringer B. Radium in the treatment of carcinoma of the bladder and prostate: review of one year's work. JAMA. 1917;68:1227–30.
45. Rosevear HM, Lightfoot AJ, O'Donnell MA, Platz CE, Loening SA, Hawtrey CE, Rubin H. Flocks and colloidal gold treatments for prostate cancer. Sci World J. 2011;11:1560–7.
46. Bagshaw MA, Ray GR, Cox RS. Selecting initial therapy for prostate cancer: radiation therapy perspective. Cancer. 1987;60:521–5.
47. Van Dyk J, Battista JJ, Bauman GS. Accuracy and uncertainty considerations in modern radiation oncology. In: The modern technology of radiation oncology. Madison: Modern Physics Publishing; 1999.
48. Stone RS, Lawrence JH, Aebersold PD. A preliminary report on the use of fast neutrons in the treatment of malignant disease. Radiology. 1940;37:322–7.
49. Body JJ, Casimiro S, Costa L. Targeting bone metastases in prostate cancer: improving clinical outcome. Nat Rev Urol. 2015;12:340–56.
50. Parker C, Nilsson S, Heinrich D, et al. Alpha emitter radium-223 and survival in metastatic prostate cancer. N Engl J Med. 2013;369:213–23.

Chapter 15
The History of Percutaneous Renal Cryoablation

Sutchin R. Patel and Stephen Y. Nakada

Introduction

The increased use of cross-sectional imaging has led to an increase in the detection of suspected renal cell carcinoma at an early stage [1]. The development of ablative techniques has led to an increase in treatment options for patients with small renal masses (≤4 cm). Percutaneous renal cryoablation has evolved into a minimally invasive treatment option for select lesions and for the high risk surgical patient. Contemporary series suggest that renal cryoablation maintains good intermediate oncologic outcomes while minimizing patient morbidity and thus has a role in the treatment of select patients with small renal masses [2].

The Development of Cryoablation

Cryoablation destroys cells by consecutive rapid freeze and thaw cycles, leading to cellular necrosis at temperatures of −20 °C or less [3]. The therapeutic use of cryoablation dates back to mid-nineteenth century England and James Arnott (1797–1883), an English physician, who was the first to use extreme cold locally for the destruction of tissue. He used "two parts finely pounded ice and one part of chloride of sodium" (a mixture of crushed ice and salt) for the palliation of tumors with resultant reduction of pain and local bleeding [4, 5]. Arnott achieved temperatures of −24 °C and treated breast cancer, uterine cancer and some skin cancers and also advocated cold treatment for acne, neuralgia and headaches. He also recognized the analgesic "benumbing" effect of cold, recommending its use to anesthetize skin before an operation [6].

S.R. Patel, M.D., F.A.C.S. (✉) • S.Y. Nakada, M.D., F.A.C.S.
Department of Urology, University of Wisconsin School of Medicine and Public Health, Madison, WI 53726, USA
e-mail: sutchin_patel@yahoo.com

S.R. Patel et al. (eds.), *The History of Technologic Advancements in Urology*,
DOI 10.1007/978-3-319-61691-9_15

Refrigerants

Despite Arnott's contributions to the field of cryoablation, salt/ice mixtures were not capable of reducing tissue temperatures to temperatures low enough to adequately treat tumors. The practical ability to clinically apply deeply cryogenic temperatures was realized when liquefied air gases became available just before 1900. Louis Paul Cailletet, in 1877, demonstrated at the French Academy of Science that oxygen and carbon monoxide could be liquefied under high pressure [7]. Campbell White, from New York, was the first to utilize refrigerants in medicine and reported success in using liquid air for the treatment of numerous conditions from lupus, herpes zoster, chancroid, warts, carbuncles and epitheliomas in 1899 [8]. Close to the time that liquid air was being used, William Pusey of Chicago advocated the use of carbon dioxide snow (carbonic acid snow) as it was easily available since it was used by manufacturers of mineral waters. The liquid carbon dioxide gas was supplied in steel cylinders under pressure and when the gas was allowed to escape, its rapid expansion led to a fall in temperature (the Joule-Thompson effect) and a fine snow was formed. The snow could easily be compressed into various shapes suitable for different treatments or applications [9]. Sir James Dewar in 1892 solved the problems of transporting and storing refrigerants such as liquid air or carbon dioxide snow by inventing a flask made of two walls of glass (or two containers, one inside the other) with a vacuum in between (which limited the transmission of heat from the outside to the inside). Cryogenic storage flasks today are called vacuum flasks or Dewar flasks in honor of Sir James Dewar [7]. Allington in 1950 was the first to use liquid nitrogen, recognizing that its properties were very similar to those of liquid air. Early treatment approaches were limited to superficial application of the cryogen, usually liquid nitrogen, by either spraying or pouring it over the lesion. These techniques limited the clinical applications of cryotherapy [10]. Dr. Irving S. Cooper, an American neurosurgeon, in 1913 designed the first liquid nitrogen probe capable of achieving temperatures of −196 °C, using it to treat Parkinson's disease by freezing the thalamus and in the treatment of previously inoperable brain tumors. His work led to an explosion of interest in liquid nitrogen and its use in many medical specialties [11]. In 1961, Cooper and Lee successfully built the first apparatus for cryotherapy and their more applicable liquid nitrogen cryogenic probe would pave the way for modern cryoablation [12].

Joule-Thomson Effect

An understanding of how we reach the temperatures during percutaneous cryoablation requires an understanding of the Joule-Thomson effect. In thermodynamics, the Joule-Thomson effect describes the temperature change of a gas or liquid when it is forced through a valve while kept insulated so that no heat is exchanged with the environment. The cooling produced via Joule-Thomson expansion makes it a valuable tool in refrigeration, air conditioning, as well as in cryogenic applications. At room temperature, all gases except hydrogen, helium and neon cool upon expansion by the Joule Thomson process. This is important in the cryoprobes we use today, as pressurized argon gas is pumped into the cryoprobe for freezing while helium gas can thus be used for thawing to create the rapid freeze and thaw cycles used in cryoablation [13].

Development of Percutaneous Cryoablation

Uchida et al. in 1995 first described percutaneous cryoablation using liquid nitrogen for the treatment of renal tumors [14]. The first initial case series for laparoscopic renal cryoablation was reported by Gill et al. [15]. With the increase in the detection of small renal masses due to the widespread use of cross-sectional imaging and the further refinements in cryotherapy technology, percutaneous renal cryoablation has an established role in the treatment of the small renal mass in select cases.

Pathophysiology of Cryoablation

Freezing provides hypothermic stress to cells as well as severe mechanical damage due to ice crystal formation. Although a thermal gradient exists within a freeze zone, there is a distinct transition between unfrozen and frozen tissue which accurately approximates the zone of lethality [16, 17]. The intensity of the freeze determines the response of the targeted tissue and ranges from an inflammatory response to cellular destruction. An inflammatory response accompanies minor freezing [16, 17]. If the freezing is severe (less than −20 °C), complete destruction of cells results due to intracellular ice crystal formation. Current cryoablation technology generates temperatures much less than −20 °C. Tissue-engineered models for renal cancer cells show that exposure to temperatures near the −30 to −40 °C range for ≥1 minute using a double freeze-thaw cycle leads to complete death [18]. Pressurized argon gas pumped into the cryoprobe is used for freezing and helium gas used for thawing via the Joule-Thompson effect [13]. Cryoablation induces cell death primarily via two mechanisms: a direct cytotoxic effect from intracellular ice crystal formation during a freeze cycle and delayed microcirculatory failure with resultant ischemia during the thaw cycle [19, 20]. Ice crystal formation removes water from the cells which in turn produces metabolic disturbances related to the freeze concentration of solutes. Ice crystals also cause mechanical damage via cell membrane disruption. The vascular stasis that develops soon after thawing is also a major mechanism of injury as it contributes to endothelial damage, thrombosis and tissue ischemia. Repetition of the rapid freeze-thaw cycles also exacerbates tissue damage [21, 22].

Post-cryoablation histopathological change follows a sequential order, from central coagulative necrosis with karyolysis, cytolysis and hemolysis surrounded by a thin peripheral freeze zone with incomplete initial cell destruction with pyknosis and less hemorrhage and congestion [19, 20]. Coagulative necrosis occurs due to the damaged endothelial cell lining of the microvasculature and increased cellular permeability which leads to edema and inflammation [2]. Shortly after thawing, the tissue appears hyperemic along this border and congestion is noted in the central zone. The freeze margin is important with regard to the therapeutic outcome. The temperatures in the freeze margin range from 0° to −20 °C at which cell survival is possible. Cell death in this region of tissue is generally due to apoptosis and secondary necrosis. Following the thaw phase there is an immediate infiltration of lymphocytes and macrophages into the necrotic tissue. The necrotic tissue is removed by the phagocytotic activity of the inflammatory cells and necrotic debris is replaced by a fibrous collagen scar over the following weeks to months [19, 20].

The ability to visualize the ice ball and thus the zone of ablation on CT during the procedure is one advantage of percutaneous renal cryoablation compared to RFA. A comparison of in vitro, ex vivo and in vivo isotherms for renal cryotherapy using 1.47 and 1.7 mm (IceRods™, Galil and PERC-17 CryoProbes™, Endocare) cryoprobes in porcine kidneys with multipoint thermal sensors found that gel and ex vivo isotherms did not predict the in vivo pattern of freezing [23]. Furthermore, the cryoprobes should be passed 5 mm beyond the tumor border to achieve suitably colder temperatures. Studies evaluating the effect of renal cryoablation on renal arterial structure have shown that ablation injury destroys arteries smaller than 180 μm but that larger arteries remain anatomically intact. It is also important to recognize that larger vessels (especially near the hilum) also serve as a "heat sink" which may increase the iceball temperatures and thus decrease cell kill in the region [21, 22]. A study of multiple cryoprobes used to treat a single lesion in a porcine model showed that the cryolesion created by three simultaneous 1.47 mm cryoprobes appeared to be larger than that of an additive effect—thus the multiple probe effect was synergistic [24]. An understanding of the physics of the cryoablation in reference to renal anatomy is thus important in order to maximize the efficacy of the procedure.

Indications and Contraindications

Optimal outcomes for renal cryoablation are dependent on appropriate lesion selection as well as careful patient selection and consideration of surgical indications and contraindications. Currently ablative techniques are used for small, enhancing renal masses (≤4 cm) in patients with advanced age and comorbid conditions. Ablation has also be advocated in patients with small renal tumors and baseline renal insufficiency, in patients with multifocal renal tumors attributable to Von Hippel-Lindau disease or in those with an absolute surgical contraindication. Some relative contraindications to ablation include large tumors (>4 cm), hilar tumors, unstable cardiovascular status and poor life expectancy. The only absolute contraindication is an uncorrected coagulopathy [25]. The American Urological Association (AUA) Guideline for Management of the Clinical T1 Renal Mass stated that thermal ablation (cryoablation or radiofrequency ablation [RFA]) via either the percutaneous and laparoscopic approach is a treatment option for the patient at high surgical risk who wants active treatment and accepts the need for long term radiographic surveillance [26]. The panel states that the standard is for percutaneous renal mass biopsy (specifically core biopsy with or without fine needle aspiration) to be performed prior to treatment to define histology and should also be considered after treatment, particularly if there is a suspicion of recurrence [26]. Prior to proceeding with renal cryoablation it is important to counsel patients about available treatment options followed by the risks of the procedure (including the risk of local recurrence and renal functional considerations), the potential need for reintervention, the need for radiographic surveillance, the potential for difficult surgical salvage in cases of tumor progression and the limitations of the current thermal ablation literature [26]. The Renal Cancer Working Group of the Young Academic Urologists Working Party of the European Association of Urology (EAU) in their review on the Current Status of Focal Cryoablation for Small Renal Masses (2016) stated that though "focal cryoablation is an established minimally invasive technique for the treatment of small renal masses, because of the lack of robust evidence is indicated in selected patients who have relative contraindications to extirpative approaches" [2]. They comment that the role of percutaneous renal cryoablation has been expanding due to its ability to reduce pain and hospitalization, the possibility of performing the procedure under sedation and that fact that it is potentially more cost effective.

Technique

Recent preoperative imaging (CT or MRI) is used in the initial surgical planning. At our institution the radiology staff will perform a planning renal ultrasound with core biopsy of the lesion prior to the day of the procedure so that pathology of the mass is known prior to ablation. Percutaneous renal cryoablation is performed in the radiology suite with both interventional radiology and urology present [27]. A survey of academic institutions in the United States in found that urologists were present at the time of the ablation in 59% of institutions and in 32% of institutions, urologists placed the needles for ablation. Nineteen percent of institutions performed a renal mass biopsy prior to the day of the procedure so that the pathology was known prior to ablation [28]. After administration of general anesthesia a foley catheter is placed and the patient is placed in the flank position and secured to the scanner table. The lesion is localized using both ultrasonography and computed tomography. If adjacent structures (colon, small bowel, pancreas) are in close proximity to the lesion or in the path of cryoprobe placement, hydrodissection is performed in order to displace adjacent organs to allow for safe probe placement and ablation [29, 30] (Fig. 15.1). In situations where the tumor cannot be approached safely, the

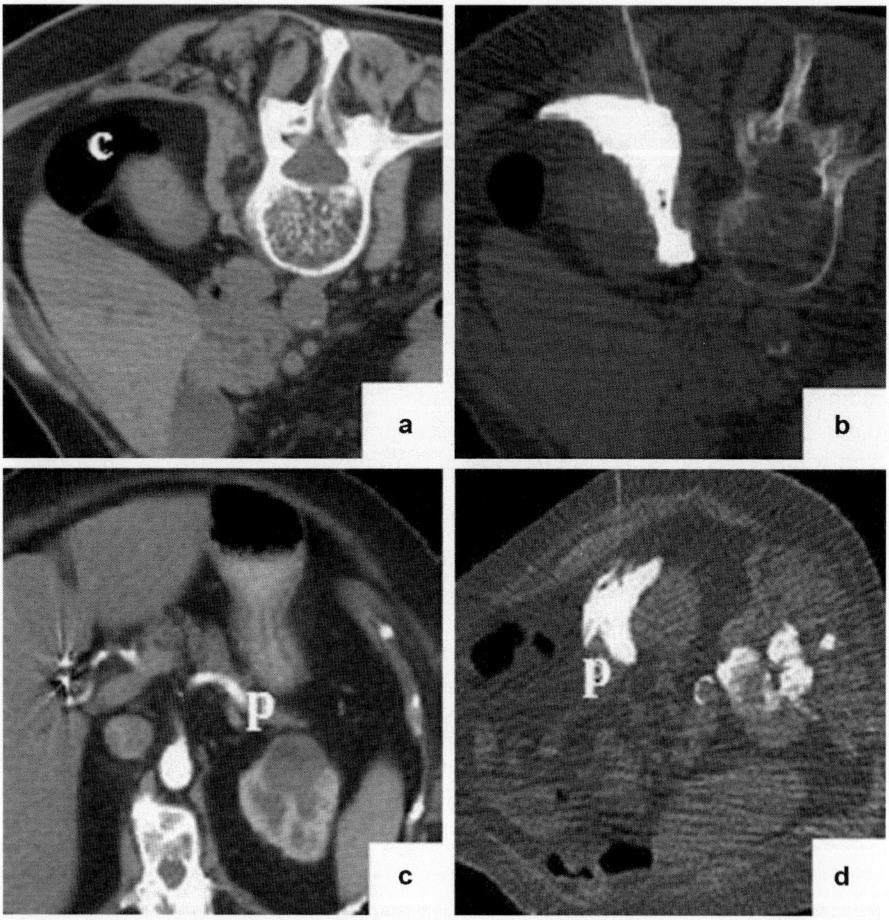

Fig. 15.1 Hydrodissection utilizing iodinated contrast medium during percutaneous renal cryoablation allows for safe mobilization of adjacent organs (**a** and **b**) Displacement of the colon (*c*) using hydrodissection with iodinated contrast (**c** and **d**) Displacement of the pancreas (*p*) using hydrodissection with iodinated contrast [30]

procedure is aborted and plans are made for an alternative management strategy. Generally two cryoablation probes (1.7 mm, Endocare) are used depending on the lesion size. After probe placement, a 10-min double freeze-thaw cycle is commenced. Both CT and US are used to monitor iceball formation. After probe removal a contrast CT is obtained in the radiology suite with delayed images (in cases when the lesion is endophytic or in close proximity to the renal pelvis) to evaluate for hematoma, an acute bleed or collecting system injury (Fig. 15.2). Patients are admitted and observed overnight. A hematocrit is drawn post-operatively and the patient is allowed to have a regular diet. Almost all of our patients are discharged home on the first postoperative day. Follow-up imaging consists of an MRI with gadolinium performed 6 months after the procedure.

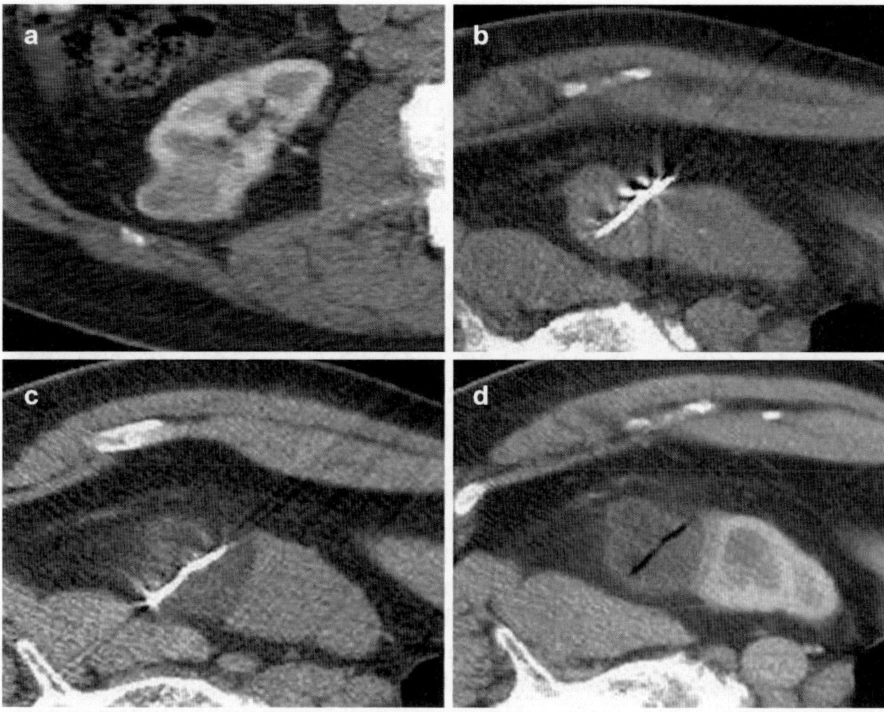

Fig. 15.2 Technique for Percutaneous Renal Cryoablation. (**a**) 3.1 cm renal mass pre-procedure imaging. (**b**) Placement of two cryoprobes under US and CT guidance. (**c**) Imaging at the end of the double freeze-thaw cycle. (**d**) Post-contrast imaging after removal of cryoprobes [44]

Outcomes

Kunkle et al. in 2008, performed a meta-analysis comparing cryoablation (19 studies, 372 lesions) to partial nephrectomy, RFA and active surveillance [31]. The authors found that patients undergoing cryoablation were significantly older than those undergoing partial nephrectomy (mean age: 65.7 vs. 60.1 years old; $p < 0.001$). The mean tumor size was significantly smaller for patients undergoing cryoablation compared to partial nephrectomy (2.56 vs. 3.40 cm; $p < 0.001$) but similar when compared to patients undergoing RFA (2.56 vs. 2.69 cm; $p = 0.40$). The mean follow-up was significantly shorter for both thermal ablation options when compared to partial nephrectomy (cryoablation, RFA, partial nephrectomy: 18.3 vs. 16.4 vs. 54.0 months respectively; $p < 0.001$), further highlighting the need for studies with longer follow-up for patients undergoing thermal ablation. When assessing local recurrence, the study found a recurrence rate of 2.6% following partial nephrectomy compared to 4.6% for cryoablation and 11.7% for RFA. Progression to metastatic disease was described in 5.6% of patients undergoing partial nephrectomy, 1.2% in patients undergoing cryoablation and 2.3% in patients undergoing RFA.

gradual shrinkage over time [46]. Gill et al. reviewed the MRI appearance of tumors treated via cryoablation in 56 patients and found gradual involution of the ablation zone by up to 75% after 3 years [47]. Stein et al. showed that in a series of 30 patients (32 cases) treated with laparoscopic renal cryoablation, 84% of treated renal masses showed no contrast enhancement at the site of treatment at 3 month imaging follow-up [48]. However 16% percent of the ablation sites showed enhancement at 3 months with three (9%) persisting by 6 months and only one displayed enhancement at 9 months. The patient with persistent enhancement at 9 months underwent a partial nephrectomy which demonstrated no recurrence of cancer. Porter et al. studied the MRI characteristics of patients undergoing renal cryoablation and also found 8 of 23 lesions imaged within 6–36 hours after ablation enhanced on MRI [49]. Seven of the eight lesions exhibited no enhancement at 6 month follow-up imaging. The authors concluded that it may thus be reasonable to wait 6 months after technically successful renal cryoablation before performing contrast-enhanced MRI. The exact cause of the persistent post-ablation enhancement in treated tumors is not known. Immediately post-ablation, tumor enhancement may be due to delayed coagulative necrosis, persistent enhancement beyond this time may be due to persistent flow in large intratumoral vessels after cryotherapy [49]. Bolte et al. assessed the MRI appearance of renal ablation sites post-cryoablation and noted peripheral rim enhancement as a common finding (7/18 patients) within 3 months of follow-up [46]. Though four of the seven patients had resolution of the rim enhancement on follow-up imaging, patients with peripheral rim enhancement with an increase in lesion size or nodular enhancement were found to have local recurrence (Fig. 15.3). Rim enhancement of these lesions may be due to viable tissue at the border of the iceball (since the peripheral edge of the ablation zone only reaches 0 °C) [46]. In cases where there is peripheral rim enhancement with an increase in lesion size or nodular enhancement of the lesion, one should consider biopsy of the ablation site. Local recurrences post-cryoablation may be treated with repeat cryoablation or surgical management [43, 50].

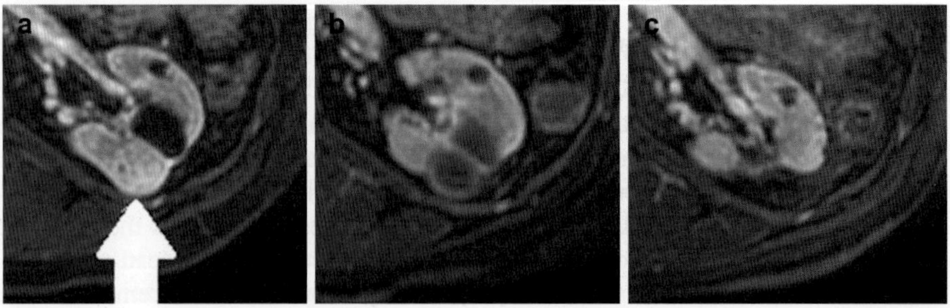

Fig. 15.3 Recurrence following Percutaneous Renal Cryoablation. (**a**) 2.6 cm renal mass in a patient with VHL. (**b**) Peripheral rim enhancement and central nodularity on superior aspect of lesion 6 months after percutaneous cryoablation. (**c**) One year following repeat percutaneous cryoablation of lesion [44]

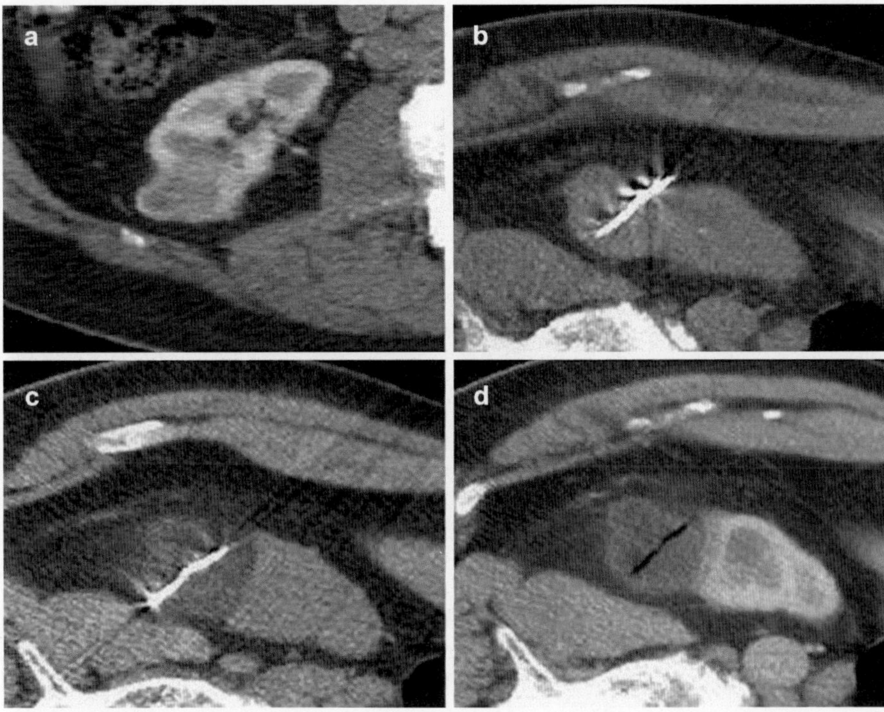

Fig. 15.2 Technique for Percutaneous Renal Cryoablation. (**a**) 3.1 cm renal mass pre-procedure imaging. (**b**) Placement of two cryoprobes under US and CT guidance. (**c**) Imaging at the end of the double freeze-thaw cycle. (**d**) Post-contrast imaging after removal of cryoprobes [44]

Outcomes

Kunkle et al. in 2008, performed a meta-analysis comparing cryoablation (19 studies, 372 lesions) to partial nephrectomy, RFA and active surveillance [31]. The authors found that patients undergoing cryoablation were significantly older than those undergoing partial nephrectomy (mean age: 65.7 vs. 60.1 years old; $p < 0.001$). The mean tumor size was significantly smaller for patients undergoing cryoablation compared to partial nephrectomy (2.56 vs. 3.40 cm; $p < 0.001$) but similar when compared to patients undergoing RFA (2.56 vs. 2.69 cm; $p = 0.40$). The mean follow-up was significantly shorter for both thermal ablation options when compared to partial nephrectomy (cryoablation, RFA, partial nephrectomy: 18.3 vs. 16.4 vs. 54.0 months respectively; $p < 0.001$), further highlighting the need for studies with longer follow-up for patients undergoing thermal ablation. When assessing local recurrence, the study found a recurrence rate of 2.6% following partial nephrectomy compared to 4.6% for cryoablation and 11.7% for RFA. Progression to metastatic disease was described in 5.6% of patients undergoing partial nephrectomy, 1.2% in patients undergoing cryoablation and 2.3% in patients undergoing RFA.

The panel for the AUA 2009 Guideline for the Management of the Clinical T1 Renal Mass performed a meta-analysis which included 15 studies (644 patients) on cryoablation compared to other treatment options including active surveillance, RFA, open partial nephrectomy (OPN), laparoscopic partial nephrectomy (LPN), open radical nephrectomy (ORN) and laparoscopic radical nephrectomy (LRN) [26]. The mean age for patients undergoing cryoablation was 67.0 years compared to 68.5, 59.5, 60.4, 62.7 and 60.7 years for patients undergoing RFA, OPN, LPN, ORN and LRN respectively. The mean tumor size for patients undergoing cryoablation was 2.6 cm compared to 2.7, 3.2, 2.6, 4.9, and 4.8 cm for patients undergoing RFA, OPN, LPN, ORN and LRN respectively. The complication rate for patients undergoing cryoablation was 4.9% (95% CI: 3.3–7.4%) compared to 6.0%, 6.3%, 9.0%, 1.3% and 3.4% for patients undergoing RFA, OPN, LPN and LRN respectively. ORN complication rates were significantly lower than all other groups ($p < 0.05$). The complication rates for cryoablation, RFA and OPN were indistinguishable ($p > 0.05$). The local recurrence free survival rates for cryoablation and RFA (90.6% and 87.0% respectively) were significantly lower than LPN, OPN, LRN and ORN (98.4%, 98.0%, 99.2%, 98.1% respectively) ($p < 0.05$).

A multi-institutional study by Johnson et al. defined the complications associated with cryoablation (139 cases) and RFA (132 cases) for small renal masses (181 percutaneous, 90 laparoscopic) [32]. The rate of major and minor complications for patients undergoing cryoablation were 1.8% (n = 2) and 9.2% (n = 17) respectively. Reported complications for cryoablation included: Minor: probe site pain or paresthesia (n = 10, 7.2%), post-operative urinary tract infection (n = 2, 1.4%), post-operative pneumonia (n = 1), minor hemorrhage (n = 1), elevated serum creatinine (n = 1), wound infection (n = 1), respiratory difficulty (n = 1); Major: significant hemorrhage (n = 1), open conversion (n = 1) due to inability to access the tumor laparoscopically. There were no deaths in patients undergoing cryoablation and the study showed a decrease in the rate of complications with increased experience. Other potentially significant complications that can occur with percutaneous renal cryoablation include: ureteral stricture—related to the proximity of the ureter to the ablation site, urine leak—as manifest by contrast extravasation outside the collecting system on the delayed phase of post-procedure CT scan imaging, bowel injury and pneumothorax—which can occur when treating upper pole renal tumors (post-procedure CT scans should include the lower lung and viewed with lung windows to exclude pneumothorax) [33–35]. Ice ball fracture is a rare complication associated with renal cryoablation that can be associated with significant hemorrhage requiring prompt intervention. Some risk factors for ice ball fractures include the use of large-diameter cryoablation probes (those used for laparoscopic cryoablation), use of multiple probes and premature removal of the cryoablation probes before the ice ball has completely thawed [36].

Contemporary clinical series have shown that flank pain (cryoprobe site pain or parethesia) continues to be the most common complication reported for renal cryoablation (9.8–10.8%) [37, 38]. In a series of 162 patients by Sidana et al. treated with renal cryoablation, the size of the lesion ($p = 0.001$), the number of cryoablation probes ($p < 0.001$) and chronic anticoagulation ($p < 0.05$) were associated with an increased incidence of significant hematoma.

Vricella et al. in a retrospective study of 52 patients treated with percutaneous renal cryoablation found that Charlson comorbidity index score ($p = 0.02$) and the number of cryoprobes used ($p < 0.005$) both significantly correlated with an increase in post-operative complications [39]. Okhunov et al. performed a retrospective analysis of 190 patients undergoing percutaneous renal cryoablation for T1a renal tumors [40]. They observed an 8.4% complication rate with 14 Clavien Grade I complications (6 large renal/retroperitoneal hematomas, 2% pneumothoraxes, 1% UTIs, 1% atrial fibrillation). There were 2 (1%) Clavien Grade II complications (intestinal perforations). Multivariable analysis showed that larger tumor dimension (OR = 2.85; $p = 0.006$) and more cryoablation probes (OR = 1.94, $p < 0.001$) were independently associated with higher risk of major complications.

The use of nephrometry scores (such as RENAL score [radius, exophytic/endophytic properties of the tumor, how close the deepest portion of the tumor is to the collecting system or renal sinus, anterior/posterior descriptor, location relative to polar line], PADUA score [pre-operative aspects and dimensions used for an anatomical score) may be helpful to predict complications after renal cryoablation, as the size of the lesion and higher nephrometry scores have been associated with a higher risk of complications [41, 42].

Ozkhunov et al. retrospectively reviewed their experience with salvage percutaneous renal cryoablation for biopsy proven renal cell carcinoma recurrence following primary cryoablation procedures [43]. Their study included 20 patients who underwent repeat cryoablation for 21 locally recurrent tumors, with a mean tumor size of 2.4 cm. All salvage cryoablation procedures were completed successfully without any complications and had a median follow-up of 30 months (range: 7–63 months). Three patients (15%) had local recurrence, occurring at 6, 13 and 35 months. Salvage percutaneous cryoablation after primary cryoablation failure is thus a feasible option with a low complication rate and acceptable short term oncologic outcomes.

Post-procedure Follow-up

The definition of therapeutic success following percutaneous renal cryoablation is based on the radiographic appearance of post-ablation axial imaging. Either contrast CT scan or MRI may be used to radiographically follow patients post-ablation [44]. Post-cryoablation lesions should decrease in size as the resultant inflammatory reaction following the thawing of the ice ball will lead to resorption of the necrotic cellular debris [45]. Though contrast enhancement of the lesion and/or growth of the lesion post-procedure can both signal local recurrence it is important to be aware that persistent contrast enhancement can be present up to 9 months post-cryoablation. Shortly after ablation, the ablated tumor may exhibit slight enlargement in size likely due to inflammation with gradual shrinkage over time [46]. Gill et al. reviewed the MRI appearance of tumors treated via cryoablation in 56 patients and found gradual involution of the ablation zone by up to 75% after 3 years [47]. Stein et al. showed that in a series of 30 patients (32 cases) treated with laparoscopic renal cryoablation, 84% of treated renal masses showed no contrast enhancement at the site of treatment at 3 month imaging follow-up [48]. However 16% percent of the ablation sites showed enhancement at 3 months with three (9%) persisting by 6 months and only one displayed enhancement at 9 months. The patient with persistent enhancement at 9 months underwent a partial nephrectomy which demonstrated no recurrence of cancer. Porter et al. studied the MRI characteristics of patients undergoing renal cryoablation and also found 8 of 23 lesions imaged within 6–36 hours after ablation enhanced on MRI [49]. Seven of the eight lesions exhibited no enhancement at 6 month follow-up imaging. The authors concluded that it may thus be reasonable to wait 6 months after technically successful renal cryoablation before performing contrast-enhanced MRI. The exact cause of the persistent post-ablation enhancement in treated tumors is not known. Immediately post-ablation, tumor enhancement may be due to delayed coagulative necrosis, persistent enhancement beyond this time may be due to persistent flow in large intratumoral vessels after cryotherapy [49]. Bolte et al. assessed the MRI appearance of renal ablation sites post-cryoablation and noted peripheral rim enhancement as a common finding (7/18 patients) within 3 months of follow-up [46]. Though four of the seven patients had resolution of the rim enhancement on follow-up imaging, patients with peripheral rim enhancement with an increase in lesion size or nodular enhancement were found to have local recurrence (Fig. 15.3). Rim enhancement of these lesions may be due to viable tissue at the border of the iceball (since the peripheral edge of the ablation zone only reaches 0 °C) [46]. In cases where there is peripheral rim enhancement with an increase in lesion size or nodular enhancement of the lesion, one should consider biopsy of the ablation site. Local recurrences post-cryoablation may be treated with repeat cryoablation or surgical management [43, 50].

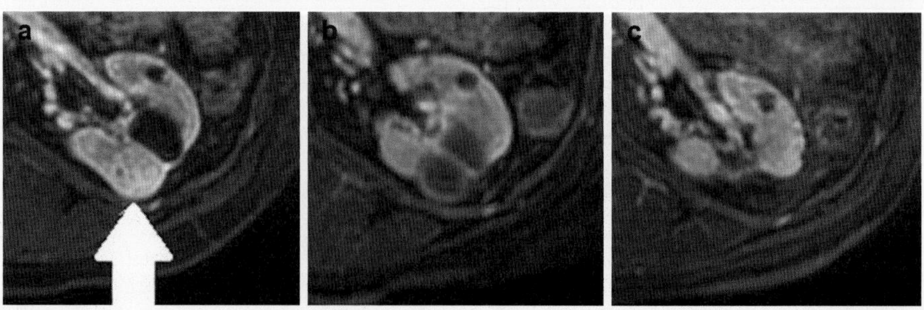

Fig. 15.3 Recurrence following Percutaneous Renal Cryoablation. (**a**) 2.6 cm renal mass in a patient with VHL. (**b**) Peripheral rim enhancement and central nodularity on superior aspect of lesion 6 months after percutaneous cryoablation. (**c**) One year following repeat percutaneous cryoablation of lesion [44]

Conclusions

We have come a long way since James Arnott's usage of a mixture of crushed ice and salt for the first therapeutic use of cryoablation. The technologic innovations in cryotherapy, the development of smaller cryoprobes as well as a better understanding of cryobiology have led to the development of percutaneous renal cryoablation. With the advantages of minimal invasiveness, reproducibility and rapid patient recovery, percutaneous renal cryoablation can be a nephron sparing alternative to partial nephrectomy for the treatment of small renal tumors in select patients. Despite promising short/intermediate term outcomes, a larger number of studies with longer follow-up are required to assess its long term efficacy.

References

1. Hollingsworth JM, Miller DC, Daignault S, Hollenbeck BK. Rising incidence of small renal masses: a need to reassess treatment effect. J Natl Cancer Inst. 2006;98:1331–4.
2. Rodriguez Faba O, Akdogan B, Marszalek M, Langenhuijsen JF, Brookman-May S, Stewart GD, Capitanio U, Sanguedolce F. Renal cancer working group of the Young Academic Urologists (YAU), working party of the European Association of Urology (EAU). Current status of focal cryoablation for small renal masses. Urology. 2016;90:9–15.
3. Chosy SG, Nakada SY, Lee FT, et al. Monitoring kidney cryosurgery: predictors of tissue necrosis in swine. J Urol. 1998;159:1370–4.
4. Arnott J. On the treatment of cancer by the regulated application of an anaesthetic temperature. London: Churchill; 1851.
5. Arnott J. Practical illustrations of the remedial efficacy of a very low or anesthetic temperature I: in cancer. Lancet. 1950;2:257–9.
6. Bird H, James Arnott MD. (Aberdeen) 1797–1883. A pioneer in refrigeration. Anaesthesia. 1949;4:10–7.
7. Cooper SM, Dawber RPR. The history of cryosurgery. J R Soc Med. 2001;94:196–201.
8. White AC. Possibilities of liquid air to the physician. JAMA. 1907;49:371–7.
9. Pusey W. The use of carbon dioxide snow in the treatment of naevi and other lesions of the skin. JAMA. 1935;49:1354–9.
10. Gage AA. Progress in cryosurgery. Cryobiology. 1992;29:300–4.
11. Das K, Benzil DL, Rovit RL, Irving S. Cooper (1922–1985): a pioneer in functional neurosurgery. J Neurosurgery. 1988;89:865–73.
12. Cooper IS, Lee A. Cryostatic congelation: a system for producing a limited controlled region of cooling or freezing of biologic tissues. J Nerv Ment Dis. 1961;133:259–63.
13. Wen CC, Nakada SY. Energy ablative techniques for treatment of small renal tumors. Curr Opin Urol. 2006;16:321–6.
14. Uchida M, Imaide Y, Sugimoto K, et al. Percutaneous cryosurgery for renal tumors. Br J Urol. 1995;75:132–6.
15. Gill IS, Novick AC, Soble JJ, et al. Laparoscopic renal cryoablation: initial clinical series. Urology. 1998;52:543–51.
16. Matin SF, Sharma P, Gill IS, Tannenbaum C, Hobart MG, Novick AC, Finke JH. Immunological response to renal cryoablation in an in vivo orthotopic renal cell carcinoma murine model. J Urol. 2010;183:333–8.
17. Nakada SY, Jerde TJ, Warner TF, Lee FT. Comparison of radiofrequency ablation, cryoablation, and nephrectomy in treating implanted vx-2 carcinoma in rabbit kidneys. J Endourol. 2004;18:501–6.

18. Baust JG, Gage AA, Bjerlund Johansen TE, Baust JM. Mechanisms of cryoablation: clinical consequences on malignant tumors. Cryobiology. 2014;68:1–11.
19. Hoffmann NE, Bischof JC. The cryobiology of cryosurgical injury. Urology. 2002;60:40–9.
20. Baust JG, Gage AA. The molecular basis of cryosurgery. BJU Int. 2005;95:1187–91.
21. Lagerveld BW, van Horssen P, Laguna Pes MP, van den Wijngaard JP, Streekstra GJ, de la Rosette JJ, Wijkstra H, Spaan JA. Immediate effect of kidney cryoablation on renal arterial structure in a porcine model studied by imaging cryomicrotome. J Urol. 2010;183:1221–6.
22. Lagerveld BW, van Horssen P, Laguna MP, can den Wijngaard JP, Wijkstra MS, de la Rosette JJ, Spaan JA. Gradient changes in porcine renal arterial vascular anatomy and blood flow after cryoablation. J Urol. 2011;186:681–6.
23. Young JL, Kolla SB, Pick DL, Sountoulides P, Kaufmann OG, Ortiz-Vanderdys CG, Huynh VB, Kaplan AG, Andrade LA, Osann KE, Louie MK, McDougall EM, Clayman RV. In vitro, ex vivo and in vivo isotherms for renal cryotherapy. J Urol. 2010;183:752–8.
24. Young JL, McCormick DW, Kolla SB, Sountoulides PG, Kaufmann OG, Ortiz-Vanderdys CG, Huynh VB, Kaplan AG, Jain NS, Pick DL, Andrade LA, Osann KE, McDougall EM, Clayman RV. Are multiple cryoprobes additive or synergistic in renal cryotherapy? Urology. 2012;79(484):e1–6.
25. Raman JD, Hall DW, Cadeddu JA. Renal ablative therapy: radiofrequency ablation and cryoablation. J Surg Oncol. 2009;100:639–44.
26. Campbell SC, Novick AC, Belldegrun A, Blute ML, Chow GK, Derweesh IH, Faraday MM, Kaouk JH, Leveillee RJ, Matin SF, Russo P, Uzzo RG. Guideline for management of the clinical T1 renal mass. J Urol. 2009;182:1271–9.
27. Hinshaw JL, Shadid AM, Nakada SY, Hedican SP, Winter TC, Lee FT. Comparison of percutaneous and laparoscopic cryoablation for the treatment of solid renal masses. AJR Am J Roentgenol. 2008;191:1159–68.
28. Patel SR, Abel EJ, Hedican SP, Nakada SY. Ablation of small renal masses: practice patterns at academic institutions in the United States. J Endourol. 2013;27:158–61.
29. Bodily KD, Atwell TD, Mandrekar JN, Farrell MA, Callstrom MR, Schmit GD, Charboneau JW. Hydrodisplacement in the percutaneous cryoablation of 50 renal tumors. AJR Am J Roentgenol. 2010;194:779–83.
30. Patel SR, Hinshaw JL, Lubner MG, Lee FT Jr, Nakada SY, Hedican SP. Hydrodissection using an iodinated contrast medium during percutaneous renal cryoablation. J Endourol. 2012;26:463–6.
31. Kunkle DA, Egleston BL, Uzzo RG. Excise, ablate or observe. The small renal mass dilemma—a meta-analysis and review. J Urol. 2008;179:1227–34.
32. Johnson DB, Solomon SB, Matsumoto ED, Kavoussi LR, Nakada SY, Moon TD, Shingleton WB, Cadeddu JA. Defining the complications of cryoablation and radiofrequency ablation of small renal tumors: a multi-institutional review. J Urol. 2004;172:874–7.
33. Wile GE, Leyendecker JR, Krehbiel KA, Dyer RB, Zagoria RJ. CT and MR imaging after image-guided thermal ablation of renal neoplasms. Radiographics. 2007;27:325–41.
34. Warlick CA, Lima GC, Allaf ME, et al. Clinical sequelae of radiographic iceball involvement of collecting system during computed tomography-guided percutaneous renal tumor cryoablation. Urology. 2006;67:918–22.
35. Brashears JH, Raj GV, Crisci A, et al. Renal cryoablation and radiofrequency ablation: an evaluation of worst case scenarios in a porcine model. J Urol. 2005;173:2160–5.
36. Schmitt GD, Atwell TD, Callstrom MR, Kurup AN, Fleming CJ, Andrews JC, Charboneau JW. Ice ball fractures during percutaneous renal cryoablation: risk factors and potential implications. J Vasc Interv Radiol. 2010;21:1309–12.
37. Sidana A, Aggarwal P, Feng Z, Georgiades CS, Trock BJ, Rodriguez R. Complications of renal cryoablation: a single center experience. J Urol. 2010;184:42–7.
38. Tsivian M, Chen VH, Kim CY, Zilberman DE, Mouraview V, Nelson RC, Albala DM, Polascik TJ. Complications of laparoscopic and percutaneous renal cryoablation in a single tertiary referral center. Eur Urol. 2010;58:142–8.

39. Vricella GJ, Haaga JR, Adler BL, Nakamoto D, Cherullo EE, Flick S, Ponsky LE. Percutaneous cryoablation of renal masses: impact of patient selection and treatment parameters on outcomes. Urology. 2011;77:649–54.
40. Okhunov Z, Moreira DM, Del Junco M, Abedi G, Lobko II, Kaler KS, Nguyen ND, Youseff R, Uchio E, Kavoussi LR, Landman J. Predictors of complications after percutaneous image-guided renal cryoablation for T1a renal cortical neoplasms. J Endourol. 2017;31:7–13.
41. Schmidt GD, Schenck LA, Thompson RH, et al. Prediting renal cryoablation complications: new risk score based on tumor size and location and patient history. Radiology. 2014;272:903–10.
42. Sisul DM, Liss MA, Palazzi KL, et al. RENAL nephrometry score is associated with complications after renal cryoablation: a multicenter analysis. Urology. 2013;81:775–80.
43. Okhunov Z, Chamberlin J, Moreira DM, George A, Babaian K, Shah P, youseff R, Kaler KS, Lobko II, Kavoussi L, Landman J. Salvage percutaneous cryoablation for locally recurrent renal-cell carcinoma after primary cryoablation. J Endourol. 2016;30:632–7.
44. Patel SR, Nakada SY. Percutaneous renal cryoablation. J Endourol (Japanese). 2011;24:164–9.
45. Kawamoto S, Solomon SB, Bluemke DA, Fishman EK. CT and MR imaging appearance of renal neoplasms after radiofrequency ablation and cryoablation. Semin Ultrasound CT MR. 2009;30:67–77.
46. Bolte SL, Ankem MK, Moon TD, Hedican SP, Lee FT, Sadowski EA, Nakada SY. Magnetic resonance imaging findings after laparoscopic renal cryoablation. Urology. 2006;67:485–9.
47. Gill IS, Remer EM, Hasan WA, Strzempkowski B, Spaliviero M, Steinberg AP, et al. Renal cryoablation: outcome at 3 years. J Urol. 2005;173:1903–7.
48. Stein AJ, Mayes JM, Mouraviev V, Chen VH, Nelson RC, Polascik TJ. Persistent contrast enhancement several months after laparoscopic cryoablation of the small renal mass may not indicate recurrent tumor. J Endourol. 2008;22:2433–9.
49. Porter CA, Woodrum DA, Callstrom MR, Schmit GD, Misra S, Charoneau JW, Atwell TD. MRI after technically successful renal cryoablation: early contrast enhancement as a common finding. AJR Am J Roentgenol. 2010;194:790–3.
50. Long L, Park S. Differences in patterns of care: reablation and nephrectomy rates after needle ablative therapy for renal masses stratified by medical specialty. J Endourol. 2009;23:421–6.

Chapter 16
Radiofrequency Ablation in the Treatment of Renal Tumors

Emily F. Kelly and Raymond J. Leveillee

Introduction

As abdominal imaging machines have become more readily available and utilized, the diagnosis of asymptomatic small renal masses (SRM) has increased. These incidental tumors account for 60% of renal cell carcinoma (RCC) diagnosis and are most often found at earlier stages and/or grades [1–3]. The incidence of RCC has been found to increase roughly 2% each year [4]. Overall, RCC is the thirteenth most common cancer worldwide and 10th most common in the Western World. In 2016, it was estimated that annually 62,700 cases and 14,240 deaths occur secondary to RCC in the United States alone [5]. Worldwide RCC accounts for the diagnosis of 270,000 cases and 116,000 deaths each year [4]. Of these patients, 20–30% of patients are found to have metastatic disease. The incidence of RCC is greatest in North America, Europe, and Australia and diagnosed least frequently in India, Africa, China, and Japan. Risk factors include smoking, increased waist-to-hip-ratio, germline mutations, and occupational exposure to trichloroethylene and perchloroethylene [4]. Two to three percent of RCC cases are familial, most commonly autosomal dominant Von-Hippel-Lindau (VHL) disease. Familial disease is frequently bilateral and multifocal, therefore correct diagnosis is essential for guiding treatment [4].

E.F. Kelly, M.D. (✉)
Department of Surgery, Division of Urology, Florida Atlantic University, Charles E. Schmidt College of Medicine, Boca Raton, FL, USA
e-mail: ekelly20@health.fau.edu

R.J. Leveillee, M.D., F.R.C.S.-G.
Department of Surgery, Division of Urology, Florida Atlantic University, Charles E. Schmidt College of Medicine, Boca Raton, FL, USA

Department of Urology, Bethesda Health Systems, Boynton Beach, FL, USA
e-mail: rleveillee@bhpgdoc.com

S.R. Patel et al. (eds.), *The History of Technologic Advancements in Urology*,
DOI 10.1007/978-3-319-61691-9_16

The Early History of RFA

Radiofrequency ablation was originally established for the ablation of aberrant cardiac pathways. Initially RFA became a treatment modality for unresectable liver tumors where significant technological advances were researched and developed and treatment protocols established [6]. Over the past two decades, the use of RFA has readily expanded. Breast, prostate, pancreatic, renal, and gynecological tumors are now commonly treated with RFA technology [7]. Recently renal ablation has acquired more acceptance in the urological community as long-term studies have shown its effectiveness in the treatment of small renal masses (SRM). This chapter will focus on the history and development of various radiofrequency ablation treatment options available.

Nephron-Sparing Surgery

Historically, RCC has been treated by radical nephrectomy (RN). Due to the increased diagnosis of lower stage/grade lesions in recent years, Nephron Sparing Surgery (NSS) has gained favor allowing for the conservation of the surrounding unaffected renal parenchyma and nephrons [2]. Options include partial nephrectomy (PN), thermal ablation (TA), and non-TA modalities. TA can be achieved through several mechanisms including RFA, cryoablation (CRY), microwave ablation (MWA), high-intensity focused ultrasound (HIFU), and laser interstitial thermotherapy [3]. Non-thermal ablation is performed less frequently via irreversible electroporation [3, 8, 9]. Of the TA modalities CRY and RFA have gained the most provider support. NSS, specifically, PN is the current standard of care for tumors found outside of the collecting system [3].

Recently, Olweny et al. showed that the 5-year oncologic outcomes of RFA vs. PN in T1a treated patients with RCC were similar, both having a cancer-specific survival rate greater than 95% [10]. However, PN still remains the standard of care secondary to the lack of studies demonstrating long-term outcomes of TA. With advances in technology and the increased availability of long-term outcome studies, TA holds a promising future for becoming the treatment of choice for solid SRM [1, 8].

Indications and Guidelines for the Use of TA

New treatment guidelines were released in 2009 by the American Urologic Association (AUA) where thermal ablation (TA) was included as a treatment "option" for all patients with SRM and T1b tumors. SRM can be defined as lesions <4 cm or clinical stage T1a, whereas T1b represents tumors >4 cm and <7 cm [11, 12]. Prior to the update, TA was "recommended" solely for the treatment of T1a tumors in patients with major co-morbidities. This category includes patients of increased age, with solitary kidneys, renal insufficiency, bilateral tumors, local reoccurrence after previous PN, patients with a genetic susceptibility for multiple tumors (VHL syndrome), and patients unable to undergo surgery [2, 8]. Now, the use of TA has expanded as a treatment "option" to all patients with T1a/b lesions including both healthy and comorbid patients [7, 11, 13, 14].

How Does RFA Work?

The fundamentals governing the mechanism of RFA are founded on the three principals of thermodynamics; conduction, convection, and radiation [15]. Conduction is defined as the movement of energy, or heat, through a solid medium. This principle provides the basis of heat-sinking, discussed later in this chapter. The end point of RFA is coagulative necrosis resulting from thermal induced cellular death and protein denaturation [7, 16].

In RFA, heat, is delivered via a monopolar probe using alternating current of 380–500 kHz from a needle electrode to grounding pads on the skin surface [8]. Success is dependent on the inverse relationship between time and temperature. As the temperature increases, the time required for complete ablation decreases [7, 8]. When the ablation zone reaches between 60 and 100 °C these changes occur instantaneously [7]. We recommend a probe design which will achieve tissue temperature of at least 60 °C to attain adequate ionic agitation for cellular death and successful ablation. A margin of at least 5 mm beyond the tumor is recommended to assure adequate treatment. Monitoring of tissue temperature and target endpoints has been the major challenge to widespread acceptance of RFA as the primary TA modality since heat cannot be monitored readily radiographically [7].

Limitations

Lorber et al. and Ferakis et al., have studied and demonstrated the relationship between tumor size and location in ablation success [17, 18]. This relationship can be best described by "heat sinking." Heat by conduction moves by way of a gradient from high temperature to low temperature, or from probe to tissue. This mechanism is increased in large tumors and vascular tumors, where the temperature gradient is increased, resulting in lower temperature at the ablation site secondary to diffusion. This results in a higher likelihood of incomplete ablation [3, 7, 8, 19]. Ferakis et al., in their series of 31 patients with 39 renal tumors ranging in size between 1.3 and 7.5 cm reported an initial ablation success of 90%. Of the tumors which reoccurred, tumor size >4 cm was found to be the number one predicting factor ($P < 0.01$, $RR = 3.31$). Furthermore, half of the centrally located tumors recurred compared to 5.9% of peripheral tumors [18]. The "heat sinking" phenomenon and determination of treatment endpoint can be overcome by the use of real-time temperature monitoring.

Improvements to Original RFA: Real-Time Temperature Monitoring

Real-time temperature monitoring allows the clinician to monitor the completeness and precision of the ablation zone, decrease the need for repeat ablation sessions, and prevent overtreatment which could damage surrounding tissue [20]. This method involves the placement of peripheral 200-μm non-conduction fiber-optic temperature probes (Lumasense, Santa Clara, CA) 5 mm from the edge of the lesion allowing for ablation to be delivered until all probes read >60 °C (Fig. 16.1). Location and histology of RCC are important since the intratumor and peritumor vascularity of the lesion can limit the effectiveness of RFA when a target endpoint is not identified [21]. Wingo and Leveillee showed that the use of temperature monitoring probes, "enhanced method," allows for successful treatment of endophytic, or centrally located tumors and expands the ablation success to allow for medium sized tumors (<5 cm) to be treated compared to the previous <4 cm recommendation. In this study 39 patients with 41 tumors were ablated under the guidance of temperature monitoring probes and followed for an average of 29 months. 92.7% of these treatments were managed successfully by a single RFA session [7]. Furthermore, Lorber et al. revealed similar results with greater than 48 months follow up in a study of 53 treatments in 50 patients with biopsy proven RCC using real-time temperature monitoring. The 5-year overall survival rate was 98%, cancer-specific survival was 100%, and reoccurrence-free survival was 92.5% [17]. Carey et al. described the use of

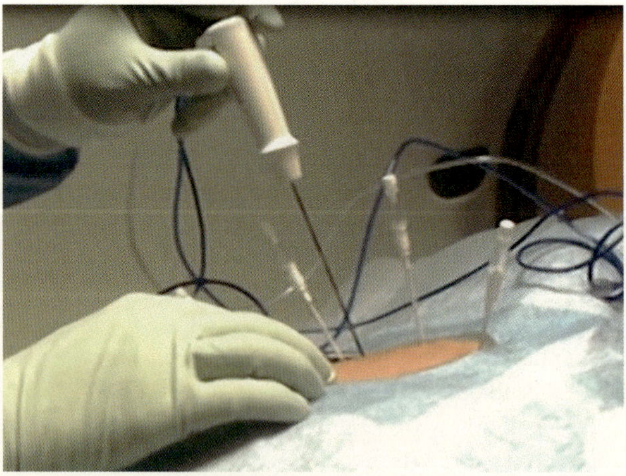

Fig. 16.1 Placement of three to four fiber-optic temperature probes (Lumasense, Santa Clara, CA) are placed at the peripheral and deep margins 5 mm from the tumor-parenchymal interface. This allows for ablation to be delivered until all probes read >60 °C. The Cool-tip® (Covidien, Valley Lab, Boulder, CO, USA) probe with hand piece is visualized in the center of the temperature probes

non-conducting temperature probes in tumors between 3 and 5 cm in 96 patients. Hundred percentage of these ablations achieved complete necrosis at the initial treatment with the real-time temperature monitors and a subsequent 95% radiographic success rate. This finding is in contrast to Gervais and colleagues, who used RFA without temperature monitoring in 39 patients with the same tumor size between 3 and 5 cm. Complete ablation was only achieved in 93.3% of patients compared to 100% of patients when temperature monitoring was deployed in Carey et al. [20]. These results demonstrate the importance of the use of temperature monitors to enhance the clinical scope of tumors which can be treated by RFA. These studies suggest that tumors up to 5 cm in diameter as well as central and hilar located masses can be treated successfully with reduced need for retreatment when aided by real-time temperature monitoring [3]. A significant drawback, however, to this technique is the additional time required for accurate temperature probe placement, a crowded field, and the paucity of availability of these probes for clinical use.

RFA Probe History

The placement of an uninsulated needle into tissue with application of RF energy leads to a significant buildup of electrical current at the metal/tissue interface (current density) and this leads to very high temperatures that exceed 100 °C. The resulting "burn" causes vaporization and charring within a few mm of the probe itself (much like a conventional "Bovie" electrocautery device). The initial plain electrode probe used for RFA (in cardiac ablation) was nothing more than a bare metal wire and was not able to accommodate rapid rises in impedance limiting ablation size. Modifications to the original probe include bipolar (bipolar electrodes), wet electrodes (saline perfusion), internal cooling (cooled electrodes), and enlargement of the field (multiple and expandable electrodes); allowing for increased target size [16].

Three RFA systems are currently available on the market in the USA and utilize either an electrical impedance-based or temperature-based treatment algorithm. Impedance-based systems include the Cool-tip® (Convidien, Boulder, CO, USA) and LeVeen® RF system 3000® (Boston Scientific, Natick, MA, USA). The Cool-tip® (Convidien, Boulder, CO, USA) utilizes a 480 kHz RF generator where the energy output is individually determined for up to three monopolar electrodes; the single electrode or cluster 3-electrode monopolar systems (Fig. 16.2). The system pump internally perfuses and chills each electrode to prevent charring of the target tissue; limiting the temperature increase to less than 25 °C at the tissue/probe interface but allowing for diffusion of current into the surrounding tissues and thereby creating frictional agitation and secondary heat [16, 22] (Fig. 16.3). The advantage of the 3-electrode monopolar system is less charring secondary to increased surface area [16]. The LeVeen® RF system 3000® (Boston Scientific, Natick, MA, USA), formerly Radiotherapeutics, incorporates an inverted dry umbrella design which

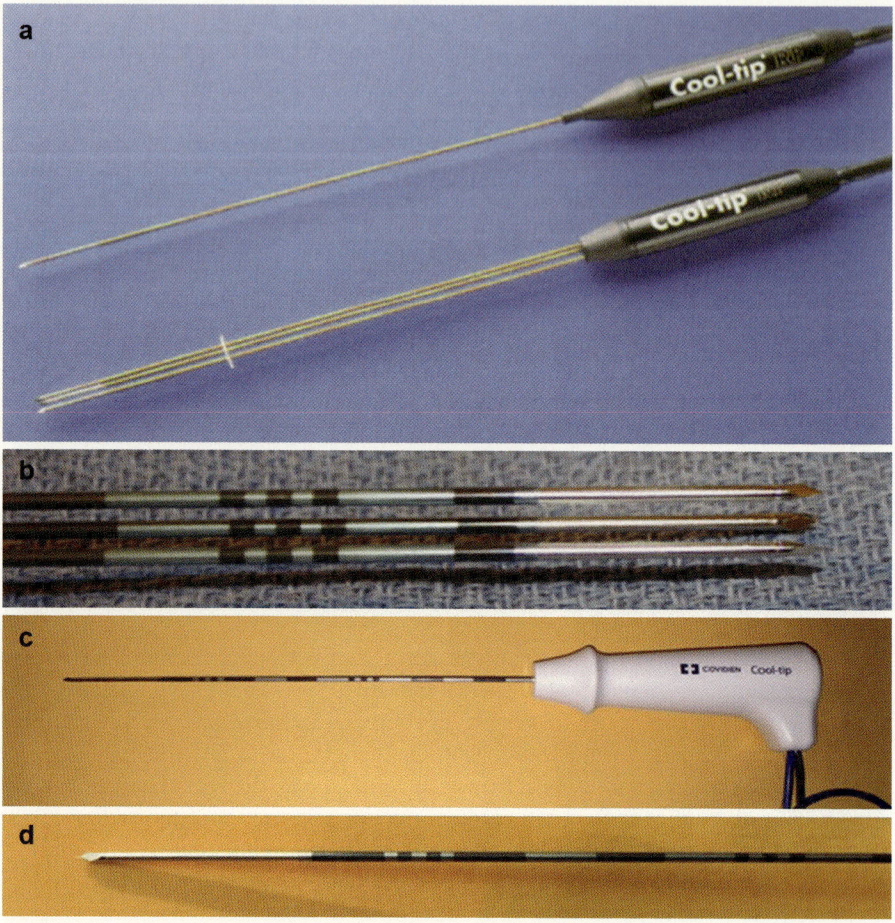

Fig. 16.2 (**a**) The 1996 Circa single-tip and cluster 3-electrode monopolar straight needles, Cool-tip® (Covidien, Valley Lab, Boulder, CO, USA) probe with hand piece. The hollow probe allows for the circulation of chilled water. (**b**) Close up of the 1996 Circa Cool-tip® 3-electrodes in one handle with the un-insulated active tip (*bracket*) and centimeter markings placed at intervals along the 10–25 cm needle shaft. This probe has a 2.5 cm emitting length. (**c**) The updated Cool-tip™ (Covidien, Medtronic, Minneapolis, MN) single straight needle provides a 17-gauge straight trocar design for accurate placement into target tissue. (**d**) Close up of the Cool-tip™ (Covidien, Medtronic, Minneapolis, MN) un-insulated active tip (*bracket*) and centimeter markings placed at intervals along the 10–25 cm needle shaft

deploys 12 tines covering a 4 cm diameter [8, 23]. This self-regulating system disperses the current over several tines and limits power output as tissue impedance rises (a Proxy for temperature) and gradually increases the power output in a technique referred to as "roll-off".

The temperature-based Starburst Radiofrequency Interstitial Tissue Ablation (RITA®) system (Angiodynamics®, Queensbury, NY, NY, USA) utilizes an

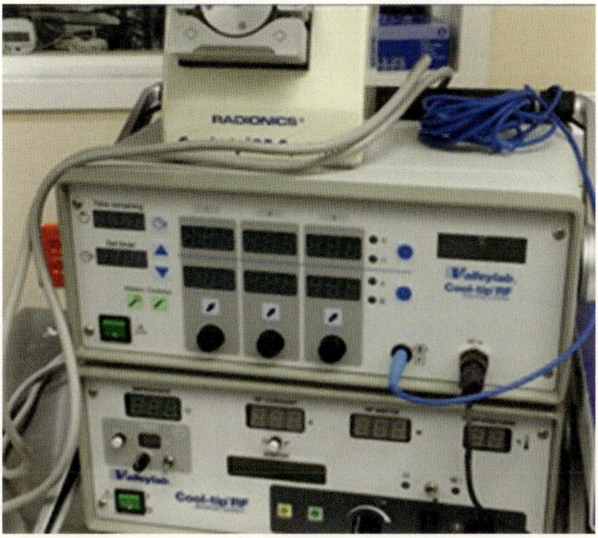

Fig. 16.3 The Cool-tip® (Covidien, Valley Lab, Boulder, CO, USA) generator. System internally perfuses and chills each electrode to prevent charring of the target tissue; limiting the temperature increase to less than 25 °C

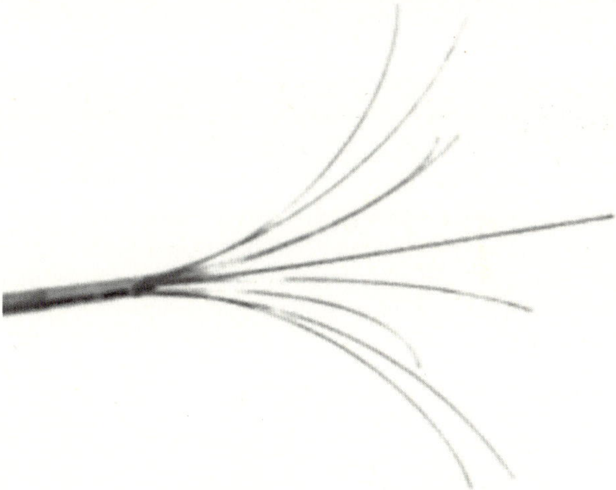

Fig. 16.4 The temperature-based Starburst Radiofrequency Interstitial Tissue Ablation (RITA®) system (Angiodynamics®, Queensbury, NY, NY, USA) utilizes an expandable (up to 9) array of small tines in a 16 gauge shaft providing up to 5 cm of deployment depth

expandable (up to 9) array of small tines in a 16 gauge shaft providing up to 5 cm of deployment depth (Fig. 16.4). Energy is delivered by a 1500 or 1500X generator. An advantage of the RITA® system is that 5 of the 9 tines are capable of intraoperative temperature recording via a thermocouple tip [23]. As the tines expand further from the shaft there is likely to be some irregular geometric shapes and one must be cautious to avoid skip lesions when utilizing the expandable devices. The Starburst system is compatible with both wet, saline infused, and the traditional dry electrodes. Dry electrodes are limited by current density requiring longer treatment times, increased electrode surface area, multi-tine electrodes, or multiple ablations [24]. Wet electrode system, allows for current density to spread via perfused conducting saline resulting in larger ablation zone size [25]. Experimentally the use of hypertonic saline (14%) provides for a more expansive and rapidly achieved ablation zone, but this concept has never been utilized commercially [26].

Animal studies with the hypertonic saline infused probes demonstrated reproducible and predictable zones of ablation in both acute and chronic studies [27]. All three of these systems can be used and system choice is dependent on physician preference [8]. A study conducted by Denys et al. compared the use of the systems mentioned above in the ablation of pig livers. The study found that the RITA® system provided the largest ablation volume and the Cool-tip® system produces an ovoid shape ablation zone, compared to other systems [25]. Lobik et al., evaluating cool tip and Rita in an experimental egg-white model determined that the former yielded "barrel shaped" lesions, whereas the expandable tined probes yield "Christmas-tree" shaped lesions [28]. Due to the fact that there are many different probe designs, and that "all RF probes are not created equal a consensus panel developed definitions to describe probe design and geometric lesion development [16].

In order to try to utilize MRI for probe placement and because MR signal can be altered by temperature in the target zone RFA specific MR-compatible devices were developed. The interface which develops between the MR machine and the RFA generator can be overcome by use of these specific MRI-compatible devices. Two MR compatible electrodes are available. First, the titanium Cool-tip RF system® (Covidien, Boulder, CO, USA) cools with circulating water which decreases the observed amount of charring within the tissue of the target thus improving results [2]. The second electrode is the nitinol StarBust Semi-Flex® (Angiodynamic®, Queensbury, NY, NY, USA) which provides a more flexible shaft for navigation to the target tissue in the MR limited gantry size and a larger ablation zone through the use of multiple active tines [2, 8] (Fig. 16.5).

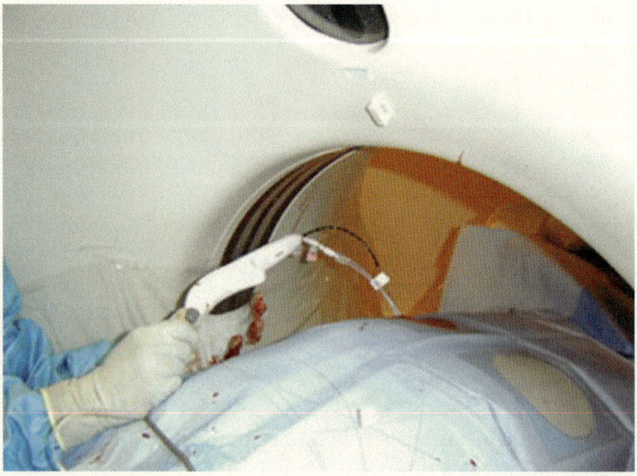

Fig. 16.5 MR-compatible StarBust Semi-Flex® (Angiodynamic®, Queensbury, NY, NY, USA) provides a flexible shaft for navigation to the target tissue in MR limited gantry size and a larger ablation zone through the use of multiple active tines

Expansion and Development of RFA: Main Delivery Mechanisms

Laparoscopic RFA

Laparoscopic US-guided RFA is utilized in anterior tumors and tumors located within 1 cm of the bowel, as described by Sterrett et al. [3]. The laparoscopic technique permits the manipulation of organs assuring that the RFA treatment is directed only toward the intended target decreasing the risk of thermal injury to the surrounding tumor free tissue. This allows for a reduction in the number of post-procedural complications resulting from thermal injury [3, 7].

First, with the patient placed on their unaffected side, small port incisions are made to allow full abdominal insufflation. Since, US imaging lacks the ability to detect heat; we recommend the placement of peripheral temperature monitors to help aid in ablation success. If temperature monitors are not utilized end goals can be monitored by pre-set impedance or temperature goals of the RFA probes depending on the system used and by direct visualization. Gas bubbles created during the ablation cycle can interfere with the US signal thus making US an unreliable way of monitoring the treatment. Three to four fiberoptic temperature probes (LumaSense, Santa Clara, CA) are placed at the peripheral and deep margins, 5 mm from boundary between the tumor and normal renal parenchyma (Fig. 16.6). Temperature probe placement is visualized under US guidance and can be aided using 5-Fr coaxial guide needle encompassed in a radiopaque sheath (Huey, Cook Vascular, Inc., Vandergrift, PA, USA) [7, 29]. Next, the RFA probe is directed toward the target tissue under US-guidance. After all temperature probes have reached the treatment

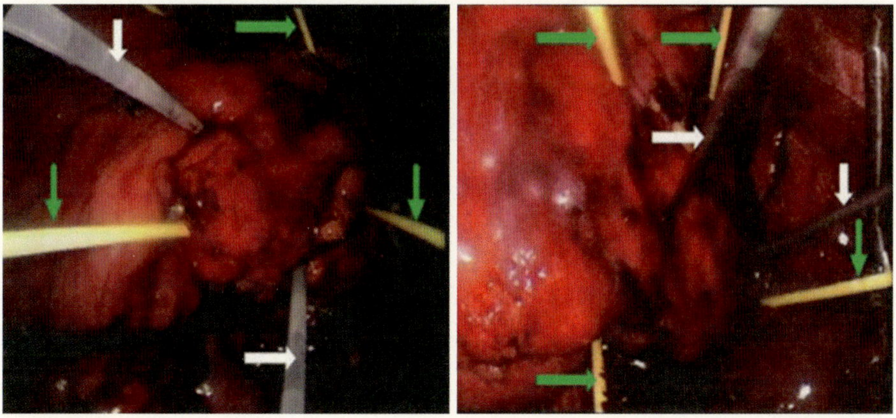

Fig. 16.6 Laparoscopic guided RFA is utilized in anterior tumors allowing for manipulation of vital surrounding organs. *Green arrows* represent fiberoptic temperature probes (LumaSense, Santa Clara, CA) placed at the peripheral and deep margins, 5 mm from boundary between the tumor and normal renal parenchyma. The *white arrow* represents the RFA probe directed toward the target tissue

goal of 60 °C, or the impedance/temperature goal has been met the RFA probe is removed, again under US guidance [3, 29].

The advantage of the laparoscopic RFA approach is the "intent to treat" described by Hui et al. and Castle et al. Percutaneous RFA can be performed by surgeons and interventionists in contrast to laparoscopic treatments which are solely performed by surgeons. The single session success rate for percutaneous approach was found to be 87% (95% CI, 82–91%) compared to 94% (95% CI, 92–96%) in the laparoscopic approach. This difference suggests that surgeons may have a more aggressive approach compared to that of interventionists [30].

Percutaneous RFA

As compared to laparoscopic RFA, the percutaneous ablation technique is best utilized for posteriorly located tumors [7]. Major delivery mechanisms include CT, MRI, cone-beam CT, and image fusion modalities; CT-guided RFA is preferred by most providers [31].

CT-RFA

CT-RFA is best utilized for posterior tumors. The patient is first placed in either the prone or lateral decubitus position. The lateral decubitus position allows for the deflation of the dependent lung decreasing movement of the kidney secondary to respiration [31]. This decreases the likelihood of pleural space injury and pneumothorax when treating upper pole masses [2, 7]. The prone position is used most often for CT-RFA of SRM. This position increases the separation between the costal margin and iliac crest allowing for a larger insertion window. However, this also increases the length of the kidney in proximity to the lung hence limiting its use for upper pole lesions [2]. CT-RFA is best performed under general anesthesia allowing manipulation of respiratory movements during probe placement [1, 7, 19].

CT-RFA is widely available decreasing the cost of the procedure [31]. CT-RFA procedures can be done at outpatient centers lowering the cost of hospital stay and resultant complications. Compared to the laparoscopic approach CT-RFA has fewer complications since laparoscopic insertion and insufflation is avoided [7]. Disadvantages include gantry-size limited access to the patient, exposure to ionizing radiation, and lack of treatment endpoint via real-time temperature monitoring [19, 31].

MR-RFA

MR-RFA was first described by Anzai et al., in 1995 for the treatment of brain tumors [32]. In 2003, Gervais and Mayo-Smith et al. reported successful MR-RFA for renal tumors [32]. In recent literature Lewin et al. provides expertise on renal

MR-RFA procedures, first introduced in 1998 [2, 7]. There are several advantages of MRI-RFA compared to CT guided treatment; most notably the lack of patient radiation exposure [2, 33]. MRI allows for increased spatial resolution and amplification of soft-tissue elements [2]. The use of MRI allows ablation of difficult-to-access lesions with trajectory limits in close vicinity to vital structures especially tumors treated near the diaphragm. These tumors are not readily accessible by CT guidance due to triangulation limits or by US due to air-artifact resulting in the increased incidence of pneumothorax [2]. More than one ablation confirmation is not possible in CT-guided RFA since contrast is needed to visualize residual tumor cells, which takes time to clear. Once contrast is injected subsequent ablation success cannot be confirmed due to the obstruction of the lingering original contrast material. As many as four ablation sessions have been reported for successful CT-RFA treatment. In contrast, MR allows for the immediate detection of post-ablation residual tumor by the presence of T2-weighted MR isointense or hyperintense signals. If residual tumor is observed, the provider can perform further ablation cycles within the same session. This eliminates the need of additional visits which would require further patient repositioning and exposure to contrast media [2, 33, 34]. It has been reported that 92–100% of MR-ablations can be achieved successfully in one session [34].

Real-time monitoring can also be achieved via MR fluoroscopy using rapid gradient echo sequences. Real-time monitoring more readily allows for the identification of a therapeutic end-point and the manipulation of the thermal ablation zone during the procedure. However, the interface of the MRI scanner presents a challenge for continuous imaging. This can be overcome by the use of intermittent MR scanning between ablations [2]. Disadvantages of MR-RFA include limited gantry size, procedure length, machine availability, equipment cost, and the need for MRI compatible sensors (as discussed earlier) [1, 31].

Cone-Beam CT

This system utilizes a large rotating C-arm and digital fluoroscopy. Manipulation of the C-arm under fluoroscopy creates a 3D model of the target allowing for precise ablation (Fig. 16.7). The trajectory is then projected onto the patient allowing for further guidance for placement of the needle along the trajectory. Once the needle is placed, further imaging is obtained via rotational angiography within seconds. This confirms needle placement and allows for further manipulation of the trajectory [1] (Fig. 16.8). A study, performed by Cheng et al., compared patient radiation exposure during cone-beam CT procedures versus conventional CT techniques in RFA ablation. Patients who underwent cone-beam ablations sustained a lower radiation dose compared to the conventional technique ($P < 0.5$), while having comparable treatment success [35]. This system is limited by respiratory movement since the point in the respiratory cycle where the images are obtained must be identical to that of needle placement. This can be overcome by having the patient hold end expiration or utilizing general anesthesia [1].

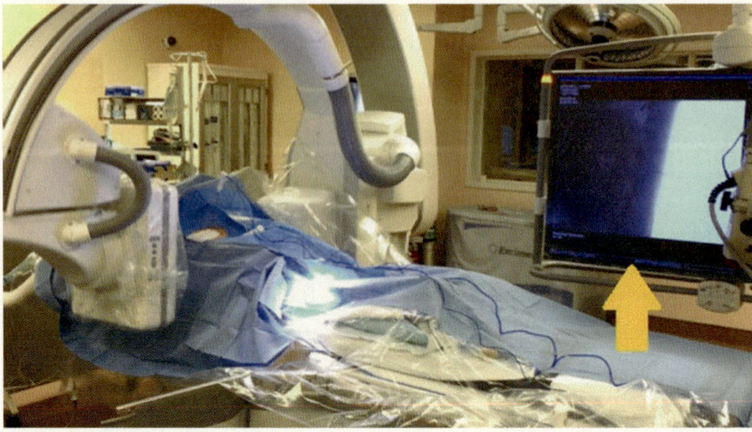

Fig. 16.7 Room set up for Cone-beam CT RFA. Notice the large gantry size allowing room for needle placement. Manipulation of the large C-arm under fluoroscopy creates a 3D model (*arrow*) of the target allowing for precise ablation

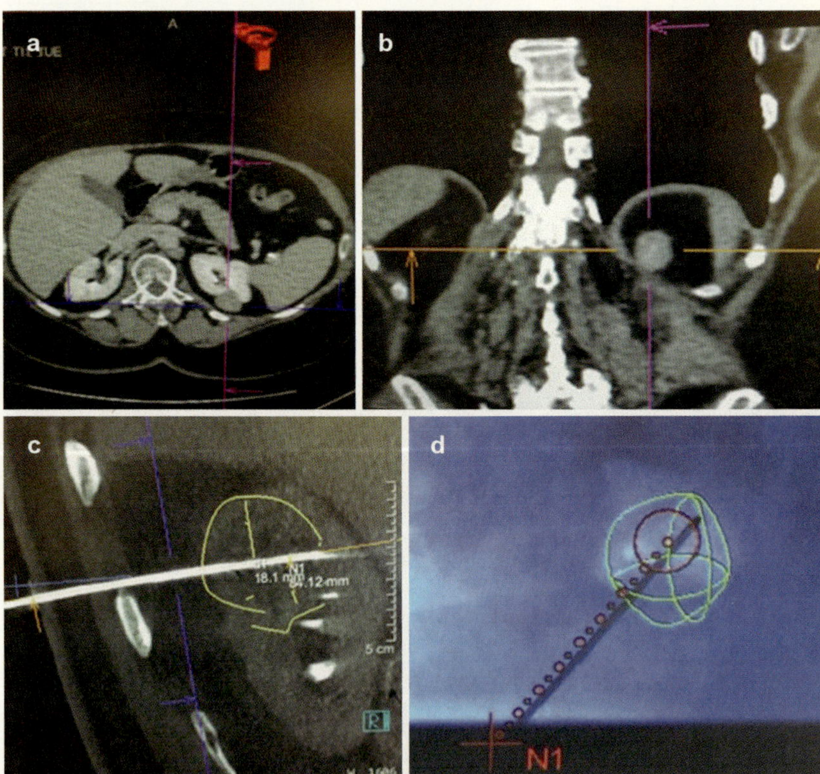

Fig. 16.8 Cone beam CT with fluoroscopic precise targeting I-guide software. (**a**) Axial view pre-planning (**b**) Coronal view pre-planning (**c**) Reimaging after needle placement in line with the needle. (**d**) Fluoroscopic confirmation of projected target

Multimodality Fusion

Amalou and Wood described a clinical trial of a patient with VHL who underwent RFA of a 3.0 cm renal tumor with multimodality fusion consisting of US, CT, EM and MRI. This fusion system is ideal for patients with renal insufficiency and elevated creatinine. The patient was not able to undergo CT-guided RFA since the non-enhanced CT did not adequately delineate the target. The EM tracking system (Northern Digital Inc., Waterloo, ON, USA), MR (Philips 3.0 T Achieva scanner, Philips Medical Systems, Best, The Netherlands), CT scan (MX 8000, Philips Medical Systems, Cleveland, OH, USA), and US contrast (Definity, Bristol Myers Squibb, N. Billerica, MA, USA) were used. A previously acquired pre-procedural enhanced CT guided the EM placement of fiducial markers. The guide needle was then advanced along the trajectory of a MR-CT fusion image with the additional guidance of US contrast resulting in a target error of 1.5 mm. The US sensor coils allowed the image to be aligned with the fused CT/MR and needle. The ablation was then guided under fusion and US. Ablation success was confirmed by a non-enhancing US contrast image. The patient's creatinine was 2.0 mg/dL prior to the procedure and 1.8 mg/dL post-ablation [36].

Training in RFA

Recently, Leveillee et al., in association with the American Urology Association published a training method for Urologists who do not have previous RFA training or who do not have access to the assistance of an Interventional Radiologist/Department. The training method utilizes non-pitted olives soaked in Isovuc (Bracco Diagnostics, Inc., New York, New York) and plumber's putty as renal ablation targets placed in fresh frozen human cadavers (Anatomic Gifts Registry, Hanover, Maryland). Urologists who participated in the protocol were able to practice CT-guided percutaneous needle placement, as well as pretreatment planning on a realistic model. Results of the training protocol demonstrated that all participants had increased confidence in performing the procedure upon completion [37] (Fig. 16.9).

Complications

The goal of NSS is to achieve at least equivalent results compared to PN and RN while affording fewer complications [3]. In comparison to surgical techniques RFA has no mortality and lower mobility; dubbed the "Band-Aid surgery" (Fig. 16.10). The reported complication rate of PN and RN is 14–26% versus a rate of 0–11% in RFA [3, 8, 34]. Infection occurs in less than 1% of ablations (cc). The Society of Interventional Radiology (SIR) has published a classification system which categorizes various complications based on long term consequence and required treatment. The basis of the system divides complications into minor (Classes A and B)

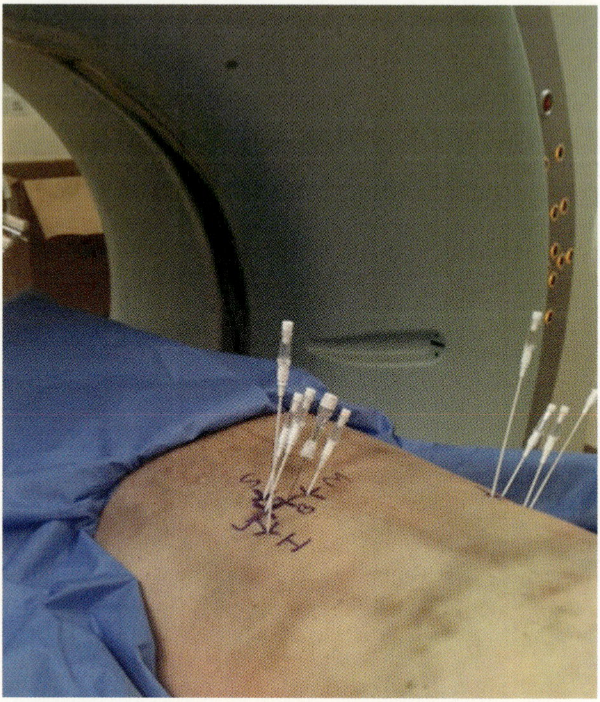

Fig. 16.9 Cadaveric model used for teaching RFA

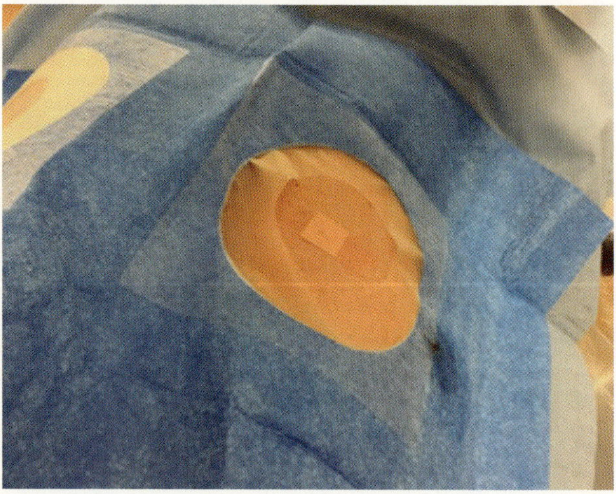

Fig. 16.10 "Band-Aid surgery"- appearance after CT-RFA renal tumor ablation

and major (Classes C-F) sub-groups; of the major complications only Class C have been reported post ablation. Minor complications require no therapy, are self-limited, and have no consequence to the patient. Major complications, in comparison require therapy and hospitalization of at least 48 hours [38].

Minor Complications

The most frequent minor complication post ablation is categorized as neuromuscular, occurring in 46% of patients. Percutaneous probe placement and manipulation leads to short-term discomfort at the insertion site. Normally the patient is afforded relief with the use of over the counter pain medications [33, 38]. Hematuria occurs in roughly 10–20% of patients arising most frequently in central ablations (p 35). Hematoma, 6–8% incidence, is clinically insignificant if less than 1 cm [8, 33]. Pneumothorax has been reported in 2–4% of ablations [38]. There is one case in the literature reporting tumor seeding of the needle track which was detected on follow-up imaging [33, 34, 38].

Major Complications

The most frequently encountered major complication is retroperitoneal hematoma, occurring in 1–8% of ablations of which only 1–2% requires transfusion. Thermal damage to surrounding tissue can result in ureteral injuries (4%), bowel perforation, the formation of perirenal abscesses, and genitofemoral nerve damage (Fig. 16.11). Thermal damage is acquired most readily in the ablation of central and anterior tumors [33, 34, 38]. In patients with upper pole renal tumors there is an increased risk of hypertensive crisis secondary to adrenal thermal damage, although never reported in the literature. Patients at risk could be considered for laparoscopic ablation. Regardless of technique these patients should be treated pre-operatively with alpha and beta-blockers taking special care to administer alpha antagonists first to avoid uncontrollable hypertension [33, 39].

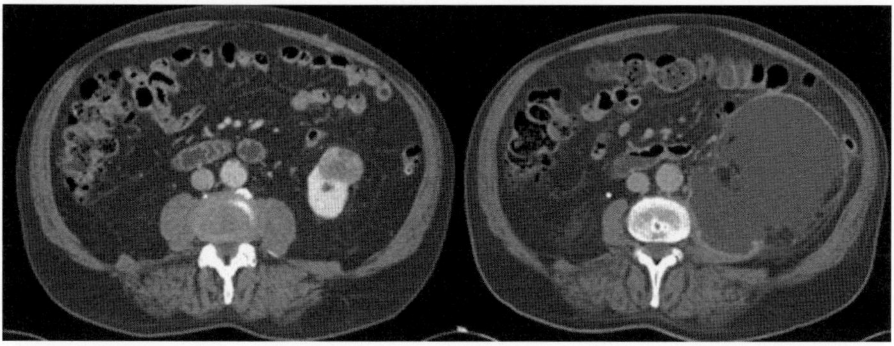

Fig. 16.11 Post-operative urinoma which developed in a 84 year-old male undergoing ablation of a 3.5 cm RCC. Four temperature probes were used all >90 °F

Ways to Decrease Incidence of Thermal Damage

As stated earlier, thermal damage post-ablation can spread via conduction to the surrounding tissue. Structures located within 1–2 cm of the ablation zone can demonstrate thermal damage post ablation [31]. The provider should be aware that conductance resulting in thermal damage can occur up to 10 mm beyond the manufacturer's published ablation zone dimension [31]. Therefore, when vital organs such as the ureter and bowel are in close proximity steps should be taken to reduce the likelihood of thermal complications. These steps include patient position, the usage of MR real-time monitoring, strait electrodes, hydrodissection, balloon displacement, and employing the RFA probe as a lever. Of these, hydrodissection is most common [31, 33, 34]. Hydrodissection involves the administration of fluid, 5% dextrose, via a percutaneous needle creating a space separating and insulating vital tissue from the ablation zone. In comparison to cryoablation, it is important that ionic solutions, a conduction media, be avoided. Complications of hydrodissection include seizure, coma, and cardiac electrical disturbances secondary to electrolyte abnormalities [31, 33, 34, 40].

Post-Ablation Follow-Up

In comparison to PN and RN, tumor cells are not resected in RFA, necessitating follow-up. The timing of serial follow-up imaging is controversial requiring clinical judgment [33, 34]. Most experts in the field perform post-ablation imaging within 1–3 months of initial ablation, 6 months, then yearly [33, 34, 38, 39]. Recurrence has been reported as late as 31 months, necessitating extended surveillance. A recommendation for length of surveillance has not been published to date. CT or MRI imaging modalities may be utilized. Some experts recommend follow-up with the same modality that aided ablation permitting comparison [31]. Contrast induced nephrotoxicity may ensue in 20–30% of patients, since many patients undergoing RFA have renal insufficiency. MRI serial imaging, however, does not expose the patient to the additive effects of ionizing radiation [2, 31, 34]. The resulting coagulation necrosis of successful RFA should enhance <10–20 HU or <15% on CT and T2 weighted MR imaging. In contrast, enhancement is expected on T1w MR films [3, 33, 34]. It is common to have limited areas of enhancement, due to fibrin or residual bleeding, within the ablation zone up to 6 months post ablation. However, after this time the size and enhancement of the lesion should decrease. If during the course of follow-up enhancement is observed or lesion size increases, recurrence should be considered and additional treatment modalities should be explored [33, 38].

36. Amalou H, Wood BJ. Multimodality fusion with MRI, CT, and ultrasound contrast for ablation of renal cell carcinoma. Case Rep Urol. 2012;2012:390912.
37. Castle SM, Gorbatiy V, Salas N, Gorin MA, Landman J, Leveillee RJ. Development and evaluation of a novel cadaveric model for performance of image-guided percutaneous renal tumor ablation. J Surg Educ. 2012;69(1):30–3.
38. De Filippo M, Bozzetti F, Martora R, et al. Radiofrequency thermal ablation of renal tumors. Radiol Med. 2014;119(7):499–511.
39. Georgiades C, Rodriguez R. Renal tumor ablation. Tech Vasc Interv Radiol. 2013;16(4):230–8.
40. Farrell MA, Charboneau JW, Callstrom MR, Reading CC, Engen DE, Blute ML. Paranephric water instillation: a technique to prevent bowel injury during percutaneous renal radiofrequency ablation. AJR Am J Roentgenol. 2003;181(5):1315–7.
41. Raman JD, Raj GV, Lucas SM, Williams SK, Lauer EM, Ahrar K, Matin SF, Leveillee RJ, Cadeddu JA. Renal functional outcomes for Tumours in a solitary kidney managed by ablative or extirpative techniques. BJU Int. 2009;105(4):496–500.
42. Raman JD, Sern JM, Zeltser I, et al. J Urol. 2008;179:2142–5.
43. Salas N, Ramanathan R, Dummett S, Leveillee RJ. Results of radiofrequency kidney tumor ablation: renal function preservation and oncologic efficacy. World J Urol. 2010;28(5):583–91.

Chapter 17
History and Development of Prostate Cryoablation

R. Joseph Babaian

The Pathophysiology of Thermal Ablation

Cryoablation is one of several therapeutic interventions that can result in thermal tissue destruction. This technique has well- documented scientific evidence supporting its efficacy as a treatment modality in the treatment of both benign and malignant diseases [1–3]. The operative mechanism produced by freezing is the extraction of heat from the targeted tissue that initiates a series of destructive events. The severity of the freezing process has long been recognized to result in a tissue response varying from inflammation to total destruction. Histologically freezing produces an area of central necrosis with a surrounding peripheral rim in which cell death is apparent [4, 5]. Successful tissue destruction resulting from cryoablation is founded on two scientific principles; first the cellular response to freezing itself and second to operative procedural factors. Freezing tissue induces cell death by setting off a cascade of events that include freeze rupture, necrosis and apoptosis. As ice forms in the targeted tissue, water is extracted from the extracellular space forming pure crystalline ice leaving behind hyperosmotic fluid in the extracellular compartment. As a consequence of this physical event, intracellular water moves to the extracellular space followed by cell shrinkage and damage to the intracellular matrix including proteins resulting from the increased salinity. In an anatomic constrained structure such as the prostate which is not totally encapsulated the expanding ice front and the spear-like ice crystals destroy both prostate cells and the capillary endothelial lining, the latter impairing the vascular tree after thawing [6]. In addition to the physical rupture of targeted tissue cells from the intracellular ice crystal formation apoptosis has been linked to thermal injury [7]. Hollister et al. have reported that after a freezing insult,

R.J. Babaian, M.D.
Department of Urology, UT M.D. Anderson Cancer Center, 7505 S. Main Street, Suite 500, Houston, TX 77030, USA
e-mail: rbabaian@mdanderson.org

S.R. Patel et al. (eds.), *The History of Technologic Advancements in Urology*,
DOI 10.1007/978-3-319-61691-9_17

prostate cancer cells die at temperatures consistent with the freeze-zone margin [8]. Induction of the apoptotic event is said to be associated with an intrinsic mitochondria induced mechanism characterized by the upregulation of cellular Bax, the pro-apoptotic protein [9]. More recently, prostate cancer cell apoptotic induction has been reported to be facilitated through an extrinsic pathway involving the interaction of tumor necrosis factor-related apoptosis-inducing ligand with its ligand in the plasma membrane [10].

The destruction of both malignant and benign tissue is dependent on a number of induced physical freeze-related associated stresses. The technical aspects of the freezing procedure namely the freeze rate, achieved nadir temperature, thaw rate and repetition of the freeze thaw cycle impact the efficacy and degree of tissue destruction. Cancer cells proximal to and those within the central necrosis zone and immediate peripheral rim are primarily killed by intracellular ice formation. The remaining viable cancer cells within the frozen prostate are proportionally destroyed as a consequence of either necrotic or apoptotic cell death depending on the extent of the stress they experience and their cell-cycle stage [11]. It is recognized that rapid freeze rates produce higher cell kill rates compared to slow freezing. Slow freezing allows cells to release intracellular water into the extracellular space reducing the formation of intracellular ice thus limiting its toxic effects. Historically, −40 °C has been the target temperature, based on evidence, it represents the lowest viability temperature of human cells [4, 8]. Prostate cancer cells have been shown to be comparatively temperature labile with a lethal temperature around −20 °C [4, 12]. Slow passive thawing performed in, *in vitro* models have confirmed enhanced prostate cancer tissue ablation compared to faster activated probe heating techniques [1]. *In vivo* and *in vitro* studies, as well as clinical experience, clearly demonstrate the superiority of the repetition of the freeze—thaw cycle in enhancing ablative efficacy [1, 13, 14]. In addition, the initial damage to the tumor vascularity decreases the second freeze cycle time and safely extends the area of central necrosis.

Cryosurgery Historical Perspective

The evolution and the utilization of "cold" temperature as a therapeutic modality has a very long history dating back to 2500 B.C. when the Egyptians used cold packs to relieve pain [15]. In 1840, cryotherapy was delivered as ice saline through tubes used to treat tumors by Arnott [16]. Oral and skin lesions were subjected to liquid gas at temperatures of −180 °C by White in 1899 [17]. Fay, a neurosurgeon, in 1938 employed the first closed cryosurgical device to treat brain tumors [18]. After WWII liquid nitrogen became available and was used to treat a myriad of conditions such as skin and neuromuscular disorders, lesions resulting from Parkinson's disease as well as brain tumors. In 1961, Cooper and Lee utilized a single insulated probe attached to a circulating pump to perform cryosurgery with the capacity to deliver liquid nitrogen at −190 °C [19].

The era of prostate cryosurgery began in 1964 when Gonder demonstrated that freezing produced tissue destruction in a canine prostate model [20]. Flocks modified the transurethral approach to deliver cryotherapy to that of the open perineal route in 1974. These experimental trials lead in 1966 to the first human prostate application of this technology [21]. Gonder reported the insertion of 1 or 2 large probes through an open perineal approach directly into the prostate and visually monitored the ice formation to determine when to terminate the treatment [22]. The next advancement came in 1974 when Megali advocated and performed a transperineal application of a single large probe using digital monitoring of the ice ball formation [23]. Due to the significant complications including urethral sloughing, recto-urethral fistula formation, incontinence, etc. this mode of therapy was not readily adopted. In 1990 the need for a multiprobe system was reported by Merry and Smidebach followed in 1994 by the conceptualization of a multiprobe system by Rubinsky and colleagues [24, 25].

As in many cases the adoption of one new technology that appears before it's time must await advances in other technological areas to rejuvenate interest, so was the case for prostate cryoablation. Two of the major limiting issues impacting prostate cryoablation were visualization of the ice ball formation and subsequently monitoring its expansion before it caused injury to adjoining structures. In 1982, the first report detailing a significant advancement regarding the monitoring of freezing in a tissue system was published [26]. Several years later the specific application utilizing transrectal ultrasound for the placement of cryoprobes into the prostate with the subsequent monitoring of the ice ball formation was reported by Onik and colleagues. [27].

Historical Evolution of Prostate Cryosurgery

The addition of cryoablation to the treatment armamentarium for both salvage and primary localized prostate cancer is based on two factors: first, the demonstration of therapeutic efficacy; and second, the significant reduction of associated complications that negatively impact quality of life and consequently, its general acceptance. The interpretation of surrogate survival data for cryosurgery has been hampered by defining how to access this treatment's efficacy and whether this modality should be held to surgical or radiation therapy definitions of biochemical failure. In the contemporary era results are determined by either achievement of a PSA value of less than or equal to 0.4 ng/mL or either the ASTRO or newer Phoenix definition for patients having undergone radiation therapy [28, 29]. The dilemma of defining PSA failure is based on the preservation of the periurethral tissue which has the potential to spare PSA producing tissue. Several investigators have shown that the lower the PSA nadir the greater is the likelihood of a negative post-treatment biopsy and stable PSA over time [30–32]. A pooled multi-institutional data registry report of 5 year biochemical free survival for patients undergoing primary cryosurgery using the Phoenix definition showed a 91%, 78% and

62% bDFS (biochemical disease free survival) in low, intermediate and high risk patients, respectively [33]. In comparison the first evidenced based definition of bDFS success (PSA < 0.4 ng/mL) reported 5 year results of 90.4%, 81.1% and 73.6% for low, intermediate and high risk patients, respectfully [28]. There are no prospective randomized trials comparing surgery and cryotherapy outcomes as primary therapies in patients with localized prostate cancer. Two prospective, randomized trials comparing cryosurgery and radiation therapy outcomes, albeit having different cT2 and cT3 patient eligibility inclusion criteria, reported opposing conclusions with respect to inferiority [34, 35]. Tables 17.1 and 17.2 summarizes bDFS in selected series of patients receiving primary and salvage cryoablation, respectively [14, 33, 36–43].

The major complications that were frequently reported in the early periods of cryosurgery for prostate cancer in the 1960s through the 1980s have been significantly reduced in both the primary and salvage settings. The contemporary reports for primary cryoablation reveal complication rates of <0.5% for rectal fistula formation [44], <8% for permanent urinary incontinence [45] and <15% for urethral sloughing when a urethral warming device is employed [46]. Erectile dysfunction remains a significant problem in patients undergoing total gland ablation in men in which the ice ball is allowed to extend to both neurovascular bundles. One year and four year potency rates of 41.4 and 51.3% have been reported with penile rehabilitation [47]. In the salvage setting complications are higher with incontinence reported in approximately 10%, urethral sloughing in 10%, rectal pain in 17% and rectal fistula in 3%. Tables 17.3 and 17.4, show the reported complications in selected series of patients undergoing primary and salvage therapy, respectively [14, 31, 35–42, 48–50].

Technologic Advances in Prostate Cryosurgery

Contemporary cryoablation for prostate cancer saw a resurgence beginning approximately 25 years ago following the first report in 1993 detailing the use of transrectal ultrasound to both monitor cryoprobe placement and ice formation within the prostate by Onik and associates [27]. The early experience focused on this modality as an option to treat patients in the salvage setting after radiation therapy and quickly expanded to include primary therapy. The initial source of cryo- thermal energy was liquid nitrogen delivered through monstrosity sized machines. The choices were limited to either the Cryotech or AccuProbe (CMS) manufactured equipment. Both machines provided the option of a maximum of only five probes all of which could be placed percutaneously via a perineal approach. The former came with a probe that was 2.6 mm at the tip and a 3.2 mm shaft while the latter was supplied with a 3.2 and 4.9 mm probe tip and shaft respectively. The CMS probes required separate skin incisions for insertion. The next major advancement was the introduction of the urethral warming device. Utilization of this transurethral catheter provided the circulation of water maintained at +43C, thus significantly reducing the incidence of

Table 17.1 Results of primary cryosurgery

					bDFS (%)			
Ref. (with actuarial data)	No. patients	Median follow-up in months (range)	Technique	PSA threshold	Low risk	Intermediate risk	High risk	nADT (%)
Bahn et al. [37] (7-year data)	590	68 (NA)	LN/Ar	<0.5 <1.0	61 87	68 79	61 71	91
Cohen et al. [39] (10-year data)	204	12.6 (9.7–15.0)	LN	ASTRO	56 (all risk groups)			0
Han et al. [38] (1-year data)	122	12 (NA)	Ar	<0.4	78	NA	71	37
Jones et al. [36] (5-year data)	1198	24 (SD ± 26)	LN/Ar	ASTRO	85	73	75	NA
Long et al. [35] (5-year data)	975	24 (SD ± 16.5)	LN/Ar	<0.5 <1.0	60 75	61 71	36 45	33

Modified from Langenhuijsen JF Eur. Urol 2009; 55: 76–86; *LN* Liquid nitrogen, *Ar* Argon

Table 17.2 Results of salvage cryosurgery

					bDFS (%)			
Ref. (with actuarial data)	No. patients	Median follow-up in months (range)	Technique	PSA threshold	Low risk	Intermediate risk	High risk	nADT (%)
Bahn et al. [43] (7-year data)	59	82 (NA)	Ar	<0.5	59 (all			NA
Chin et al. [40] (5-year data)	118	19 (3–54)	Ar	<0.5	NA	NA	34	60
Ismail et al. [41] (5-year data)	100	33 (mean) (12–79)	Ar	<0.5	73	45	11	46
Ng et al. [42] (8-year data)	187	39 (mean) (NA)	Ar	Houston	56	NA	14	71
Pisters et al. [14] (5-year data)	279	22 (SD ± 25)	LN/Ar	ASTRO Phoenix	59 (all risk groups) 55 (all risk groups)			NA

Modified from Langenjuijsen JF Eur. Urol 2009; 55: 76–86; *LN* Liquid nitrogen, *Ar* Argon, *bDFS* Biochemical disease-free survival

Table 17.3 Complications (%) after primary cryosurgery

Ref.	No. patients	Technique	Fistula	Retention	Incontinence	Impotence	Perineal pain
Badalament et al. [49]	290	Cryocare	0.4	NA	4.3	85	12
Bahn et al. [37]	590	LN/Ar	0.004	5.5	4.3	95	NA
Cohen et al. [39]	239	Cryocare Seednet	2.2	3	0.4	4	0.4
Han et al. [38]	122	AR	0	NA	3	87	6
Jones et al. [36]	1198	LN/Ar	0.4	NA	2.9	91	NA
Long et al. [35]	975	LN/Ar	0.4	10	7.5	93	NA
Shinohara et al. [31]	102	NA	1	23	15	86	3
Wake et al. [48]	106	Cryocare	0	22	8	NA	NA

Table 17.4 Complications (%) after salvage cryosurgery

Ref.	No. patients	Technique	Fistula	Retention	Incontience	Impotence	Perineal pain
Chin et al. [40]	118	Ar	3.3	8.5	6.7	NA	NA
Ismail et al. [41]	100	Ar	1	2	13	86	4
Katz et al.[50]	157	Cryocare seednet	0	5.8/1.9	9.7	NA	12.8
Ng et al. [42]	187	Ar	2	21	3	NA	14
Pisters et al. [14]	279	LN/Ar	1.2	NA	4.4	NA	NA

Modified from Langenhuijsen JF et al. Eur. Urol 2009; 58: 76–86; *LN* Liquid nitrogen, *Ar* Argon

urethral sloughing and resulting urinary retention. This device required meticulous attention since it created an accompanying heat sink that could potentially impact prostatic tissue destruction.

Unfortunately, this device was removed from the market place by the FDA leading to the development of less effective homemade replacement devices and an increase in the incidence of urethral sloughing. Eventually, the urethral warming device received FDA approval and continues to be used to this day.

The mid to late 1990s saw many technological advances in the field of prostate cryosurgery which dramatically changed the adverse reputation that had become associated with this treatment modality. Not only was there a significant reduction in the major complication rates but experience lead to the development of more appropriate patient selection criteria. It had long been appreciated that the temperature to achieve lethal ice to reliably destroy prostate cells was around −40 °C [51]. The problem was how to ascertain the exact temperature within the ice ball since the monitoring process was limited to the visual assessment of ice formation [52]. Temperature monitoring was further complicated by the knowledge that the temperature at the interface between tissue and ice formation as seen by ultrasound was 0 °C. The introduction of thermocouples that could be placed percutaneously into the prostate under ultrasound guidance provided valuable information that could be used to achieve lethal ice formation homogeneously throughout the target area [53, 54]. The original thermocouples with only a single terminal point sensor provided limited feedback data with respect to the achieved temperature along the cryoprobe shaft. This information gap has been addressed with the introduction of re-useable multi-point sensing device inserted through a disposable 17 gauge sheath capable of recording temperature at either 4 or 8 points 10 or 5 mm apart, respectively [52]. A significant technological advancement occurred with the introduction of argon gas freezing equipment which represents the mainstay of current delivery systems for cryoablation. This freezing system takes advantage of the Joule-Thompson principle whereby pressurized argon gas is forced through small caliber tubes that allows for rapid temperature drops secondary to the free expansion of the gas. This new system has several advantages over the original liquid nitrogen equipment. It provides faster freezing rates which in turn mechanistically makes the ice formation process more lethal in the destruction of tissue. Safety is also improved because freezing can be more quickly terminated providing more control of the extent of the tissue ablation by reducing unintended tissue injury associated with the delay in response time after shutting down active freezing.

These newer delivery systems often referred to as the third generation offered another opportunity for technological improvement, namely cryoprobe enhancement. The caliber of the probes was reduced from 4.9 to 2.4 mm and smaller (17 gauge). The advantage of these was the ability to place them percutaneously, either free hand or through a brachytherapy perineal template without a skin incision, as well as the placement of an increased number of probes. An added feature of these 3rd generation machines is the capability of active thawing using Helium gas heated to 67 °C. Lee and colleagues reported the advantage of placing 6–8 probes compared to the limit of 5 imposed by the original liquid nitrogen equipment [53]. This incremental enhancement produced a more homogeneous freezing throughout the prostate. Further attempts to increase the number of probes with the intent to improve outcome have produced controversial interpretations based on PSA results [54]. Knowledge of the characterization of the ice created by the various cryoprobes is critical to the outcome of tissue destruction. Another procedural advance was described in 2000 detailing the separation of the rectum from Denonvillier's fascia using an injection of normal saline [55]. This maneuver is touted to decrease the fear of rectal injury, provide enhanced lethal ice delivery to encompass all the posterior prostatic tissue including the fibromuscular rim and faster freezing. This maneuver has also been shown to work effectively in patients who have received prior radiation therapy [55].

Technology in the field of software development has continued to evolve to the point that standardization of treatment planning programs providing both the optimum location and placement guidance of the ideal number of cryoprobes is available. In addition, the software has the capacity to automatically control the cryoprobes as well as to contour the formation of the ice ball. As a consequence, this new technology may help standardize a procedure that has traditionally been highly operator dependent and it may reduce cryotherapy morbidity.

Future Directions

In an era where minimally invasive multimodal or combination therapy is the prevailing interventional approach to enhance outcome, there is fertile opportunities to explore cryosurgery as one of the component pieces. Specifically, combining cryoablation with chemotherapy, immunotherapy and either cryo- enhancing or protective compounds should be explored. The utilization of focal cryoablation and the technical ability to contour lethal ice formation minimizing adjacent tissue injury provides another opportunity for continued future research of this modality.

References

1. Baust JG, Gage AA, Klossner D, Clark D, Miller R, Cohen J, et al. Issues critical to the successful application of cryosurgical ablation of the prostate. Technol Cancer Res Treat. 2007;6:97–109.
2. Gage AA, Baust JG. Cryosurgery of tumors. J Am Coll Surg. 2007;201:342–56.
3. Hoffmann NE, Bischof JC. The cryobiology of cryosurgical injury. Urology. 2002;60:40–9.
4. Gage AA, Baust J. Mechanism if tissue injury in cryosurgery. Cryobiology. 1998;37:171–86.
5. Larson TR, Robertson DW, Corcia A, Bostwich DG. In vivo interstitial temperature mapping of human prostate during cryosurgery with correlation to histopathologic outcomes. Urology. 2000;55(4):547–52.
6. Ayala AG, Ro JY, Babaian RJ, Troncoso P, Grignon D. The prostate capsule: does it exist? Its importance in staging and treatment of prostatic carcinoma. Am J Surg Pathol. 1989;13(1):21–7.
7. Baust JG, Gage AA, Clarke D, Baust JM, Van Buskirk R. Cryosurgery – a putative approach to molecular-based optimization. Cryobiology. 2004;48:190–204.
8. Hollister WR, Mathew AJ, Baust JG, Van Buskirk RG. Effects of freezing on cell viability and mechanism of cell death in a human prostate cancer cell line. Mol Urol. 1998;2:13–8.
9. Clark K, Baust JM, Van Buskirk RG, Baust JG. Addition of anti-cancer agents enhancing freezing-induced prostate cancer cell death: implication of mitochondrial involvement. Cryobiology. 2004;49:45–61.
10. Clark DM, Rubilitto AT, Van Buskirk RG, Baust JG, Gage AA, Baust JM. Targeted induction of apoptosis via TRAIL and cryoablation: a novel strategy for the treatment of prostate cancer. Prostate Cancer Prostatic Dis. 2007;10(2):175–845.
11. Baust JG, Gage AA. The molecular basis of cryosurgery. BJU Int. 2005;95:1187–91.
12. Klossner DP, Baust JM, Van Buskirk RG, Gage AA, Baust JG. Cryoablative response of prostate cancer cells is influenced by androgen receptor expression. BJU Int. 2008;101:1310–6.
13. Shinohara K, Connolly JA, Presti JC, Carroll PR. Cryosurgical treatment of prostate cancer (stages T1 to T4): preliminary results. J Urol. 1996;156:115–20.
14. Pisters LL v, Eschenbach AC, Scott SM, Swanson DA, Dinney CP, Pettaway CA, et al. The efficacy and complications of salvage cryotherapy of the prostate. J Urol. 1997;157:921–5.
15. Schmidt JD, Doyle J, Larison S. Prostate cryoablation: update 1998. CA Cancer J Clin. 1998;48(4):239–53.
16. Arnott J. Practical illustrations of the remedial efficacy of a very low or anesthetic temperature. Lancet. 1850;2:257–9.
17. White AC. Possibilities of liquid air to the physician. JAMA. 1901;36:426–8.
18. Neel HB 3rd. Cryosurgery for the treatment of cancer. Laryngoscope. 1980;90:1–48.
19. Cooper IS, Lee A. Cryothalamectomy-hypothermic coagulation: a technical advance in basal ganglia surgery: preliminary report. J Am Geriatr Soc. 1961;9:714–8.
20. Gonder MJ, Soanes WA, Smith V. Experimental prostate surgery. Investig Urol. 1964;1:610–9.
21. Flocks RH, Nelson CM, Boatman DL. Perineal cryosurgery for prostatic carcinoma. J Urol. 1972;108:933–5.
22. Gonder MJ, Soanes WA, Shulman S. Cryosurgical treatment of the prostate. Investig Urol. 1966;3:372–8.
23. Megali MR, Gursel EO, Veenema RJ. Closed perineal cryosurgery in prostate cancer. New probe and technique. Urology. 1974;4(2):220–2.
24. Merry M, Smidebush M. Apparatus for cryosurgery. 1990. US Patent 4,946,460.
25. Rubinsky B, Onik G, Finkelstein JJ, Neu D, Jones S. Cryosurgical system for destroying tumors by freezing. 1994. US Patent 5,334,181.
26. Ando K. Cystoprostatectomy under control of ultrasono-tomagraphy. Presented at the 14th Congress of International Urologic Society. 1982.

27. Onik GM, Cohen JK, Reyes GD, Rubinsky B, Chang Z, Baust J. Transrectal ultrasound guided percutaneous radical cryosurgical ablation of the prostate. Cancer. 1993;72:1291–9.
28. Levy DA, Ross AE, El Shafei A, Krishnan N, Hatem A, Jones JS. Definition of biochemical success following primary whole gland prostate cryoablation. J Urol. 2014;192(5):1380–4.
29. Roach M 3rd, Hank G, Thames H Jr, Shellhammer P, Shipley WU, Sokol GH, Sandler H. Defining biochemical failure following radiotherapy with or without hormonal therapy in men with clinically localized prostate cancer: recommendation of the RTOG-ASTRO Phoenix Consensus Conference. Int J Radiat Oncol Biol Phys. 2006;65(4):965–74.
30. Ellis DS. Cryosurgery as primary treatment for localized prostate cancer; a community experience. Urology. 2002;60(2 Suppl 1):34–9.
31. Shinohara K, Rhee B, Presti JC Jr, Carroll PR. Cryosurgical ablation of prostate cancer: patterns of cancer recurrence. J Urol. 1997;158:2206–9.
32. Benoit RM, Cohen JK, Miller RJ Jr. Cryosurgery for prostate cancer: new technology and indications. Curr Urol Rep. 2000;1:41–7.
33. Jones JS, Rewcastle JC, Donnelly BJ, Lugnani FM, Pisters LL, Katz AE. Whole gland primary prostate cryoablation: initial results from Cryo-ON line data registry. J Urol. 2008;180:554–8.
34. Donnelly BJ, Saliken JC, Brasher PMA, Ernst SC, Rewcastle JC, Lau H, et al. A randomized trial of external radiotherapy versus cryoablation in patients with localized prostate cancer. Cancer. 2010;116:323–30.
35. Chin JL, Al-Zahrani AA, Autran-Gomez AM, Williams AK, Bauman G. Extended follow-up oncologic outcome of randomized trial between cryoablation and external beam therapy for locally advanced prostate cancer (T2a-T3b). J Urol. 2012;188:1170–5.
36. Long JP, Bahn D, Lee F, Shinohara K, Chinn DO, Macaluso JN Jr. Five-year retrospective, multi-institutional pooled analysis of cancer- related outcomes after cryoablation of the prostate. Urology. 2001;57:518–23.
37. Bahn DK, Lee F, Badalament R, Kumar A, Greski J, Chernick M. Targeted cryoablation of the prostate: 7-year outcomes in the primary treatment of prostate cancer. Urology. 2002;60:3–11.
38. Han KR, Cohen JK, Miller RJ, et al. Treatment of organ confined prostate cancer with third generation cryosurgery: preliminary multicenter experience. J Urol. 2003;170:1126–30.
39. Cohen JK, Miller jr RJ, Ahmed S, Lotz MJ, Baust J. Ten year biochemical disease control for patients with prostate cancer treated with cryosurgery as primary therapy. Urology. 2008;71:515–8.
40. Chin JL, Pautler SE, Mouraviev V, Touma N, Moore K, Downey DB. Results of salvage cryoablation of the prostate after radiation; identifying predictors of treatment failure and complications. J Urol. 2001;165:1937–41.
41. Ismail M, Ahmed S, Kastner C, Davies J. Salvage cryotherapy for recurrent prostate cancer after radiation failure: a prospective case series of first 100 patients. BJU Int. 2007;100:760–4.
42. Ng CK, Moussa M, Downey DB, Chin JL. Salvage cryoablation of the prostate: follow-up and analysis of predictive factors for outcome. J Urol. 2007;178:1253–7.
43. Bahn DK, Lee F, Silvermann P, et al. Salvage cryotherapy for recurrent prostate cancer after radiation therapy: a seven year follow-up. Clin Prostate Cancer. 2003;2:111–4.
44. Prepelica KL, Okeke Z, Murphy A, Katz AE. Cryosurgical ablation of the prostate: high risk patient outcomes. Cancer. 2005;103:1625–30.
45. De La Tallie A, Benson MC, Bagiella E, Burkhardt M, Shasigh A, Olsson CA, et al. Cryoablation for localized prostate cancer using an argon-based system: complication rates and biochemical recurrence. BJU Int. 2000;85:281–6.
46. Cohen JK, Miller RJ, Shuman BA. Urethral warming catheter for use during cryoablation of the prostate. Urology. 1995;45:861–4.
47. Ellis DS, Manny TB Jr, Rewcastle JC. Cryoablation as primary treatment for localized prostate cancer followed by penile rehabilitation. Urology. 2007;69:306–10.
48. Wake RW, Hollabaugh RS Jr, Bond KH. Cryoablation of the prostate for localized adenocarcinoma: a preliminary experience. J Urol. 1996;155:1663–6.

49. Badalament RA, Bahn DK, Kim H, Kumar A, Bahn JM, Lee F. Patient-reported complications after cryoablation therapy for prostate cancer. Urology. 1999;54:295–300.
50. Katz AE, Preplica KL, Masson P, Benson MC, McKierman JM. Salvage cryosurgical ablation of the prostate (TCAP) for patients failing radiation: 10 year experience. J Urol. 2005;173:450. (abstract 1662)
51. Tatsutani K, Rubinsky B, Onik GM, et al. Effect of thermal variables on frozen human primary prostatic adenocarcinoma cells. Urology. 1996;48:441–7.
52. Gowardhan B, Greene D. Cryotherapy for the prostate: in vitro and clinical study of two new developments; advanced cryoneedles and a temperature monitoring system. BJU Int. 2007;100:295–302.
53. Lee F, Bahn DK, Badalament RA, et al. Cryosurgery for prostate cancer; improved glandular ablation by use of 6–8 cryoprobes. Urology. 1999;54:135–40.
54. Moore Y, Sofer P. Successful treatment of locally confined prostate cancer with the seed net system: preliminary multi-center results. Clinical application notes Feb 2001. Available through Galil Medical, Haifa. 2001. http//Galilmedicalcom. Accessed 7 Nov 2001.
55. Onik G, Narayan P, Brunelle R, et al. Saline injection into Denonvilliers' fascia during prostate cryosurgery. J Min Ther Relat Tech. 2009;9:423–7.

Chapter 18
History of Laparoscopic Renal Surgery

Louis R. Kavoussi

The first laparoscopic renal procedure was performed at Washington University in St. Louis in the late spring of 1990 [1]. This approach was conceived and engineered by Dr. Ralph Clayman. For several years leading up to the event, Dr. Clayman had a laparoscopic set sitting in the corner of his office. Many a resident who sat in the office heard Dr. Clayman opine that someday that equipment would be used to remove a solid organ. They smiled politely although most thought it was an impossible harebrained scheme.

By 1990 laparoscopy had been around for over 80 years [2]. The technique was first introduced by gynecologists for diagnosing pelvic pathology. For over 60 decades, very little interventional work was attempted with this equipment. The available tools were very rudimentary, and allowed for potentially moving ovaries away or placing a clip on the fallopian tube. With the advent of laparoscopic cholecystectomy and advances in the camera technology, the environment was ripe for more advanced intervention [3].

In the late 1970s, Dr. Kurt Semm, a gynecologist at the University of Kiel began developing instruments for intervention [4]. He had some very basic equipment constructed for oophorectomy and myomectomy. In 1982, he performed a laparoscopic appendectomy, and this set off a challenge in surgical culture. For the majority of the twentieth century, surgeons focused on techniques that decreased mortality and morbidity. With these successes came a change in societal thinking and technological advances began allowing focus on addressing secondary concerns with patients such is postoperative discomfort, recuperation, and cosmesis.

A major breakthrough occurred in of 1985 when Erich Mühe performed the first laparoscopic cholecystectomy, in 2 h [5]. Report of this case quickly spread throughout Germany and France, and eventually around the world. Indeed within 2–3 years

L.R. Kavoussi, M.D.
Smith Institute for Urology, Hofstra Northwell School of Medicine,
Lake Success, NY 11042, USA
e-mail: LKavoussi@NSHS.edu

S.R. Patel et al. (eds.), *The History of Technologic Advancements in Urology*,
DOI 10.1007/978-3-319-61691-9_18

of its introduction at the SAGES meeting in 1988, laparoscopic cholecystectomy became the preferred approach in the United States.

Laparoscopic cholecystectomy was the accelerant for the development improved manipulative equipment. Instrument companies focused on producing novel devices as well as those that mirrored traditional open instruments. A variety of graspers, dissecting and hemostatic tools were born. On the disposable front, companies worked on developing automated clip systems and staples.

In parallel with instrument development were significant efforts aimed at improving video camera technology. Traditionally, endoscopy was performed via direct ocular vision through a rigid lens. The surgeon would hold a lens to view the abdomen in one hand and operate with a single hand. The development of video chips revolutionized endoscopic surgery. Video cameras allowed images to be viewed on a screen, thus allowing assistant to hold the camera and thus freeing up both the surgeon's hands to hold instruments. The advent of the laparoscopic cholecystectomy both encouraged and was a product of patient centered surgery. The acceptance of laparoscopic cholecystectomy was astoundingly rapid. The preferred adaptation of this technique was a tour-de-force in patient's ability to change global clinical care.

In urology through the 1980s, there were also technical revolutions taking place. Up until that point, the management of stone disease was for the most part via open surgical extrication or blind basketing. Advances in endoscopic technology and equipment gave birth to minimally invasive approaches such as ureteroscopy, percutaneous stone removal, and extracorporeal shock wave lithotripsy. There was the birth of minimally invasive urologists known as endourologists. They took very seriously, the patient's desires to address secondary issues and put tremendous amount of research and innovation into making surgery less of a burden.

One of the young leaders of the Endourologic Society was Ralph Clayman. Ralph was on faculty at Washington University in Saint Louis. Arthur Smith, who many consider one of the fathers of Endourology, had mentored him at the University of Minnesota. Ralph subsequently moved to Dallas as an American Urological Association Cancer Research Fellow, however, his skill in percutaneous stone removal made him more valuable in teaching residents, fellows, and staff modern techniques for approaching stone disease. Following completion of his fellowship, he took a position at Washington University in Saint Louis in 1985.

Dr. Clayman was an incredibly innovative individual. He had come up with a number of novel approaches and devices to improve endoscopy and ureteroscopy. He was very much intrigued by the potential benefits of laparoscopy to urology. He was able to convince Stortz Incorporated to loan him a laparoscopic cholecystectomy set, which he set aside in the corner of his office. To any resident who entered his office, he would regale them of his vision of removing the kidney laparoscopically. Many of the residents including myself dismissed this as fantasy.

In parallel with the events, the University of San Antonio, Texas, recruited Thierry Vancaillie, from Europe who was an expert in gynecologic laparoscopy. He spent some time at a small hospital outside of San Antonio, Southeast Baptist Hospital. One day while he was sitting in the doctor's lounge, he met William

Schuessler, a urologist. Dr. Schuessler was not an academic urologist, but a community urologist. They began talking, and the question came up as to whether there would be utility in performing pelvic lymph node removal for staging patients with prostate cancer. At that time brachytherapy was a common modality for treating prostate cancer and imaging was insufficient to determine if patients had pelvic lymphatic involvement. A minimally invasive method to determine node status was believed to have utility in determining which patients may not benefit from local therapy.

The team embarked on a series of laparoscopic node dissections and presented the technique at the 1990 meeting of the American Urological Association. In the audience was Dr. Ralph Clayman, who now saw that the timing was right to perform a laparoscopic nephrectomy. Upon returning to St. Louis, he assembled a team of individuals to attempt this in the laboratory. Dr. Nathaniel Soper was a young general surgeon, who had been performing laparoscopic cholecystectomies. He gave insight into creation of the pneumoperitoneum and trocar placement. Also, working in the laboratory were myself, a young junior partner of Dr. Clayman, who was just recently out of residency as well as Dr. Sherburne Figenshau, who was doing a year of research in the laboratory with Dr. Clayman.

Utilizing the borrowed laparoscopic set and discarded instruments from the operating room the team was able to perform a laparoscopic dissection, isolation and detachment of the kidney in a live porcine model in about 4 h. The problems still remained on how to remove the solid organ through a port site incision.

Dr. Clayman had contacts at Cook Urological in Spencer Indiana. Engineers agreed to drive down for each of the evenings when dissections were performed to help solve this problem. The first issue was developing an impermeable tough entrapment sac. This was perceived as needed to prevent tumor spillage. Butterfly net plastic entrapment sacs were commercially available. They were quite sufficient for removing gallstones, ovaries, and gallbladders were not tough enough to allow in-vivo fragmentation of the kidney.

A variety of different commercially available products were considered to create the entrapment sac. A team member scoured a local K-Mart to look at the sandwich and freezer bags to see if there was anything suitable. One evening, Dr. Clayman brought in a bright red bag that was very tough and durable, and appeared to be watertight. The dissected kidney was maneuvered into the bag and subsequently morcellated without any spillage. He then revealed that this bag was made of his Patagonia running shorts. He had been out for a run in the rain and noticed the water beading up on his shorts. The material seemed tough enough so he brought the running shorts into work and had his secretary Fran sew them into bags to be used in the laboratory. The engineers in Cook subsequently took this material and used it as a guide to develop a commercially viable entrapment sac.

The second part of extraction required the development of a tissue morcellator. This device had to break up the kidney without disrupting the integrity of the sac. It also had to be able to evacuate the fragments. Again the engineers from Cook Inc. came through. Ed Pingleton and colleagues developed a device in their garage out of parts picked up from a hardware store that fit the bill perfectly.

By June after doing five porcine sessions, the team was prepared to attempt this on a human. The patient, an 85 year old woman, had a 3 cm asymptomatic right middle lower pole renal mass discovered on CT scan for a trauma work-up. Following Investigation Review Board approval, the patient underwent preoperative embolization with ethanol under intravenous sedation. She was taken to the operating room, a ureteral catheter was inserted to help identify the ureter, and five laparoscopic ports were used for dissection. The operating team consisted of Ralph Clayman as surgeon, Lou Kavoussi as first assistant and Sherb Figenshau as the cameraman. Nate Soper helped with access as this was the first laparoscopic case on a human any of the team members performed.

The kidney was successfully dissected, and removed by morcellation. In total, the operation lasted 7 h, and the patient was discharged on post-operative day 6. She stayed in the hospital so long because she developed congestive heart failure. This was a result of replacing fluid in the OR as if this were an open case. With laparoscopy there is much less insensible fluid loss. Of note, the pathology revealed an oncocytoma.

The case chronicled as a letter in the *New England Journal of Medicine* in 1991, generated tremendous amount of interest [1]. There was an explosion of laparoscopic courses offered throughout the country tendering experience in pelvic lymphadenectomy as well as nephrectomy. There were many lectures given on laparoscopic nephrectomy by individuals, who had never seen or performed one, except for the video footage from the initial cases at Washington University and the initial report.

For several years there was significant pushback regarding its efficacy in treating malignancy. Careful data collection over time bore out equivalent oncologic outcomes compared with open surgery. The pathologic outcomes were the same over time with less morbidity compared to traditional surgery. Eventually, the laparoscopic approach for kidney removal supplanted open surgery in the majority of patients.

Laparoscopic nephrectomy served as a springboard for other urologic procedures. Laparoscopic partial nephrectomy, cyst ablation, pyelolithotomy, pyeloplasty and donor nephrectomy to name a few, eventually were developed, and also have become the preferred approach to open surgery. In 1995 a paper published by Winfield et al. described their success of laparoscopic partial nephrectomy in four patients [6]. Shortly thereafter, the first laparoscopic live donor nephrectomy was performed by Dr. Kavoussi [7]. As the technique was refined, the average operative time and length of stay both improved, and exploration of other laparoscopic urologic surgeries such as laparoscopic nephroureterectomy and retroperitoneal lymph node dissection began to emerge. Initially the laparoscopic nephrectomy was slow to be adopted widely, secondary to increased operative time and the significant learning curve. The benefit of laparoscopic surgery, however, included significantly reduced postoperative analgesia requirements (ninefold) and intraoperative blood loss [8]. Eventually with more widespread adoption and the increased benefits, laparoscopic radical nephrectomy became the gold standard for renal tumors not amenable to partial nephrectomy.

Laparoscopic renal surgery is far from perfect. The incidence of renal incidentaloma is on the rise with an aging and increasingly morbid population. Goals for the future of renal surgery should include improving outcomes, decreasing morbidity and mortality, and decreasing length of recovery in a cost effective manner.

As technology expands, so will the capabilities of LESS and NOTES as new instruments are designed. Robotic technology has allowed more surgeons with limited laparoscopic skills to offer patients a minimally invasive approach to their pathology. Future robots will decrease variability of performance with decreased learning curve in an effort to improve and standardize patient outcomes. The primary limitation of LESS currently involves the ability to dissect with the close proximity of instruments. Newer robots will have better flexibility and ability to perform from a single port site.

An emerging trend is computer-assisted surgery (CAS), which is the integration of computer technology for pre-surgical planning and guidance, and includes the fields of surgical robots as well as image-guided system (IGS) and augmented reality (AR). Future robotic applications include image-guided robots that through the use of CT, MRI, or ultrasound, aid in safely introducing instruments or needles into the kidney [9]. Such systems would help in reducing inadvertent organ injury such as obtaining percutaneous access for nephrolithotomy. With an increasing push to perform LESS and NOTES, AR technology can help in identifying organs as well as orientating structures and position from novel approaches [9]. Such technology would also allow for improved identification of renal masses with the aim of increasing complete tumor resection rate while minimizing removal of healthy renal parenchyma.

Lastly, the future of advancements in laparoscopic renal surgery consists of improving and standardizing training in an effort to reduce adverse surgical events and improve outcomes. The GOALS score, short for Global Operative Assessment of Laparoscopic Skills, is a validated global rating scale for laparoscopy and consists of five categories: depth perception, bimanual dexterity, efficiency, tissue handling, and autonomy, that are evaluated by a blinded observer [10]. Multiple studies have attempted to investigate the best method for introducing new trainees to laparoscopy, and how to best shorten the learning curve and minimize adverse events. In a recent blinded, three-arm study of general surgery resident, 30 residents were assigned to one of three groups. The control group had a traditional intraoperative laparoscopic learning model in which the surgeon taught the trainee intraoperatively. The second group received intensive simulated training prior to real life exposure, and the third group was a blend between the first two groups. In their investigation, they found the second group to have the shortest learning curve on GOALS assessment, and they were able to perform their procedures more quickly and accurately with decreased adverse events compared to the other two groups [10]. From this study, the author argues that simulation modules are an important curriculum component prior to "hands on" operative experience, although larger studies are needed.

Over the last 30 years, laparoscopic renal surgery has evolved in technology and technique. With the introduction of robotics and new instruments, renal surgery has become less invasive, while improving operative outcomes. As new technology develops, the envelope will continue to be pushed by urologists with the hope of eventually eliminating surgical morbidity completely while increasing cure.

References

1. Clayman RV, Kavoussi LR, Soper NJ, et al. Laparoscopic nephrectomy. N Engl J Med. 1991;324:1370–1.
2. Lau WY, Leow CK, Li AK. History of endoscopic and laparoscopic surgery. World J Surg. 1997;21:444–53.
3. Himal HS. Minimally invasive (laparoscopic) surgery. Surg Endosc. 2002;16:1647–52.
4. Semm K. Endoscopic appendectomy. Endoscopy. 1983;15:59–64.
5. Blum C, Adams D. Who did the first laparoscopic cholecystectomy. J Minim Access Surg. 2011;7:165–8.
6. Winfield HN, Donovan JF, Lund GO, Kreder KJ, Stanley KE, Brown BP, et al. Laparoscopic partial nephrectomy: initial experience and comparison to the open surgical approach. J Urol. 1995;153:1409–14.
7. Ratner LE, Ciseck LJ, Moore RG, et al. Laparoscopic live donor nephrectomy. Transplantation. 1995;60:1047–9.
8. Kerbl DC, Mcdougall EM, Clayman RV, Mucksavage P. A history and evolution of laparoscopic nephrectomy: perspectives from the past and future directions in the surgical management of renal tumors. J Urol. 2011;185:1150–4.
9. Micali S, Pini G, Teber D, Sighinolfi MC, De Stefani S, Bianchi G, et al. New trends in minimally invasive urological surgery: what is beyond the robot? World J Urol. 2013;31:505–13.
10. De Win G, Van Bruwaene S, Kulkarni J, Van Calster B, Aggarwal R, Allen C, et al. An evidence-based laparoscopic simulation curriculum shortens the clinical learning curve and reduces surgical adverse events. Adv Med Educ Pract. 2016;7:357–70.

Chapter 19
The Development of Hand-Assist Laparoscopy

John Roger Bell and Stephen Y. Nakada

Introduction

Urologic surgery has experienced many technologic breakthroughs throughout history, however, one of the most significant in recent years was the development of laparoscopic surgery. This technique has allowed urologists to perform nephrectomy through a minimally invasive approach. This has resulted in urologists being able to perform a number of operations for both benign and malignant urologic renal conditions with less post-operative pain, faster recovery and equivalent outcomes compared to the open approach. It is widely accepted as a surgical option now and many do not appreciate the controversies and challenges that surrounded the development of the hand-assisted laparoscopic surgery (HALS). In this chapter, we will review the history of the development of HALS and the early challenges and the techniques and technologic innovation that led to the approach it is today.

History and Rationale of the Hand-Assisted Approach

The first laparoscopic nephrectomy in a human was performed on June 25, 1990 by Ralph Clayman and colleagues at Washington University in St. Louis, MO [1, 2]. Following this innovation, many laparoscopic surgeries followed that continued to refine the initial techniques as well as pursue new applications for this technique [3] (Table 19.1). Laparoscopic surgery proved to have many advantages over traditional open surgery including improved post-operative pain and convalescence [4, 5]. Although there were advantages in using a laparoscopic approach, urologists

J.R. Bell, M.D. • S.Y. Nakada, M.D., F.A.C.S. (✉)
Department of Urology, University of Wisconsin School of Medicine and Public Health, Madison, WI, USA
e-mail: nakada@urology.wisc.edu

S.R. Patel et al. (eds.), *The History of Technologic Advancements in Urology*, DOI 10.1007/978-3-319-61691-9_19

Table 19.1 Hand-assisted laparoscopy timeline in urology

1993	First reported case of HAL while performing splenectomy	Boland et al. [31]
1994	First HAL nephrectomy	Tierney et al. [32]
1996	HAL nephrectomy in a pig using PneumoSleeve	Bannenberg et al. [15]
1997	HAL nephrectomy using PneumoSleeve	Nakada et al. [17]
1997	HAL nephroureterorectomy	Keeley et al. [33]
1998	HAL donor nephrectomy	Wolf et al. [9]
2001	HAL partial nephrectomy	Stifelman et al. [7]

were slow to adopt this technique due to several concerns. Standard laparoscopic nephrectomy significantly decreased tactile feedback and replaced the surgeon's dexterous hands with instruments that were far less agile. This decreased tactile sense was an obvious concern to urologists as they felt they had lost a key component of surgical technique not being able to palpate the tissues and assist in blunt dissection of tissue planes. Laparoscopic instruments did not allow for articulation, which limited the ability to perform certain urologic surgeries. In addition, operative times were longer for early laparoscopic surgeries when compared to open surgery (the initial surgery lasted almost 7 h). The loss of three-dimensional vision was another significant concern to surgeons who feared this would negatively affect surgical outcomes. Finally, as is the case with any new technique many urologists were concerned about the learning curve and the outcomes on the early patients [3, 5].

Several innovative urologists began thinking about ways to address these concerns and to make this technique more user friendly. The solution to many of these concerns was to allow the surgeon to use one hand in conjunction with the laparoscopic instruments in order to perform the procedure. This became known as HALS.

HALS allowed the urologist to palpate, identify, and retract during the dissection in order to protect against injury to surrounding structures such as the liver, spleen, bowel and adrenal glands as well as to improve exposure. This technique empowered urologists to more confidently proceed with the renal procedures and reduce the operative time. The intraoperative hand allowed the urologist to regain tactile feedback that had been "lost" during standard laparoscopic procedures. This could be used to better identify structures such as the renal artery during the hilar dissection. The intraoperative hand could also be used to provide a safe amount of traction, such as when reflecting the bowel or when lifting the kidney to identify the hilum. This was felt to be safer by many urologists as the surgeon could better assess how much traction was being placed on tissues when compared to standard laparoscopic instruments. The intraoperative hand could separate natural planes efficiently and allowed the urologist proprioception and provided a reference for improved depth perception during surgery. Typically, the surgeon would introduce

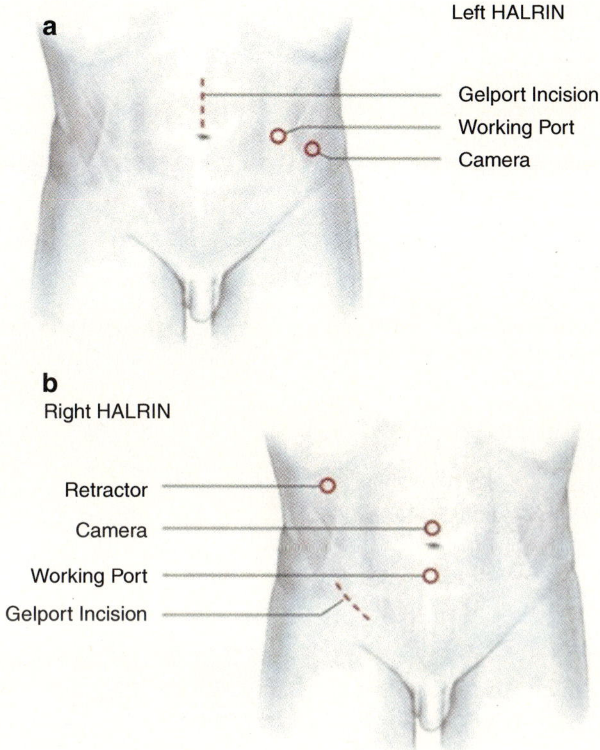

Fig. 19.1 Possible port configurations for hand-assisted laparoscopic nephrectomy. Configurations for left (**a**) and right (**b**) sided hand-assisted laparoscopic nephrectomy are shown. These depictions assume a right-hand dominant surgeon such that the non-dominant hand is used to insert into the abdomen while the dominant hand is used to control laparoscopic instruments during dissection (Used with permission from Sterret and Nakada. Hand-Assisted Radical Laparoscopic Nephrectomy. BJUI 2008 Aug; 102(3):404–15)

the non-dominant hand into the abdomen and reserve the dominant hand for control of various laparoscopic instruments during the procedure (Fig. 19.1).

In addition to several intraoperative advantages, HALS facilitated intact removal of operative specimens without morcellation, as the specimen could be removed via the existing hand port incision (Fig. 19.2). This was a particular concern in cases of suspected or known malignancies where specimen morcellation by some, was "neither appealing nor desirable" [6]. The HAL approach significantly expanded the possibilities of minimally invasive surgery by allowing the surgeon to perform advanced maneuvers. Urologists were now able to identify vascular thrombi and manipulate them towards to kidney. Laparoscopic suturing was easier with the hand-assisted approach. Partial nephrectomies were performed using the operative hand to manually compress the kidney in the same method as is done during open surgery [7]. HAL was also used to perform nephroureterectomies, donor nephrectomies, tumor thrombus removal and perform procedures in morbidly obese patients [8–11]. Even though HALS did not create true three-dimensional imaging during surgery, it provided many other benefits over standard laparoscopy. These advantages translated into shorter operative times which enticed urologists to use HALS and also provide a bridge between open surgery and laparoscopy [5].

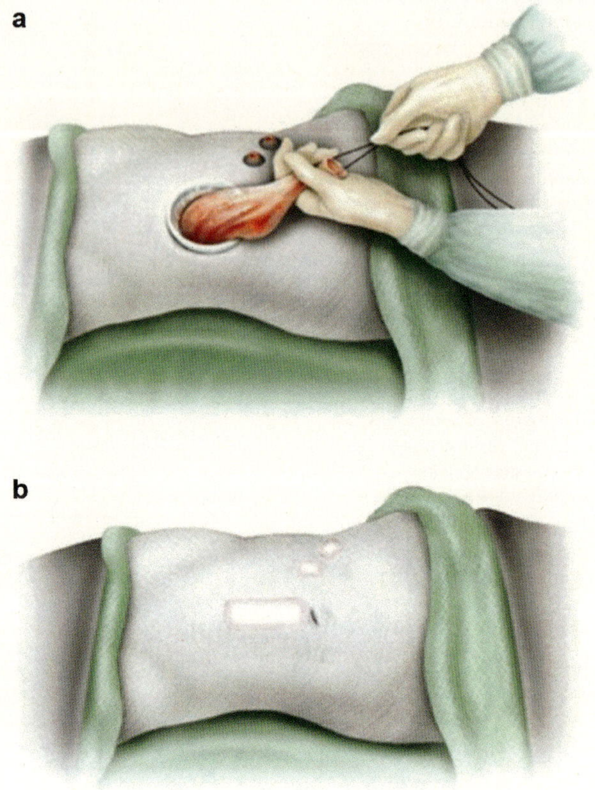

Fig. 19.2 Intact specimen extraction through a hand assist device. (**a**) The use of the hand assist devices offered many advantages during the surgical procedure. Another advantage was the ability to easily and quickly remove intact specimens. (**b**) The incision used to place the hand assist device therefore doubled as the extraction site (Used with permission from Sterret and Nakada. Hand-Assisted Radical Laparoscopic Nephrectomy. BJUI 2008 Aug; 102(3):404–15).

History of the Development of Hand-Assisted Laparoscopy

The first reported case of manual assistance during a laparoscopic surgery is credited to Drs. Edward Tiley and James Boland, Roberto Kusminsky, and James Tierney. They were performing a laparoscopic splenectomy in May 1992 when they encountered bleeding from a short gastric vessel. During this episode, a small incision was made and a surgeon's hand was introduced to help control the bleeding. The resulting incision was then used to deliver the intact spleen after dissection was complete. This successful operation led these surgeons to use this approach during subsequent surgeries. The group performed another HAL splenectomy by making a pfannenstiel incision, then the hand was inserted using a long obstetrical glove [12]. The group referred to this technique as laparoscopic minilaparotomy [13]. Their technique involved inserting a laparoscopic camera into the abdomen to visually assess the abdomen. The group reported that patients were tolerating diet and ambulating within 24–72 h in comparison to 6.5 days that was reported as the average for open surgical laparotomy. Tschada et al. then reported their use of "manual assistance" during a report of laparoscopic nephrectomies in 1995 [14]. In this abstract, the operative times for manual assistance cases were shorter compared to traditional laparoscopic cases (2.5–5 h vs. 4–6 h).

The incorporation of the surgeon's hand into the operation certainly had significant advantages. During the initial surgery by Boland and colleagues it certainly allowed for important and expedient control of bleeding during the operation. Yet, the technique of inserting just the surgeon's hand through an incision proved to have several disadvantages for the surgeon. First, the incision was sized to one particular surgeon meaning that if any other surgeon was involved in the procedure, the incision would have to be modified. This would be a particular problem if the initial incision was larger than a subsequent surgeon's hand as the pneumoperitoneum would leak around the surgeon's hand. Another limitation of this approach was that other instruments could not be placed through this incision as again, pneumoperitoneum would be lost by inserting a smaller instrument through this larger incision. Furthermore, many surgeons reported hand cramping during surgeries and would at times have to remove their hand to allow it to recover before continuing the operation [15].

One solution to these problems was the development of a port or sleeve type device that allowed a surgeon to insert and withdraw and even change operators while maintaining pneumoperitoneum. Although early devices did not always succeed in accomplishing these tasks, they paved the way for further innovation. The first device to be used was called the PnuemoSleeve (Dexterity, Atlanta, GA). Porcine surgeries were done in order to establish efficacy by Bannenberg et al. [15, 16]. These experiments allowed the surgeons to decrease operative time, allow for the exchange of hands and even allow the use of traditional open instruments to be used during the procedure. In one of the surgeries, the authors described the purposeful cutting of a renal vein to test the ability to control this with the intraoperative hand. They reported that this was "easily controlled by pressure with the thumb and forefinger while retracting the kidney laterally." Clips were placed after the bleeding vessel was secured to ligate the bleeding vessel [15]. These animal studies then paved the way for use in humans using the PnuemoSleeve.

The first hand-assisted laparoscopic nephrectomy in a human using a hand-assist device (PneumoSleeve) was performed by Drs. Stephen Nakada and Timothy Moon at the University of Wisconsin in April of 1997 (Fig. 19.3). The patient was a 60 year-old woman with multiple sclerosis and recurrent stone disease who developed end-stage renal failure requiring hemodialysis. She had recurrent episodes of pyelonephritis and chronic right flank pain and had a past surgical history that included an open right pyelolithotomy and appendectomy. She had a right-sided nephrostomy tube in place at the time of surgery. The primary surgeon was left-handed and therefore the PneumoSleeve was placed in the midline just superior to the umbilicus by making a 7 cm incision. Two additional 12 mm ports were placed and a 5 mm port was used for the liver retractor. The specimen was removed intact through the midline incision. The surgery lasted 4 h and 18 min with 100 cc of blood loss. The patient was discharged on postoperative day 3 and returned to normal activity within

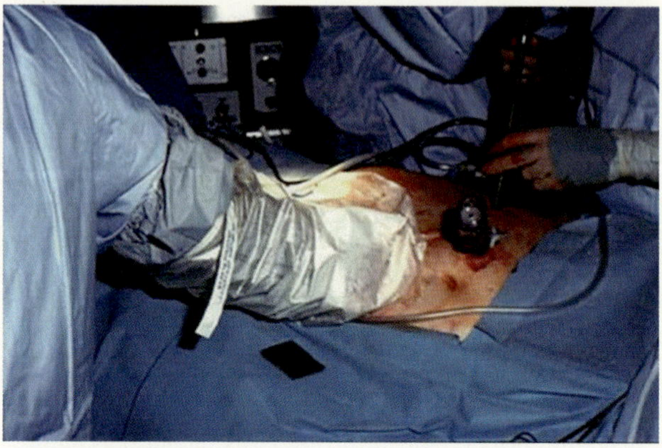

Fig. 19.3 Operative photograph of the first hand-assisted laparoscopic nephrectomy using the PneumoSleeve. Drs. Stephen Nakada and Timothy Moon are shown here performing the first hand-assisted laparoscopic nephrectomy using a hand assist device (PneumoSleeve) in 1997. The surgery lasted just over 4 h and the patient was discharged home on post-operative day 3. [Photo courtesy of Dr. Stephen Nakada]

7 days. Subsequently a HALS radical nephrectomy was performed on a 4 cm RCC successfully by that same surgical team [17].

Hand Port Devices and Development

The development of the hand-assist devices (HADs) were paramount to the widespread application of HAL. These offered the ability to for the surgeon to insert and withdraw his hand through the procedure and for the exchange of surgeons to occur. They allowed the introduction and removal of other laparoscopic and traditional surgical instruments as well as sponges into the abdomen and withdraw them without losing pneumoperitoneum. We have already briefly introduced the PneumoSleeve as the first product of this type. Several other products were subsequently developed that allowed surgeons to accomplish these goals. HADs are generally divided into first and second-generation devices. The first generation devices included the HandPort, the IntroMit, and the PneumoSleeve. Second generation devices include the LapDisc, the OmniPort and the Gelport [18]. We will discuss these devices including their advantages and limitations in the following section.

The PneumoSleeve (Dexterity, Atlanta, GA) was the first device available in the United States [17, 19, 20]. The device used an adhesive plate that attached to the abdominal wall (Fig. 19.4). The surgeon then wore a sleeve that attached to the abdominal wall thus creating the seal. The set included an adhesive locking ring, a paper template, a protector-retractor, two sleeves, the Pneumo Dome. The laparoscopic ports were first placed and the location of the PneumoSleeve was inspected. The adherent base is placed on the abdomen. The paper template was then used to

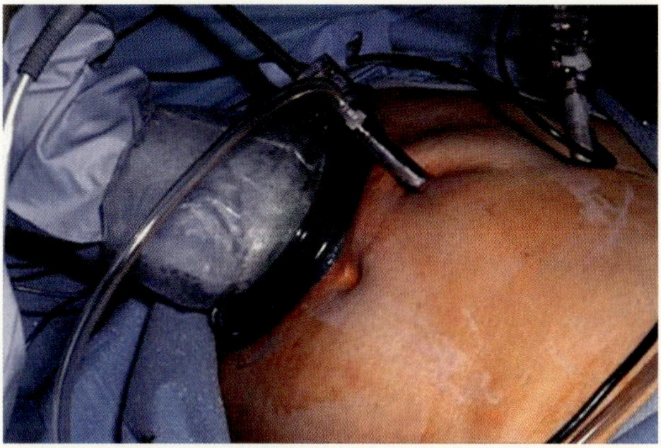

Fig. 19.4 Intraoperative photograph of a PneumoSleeve in use during a hand-assisted laparoscopic nephrectomy. The PneumoSleeve consisted of an internal protractor-retractor sleeve (not shown). A plastic base attached to the patient and the Pneumo Dome was secured to the base as well as to the surgeon's hand. [Photo courtesy of Dr. Stephen Nakada]

mark the planned incision. The size of the incision was based on the surgeon's hand size. The protractor-retractor was inserted through the incision with the inner ring placed just inside the peritoneal cavity. This component served as a wound protector and helped to retract the edges to facilitate insertion of the surgeon's hand through the wound. The sleeve component was then placed over the surgeon's fingers. A dark glove was typically placed over the surgeon's hand as light colored gloves tended to reflect too much light which obscured the surgeon's visualization. The sleeve was then locked to the adherent base on the abdomen. Pneumoperitoneum is lost during the insertion process, however after the ring is locked it can be re-established [20–22].

One of the main complaints of the PneumoSleeve was the relatively frequent loss of pneumoperitoneum. There were several reasons this might occur. One was that the base would often loose its adhesive attachment to the patient during the case with resultant loss of pneumoperitoneum. Some surgeons suggested meticulous skin preparation as well as placing a separate clear adhesive drape to the skin and then placing the adherent base to this drape. The sleeve was long and somewhat redundant putting it at risk of perforation during the insertion of other instruments which would result in a loss of pneumoperitoneum [22]. The device was somewhat cumbersome to attach to the surgeon which meant a somewhat laborious process to switch operators. The PneumoSleeve took approximately 40 min to apply and had a cost of about $400 [5, 17].

The Hand-Port (Smith & Nephew Endoscopy, Andover, MA) was a two-piece device that consisted of a base plate that attached to the patient and a sleeve worn by the surgeon that attached to the base plate. It was approved for use in the United States in 1999. The system was packaged with the base retractor, bracelet, sleeve, and HandPort cap. This device did not require adhesive in order to attach to the patient. An incision was made and the base plate was inserted through the patient's incision and into the operative field. The surgeon then placed a plastic sleeve around his arm and secured this with a bracelet. A second dark glove was then placed over the sleeve and the bracelet. The sleeve was then secured to the baseplate thus creating the closed system. The baseplate contained an inflatable rim that was inflated with a bulb inflator to seal the inner ring against the abdominal wall. The most common problem with this device, was that the baseplate would "pop out" from the operative field resulting in a loss of pneumoperitoneum. This device was often inserted after pneumoperitoneum had been established, however, it could also be placed prior to establishing insufflation [21, 22].

A number of surgeries were used to evaluate the HandPort device by a multi-institutional team of surgeons [23]. This included 68 HAL surgeries of various types including 7 living-related donor nephrectomies. During these cases, the mean operative time was 277 min with none of them requiring conversion to open procedure. The mean length of stay was 4.3 days with a warm ischemia time of less than 1 min in the partial nephrectomies. During these 68 surgeries, physicians reported mild hand fatigue in 14 of these surgeries (20.6%) and severe hand cramping in 2 of these surgeries (2.9%). Seventeen of these surgeries (25%) demonstrated some amount of pneumoperitoneum leak [20, 21, 23].

In a survey among training urologists, the first generation devices scored less than 8.1 out of 10 in all categories studied and had an overall satisfaction rating of 7.7/10. The largest drawbacks were their tendency to leak pneumoperitoneum and the need to attach to the surgeon, patient or both. In this study, none of these devices were superior to the other in terms of overall satisfaction, however, the PneumoSleeve and the IntroMit did tend to contain the pneumoperitoneum better than the HandPort [20]. Based on the experience with the first generation devices, a second generation of devices was developed in an attempt to improve upon the previous design.

The second-generation devices featured a design that did not require the surgeon to double glove, use sleeves, use adhesives to attach component to the patient and did not require elements of the device to attach to the surgeon [18]. This design allowed for easier and more secure placement and allowed for ease on inserting and withdrawing hands as well as other surgical devices. The second-generation devices were the OmniPort, LapDisc, and the GelPort.

The OmniPort (Weck Surgical, Research Triangle Park, NC) was a one-piece device that had some design similarities to the IntroMit. It was a clear, inflatable, one-piece device where one portion spanned the height of the wound and another portion extended above the patient's skin. The portion of the sleeve that extended above the patient's skin was inflated with a bulb inflation device to create a seal around the surgeon's hand in order to contain pneumoperitoneum. However, with this design, every time the surgeon removed his hand, the device would need to be deflated and subsequently re-inflated which resulted in the disruption of pneumoperitoneum. The average cost of this device in 2004 was $440.18.

The LapDisc (Ethicon Endosurgical, Cincinnati, OH) consisted of a sleeve with two discs on either end of the cylindrical device. This device was inserted into the incision with one disc against the anterior peritoneum and the other extending out of the incision. This sleeve was covered with a thin-plastic material that would be rotated in order to create a concentric seal around the surgeon's hand. The device had a smaller footprint at only 12 cm in diameter, making it more attractive for use in thin patients. However, one drawback of this device was the relatively short sleeve height, making it difficult to use in obese patients. The average cost for the device in 2004 was $440.18.

GelPort (Applied Medical, Rancho Santa Margarita, CA) is made of a soft, gel-like material that can expand to allow the insertion of the surgeon's hand and then seal when the hand is withdrawn. It is placed by first making an incision through the skin, subcutaneous tissue, fascia and peritoneum that is large enough to accommodate the surgeon's hand. The GelPort has a cylindrical sleeve that is made of a soft, clear plastic and contains a plastic ring at each end. The inner ring is a malleable plastic ring that is inserted into the incision with the ring inside of the abdominal cavity. The other ring is rolled to tighten the sleeve against the incision. This makes it where the two rings are flush with the patient's skin and anterior peritoneum. The gel cap is then clamped on the external ring thus forming a seal. One downside of the device is the external ring has a diameter of 16 cm that made it more difficult to use on patients who are thin or have small torsos. The average cost for the device in 2004 was $500 and included the GelPort, 4 trocars and a clip applier [18]. The average time to apply was 5 min [24]. Another application of this device was the ability to introduce ports and instruments directly through the GelPort without causing significant degradation to the device and without the loss of pneumoperitoneum [25].

The second-generation devices were compared to each other in a similar fashion as the first-generation devices. Urologists with no laparoscopic experience underwent training and evaluated the second-generation devices in a porcine model. This study found that the Gelport performed better in all measured categories when compared to the first generation devices and generally was rated higher than the OmniPort or LapDisc [18].

Outcomes of Renal Hand-Assisted Laparoscopy

Nakada et al. found similar operative times when compared to open renal surgery with a lower length of stay, faster return to activities and lower blood loss [4]. Shuford et al. found that the length of stay was the same between LRN and HALRN and both modalities were shorter than open radical nephrectomy. HALRN showed a lower transfusion rate when compared to open nephrectomy and was not statistically different than LRN. There was no statistical difference in overall complication rate when comparing the three surgical modalities [26]. Wolf et al. compared standard laparoscopic renal surgery versus HAL and found no difference in time to oral intake, length of stay, post-operative narcotic usage, time to return to normal activity and post-operative pain scores. However, the mean operative time was 199 min shorter in the HAL versus the standard laparoscopy group [5].

Complications of Hand-Assisted Laparoscopy

Several studies reported a similar rate of transfusion, wound infection, post-operative ileus, bowel obstruction, incisional hernia, DVT, PE, MI, PNA, and urinary retention [26–28]. Pareek et al. performed a meta-analysis on the complication rate of laparoscopic versus HAL renal surgery. This study found no significant difference between the two in regards to overall complication rate. Not surprisingly, the incisional hernia rates were actually slightly higher in the laparoscopic cases. The HAL cases did demonstrate a higher rate of post-operative wound infection [29]. Nelson and Wolf reported no difference in the rate of complications, hospital cost, length of stay, return to activity or post-operative pain between HALRN versus LRN. They also found shorter operative times for HALRN [30].

Conclusions

The choice of surgical procedure is based on a multitude of factors including patient and tumor characteristics, surgeon experience and preference, device availability and patient preferences. Certainly the robotic approach has added another important modality in the surgical treatment of renal pathology. However, laparoscopy still has an important role as it is generally faster and is certainly less expensive than the robotic approaches. The laparoscopic technique revolutionized urologic surgery by reducing post-operative pain and convalescence. However, the purely laparoscopic approach did have limitations and drawbacks. The hand-assisted technique tremendously expanded the surgical possibilities without increasing the morbidity of the procedure. It allowed urologists to make the transition to laparoscopic surgery and has truly been a landmark development in the history of urology.

References

1. Clayman RV, Kavoussi LR, Soper NJ. Laparoscopic nephrectomy. N Engl J Med. 1991;324:1370–1.
2. Clayman RV, Kavoussi LR, Soper NJ, et al. Laparoscopic nephrectomy: initial case report. J Urol. 1991;146:278–82.
3. Clayman RV, Kavoussi LR, McDougall EM, et al. Laparoscopic nephrectomy: a review of 16 cases. Surg Laparosc Endosc. 1992;2:29–34.
4. Nakada SY, Fadden P, Jarrard DF, et al. Hand-assisted laparoscopic radical nephrectomy: comparison to open radical nephrectomy. Urology. 2001;58:517–20.
5. Wolf JS, Moon TD, Nakada SY. Hand assisted laparoscopic nephrectomy: comparison to standard laparoscopic nephrectomy. J Urol. 1998;160:22–7.
6. Kusminsky RE, Boland JP, Tiley EH, et al. Hand-assisted laparoscopic splenectomy. Surg Laparosc Endosc. 1995;5:463–7.
7. Stifelman MD, Sosa RE, Nakada SY, et al. Hand-assisted laparoscopic partial nephrectomy. J Endourol. 2001;15:161–4.

8. Stifelman MD, Sosa RE, Andrade A, et al. Hand-assisted laparoscopic nephroureterectomy for the treatment of transitional cell carcinoma of the upper urinary tract. Urology. 2000;56:741–7.
9. Wolf JS, Tchetgen M-B, Merion RM. Hand-assisted laparoscopic live donor nephrectomy. Urology. 1998;52:885–7.
10. Sundaram CP, Rehman J, Landman J, et al. Hand assisted laparoscopic radical nephrectomy for renal cell carcinoma with inferior vena caval thrombus. J Urol. 2002;168:176–9.
11. Hedican SP, Moon TD, Lowry PS, et al. Hand-assisted laparoscopic renal surgery in the morbidly and profoundly obese. J Endourol. 2004;18:241–4.
12. Boland JP, Kusminsky RE, Tiley EH, et al. Evolution of hand-assisted laparoscopic surgery. J Endourol. 2005;19:133–5.
13. Kusminsky RE, Tiley EH, Lucente FC, et al. Laparoscopic staging laparotomy with intra-abdominal manipulation. Surg Laparosc Endosc. 1994;4:103–5.
14. Tschada R, Rassweiler J, Schmeller N, et al. Laparoscopic tumor nephrectomy-the German experiences (abstract). J Urol. 1995;153(Suppl):479A.
15. Bannenberg JJG, Meijer DW, Bannenberg JH, et al. Hand-assisted laparoscopic nephrectomy in the pig: initial report. Minim Invasive Ther Allied Technol. 1996;5:483–7.
16. Bannenberg J, Meijer D, Leahy P, et al. A new method for laparoscopic nephrectomy. Min Invas Ther. 1994;3(Suppl. 1):73.
17. Nakada SY, Moon TD, Gist M, et al. Use of the pneumo sleeve as an adjunct in laparoscopic nephrectomy. Urology. 1997;49:612–3.
18. Patel R, Stifelman MD. Hand-assisted laparoscopic devices: the second generation. J Endourol. 2004;18:649–53.
19. Lowry PS, Nakada SY. Hand-assisted laparoscopic radical nephrectomy. J Endourol. 2004;18:337–44.
20. Stifelman M, Nieder AM. Prospective comparison of hand-assisted laparoscopic devices. Urology. 2002;59:668–72.
21. Seifman BD, Wolf JS Jr. Technical advances in laparoscopy: hand assistance, retractors, and the pneumodissector. J Endourol. 2000;14:921–8.
22. McGinnis DE, Gomella LG, Strup SE. Comparison and clinical evaluation of hand-assist devices for hand-assisted laparoscopy. Tech Urol. 2001;7:57–61.
23. Litwin DE, Darzi A, Jakimowicz J, et al. Hand-assisted laparoscopic surgery (HALS) with the HandPort system: initial experience with 68 patients. Ann Surg. 2000;231:715–23.
24. Rane A, Dasgupta P. Prospective experience with a second-generation hand-assisted laparoscopic device and comparison with first-generation devices. J Endourol. 2003;17:895–7.
25. Lee DI, Landman J. Novel approach to minimizing trocar sites during challenging hand-assisted laparoscopic surgery utilizing the Gelport: trans-gel instrument insertion and utilization. J Endourol. 2003;17:69–71.
26. Shuford MD, McDougall EM, Chang SS, et al. Complications of contemporary radical nephrectomy: comparison of open vs. laparoscopic approach. Urol Oncol. 2004;22:121–6.
27. Moore NW, Nakada SY, Hedican SP, et al. Complications of hand-assisted laparoscopic renal surgery: single-center ten-year experience. Urology. 2011;77:1353–8.
28. Ono Y, Kinukawa T, Hattori R, et al. Laparoscopic radical nephrectomy for renal cell carcinoma: a five-year experience. Urology. 1999;53:280–6.
29. Pareek G, Hedican SP, Gee JR, et al. Meta-analysis of the complications of laparoscopic renal surgery: comparison of procedures and techniques. J Urol. 2006;175:1208–13.
30. Nelson CP, Wolf JS. Comparison of hand assisted versus standard laparoscopic radical nephrectomy for suspected renal cell carcinoma. J Urol. 2002;167:1989–94.
31. Boland J, Kusminsky RE, Tiley EH. Laparoscopic mini-laparotomy with manipulation: the middle path. Minim Invasive Ther. 1993;2:63–7.
32. Tierney J, Oliver S, Kusminsky R, et al. Laparoscopic radical nephrectomy with intra-abdominal manipulation. Minim Invasive Ther. 1994;3:303–5.
33. Keeley FX, Sharma NK, Tolley DA. Hand-assisted laparoscopic nephroureterectomy. BJU Int. 1999;83:504–5.

Chapter 20
History and Development of Robotics in Urology

Gabriel Ogaya-Pinies, Hariharan Palayapalayam Ganapathi, Travis Rogers, and Vipul Patel

Background

The first robot was designed and possibly constructed by Leonardo da Vinci around the year 1495. Leonardo's robot is a nickname given to a humanoid automaton which is believed to be the result of Leonardo's anatomical research in the Canon of Proportions as described in the *Vitruvian Man* (Fig. 20.1). The design notes for this model appear in sketchbooks that were rediscovered in the 1950s and this prototype was reconstructed in 2002 and was able to make several human-like motions, including sitting and moving its arms, neck and jaw [1].

However the word robot wasn't coined until 1923 by Karel Capek and comes from the Czech word "robota" which means slave labor. In his science fiction book "Rossum's Universal Robots" an inventor creates robots as a cheap labor force. However, the story turns sinister when these robots become highly intelligent and capable of feelings, realizing that they are superior to humans. They declare war on humans and try to eliminate the entire human race from the face of the earth [2].

Modern industrial robots however, did not appear until the 1950s, when Unimation (Universal Automation), a company created by Devol and Engelberg, developed the Unimate, a jointed industrial robot arm used by General Motors assembly lines [3]. The success of robotics in industry is due in large part to their versatility and capability. Robots are able to perform multiple tasks that are often unpleasant and dangerous for humans and range from requiring tremendous strengths to millimetric precision. It was not until the 1980s that robots became part of the surgical field. The National Aeronautics and Space Administration Ames Research Center investigated virtual reality systems in collaboration with mechanical engineers at the Stanford Research Institute (SRI). They were interested in robotic technologies to develop a

G. Ogaya-Pinies, M.D. • H.P. Ganapathi, M.D. • T.R. Rogers, M.D. • V. Patel, M.D. (✉)
Global Robotics Institute, Celebration, FL, USA

Florida Hospital Celebration Health, Celebration, FL, USA
e-mail: vpatel2171@aol.com

S.R. Patel et al. (eds.), *The History of Technologic Advancements in Urology*,
DOI 10.1007/978-3-319-61691-9_20

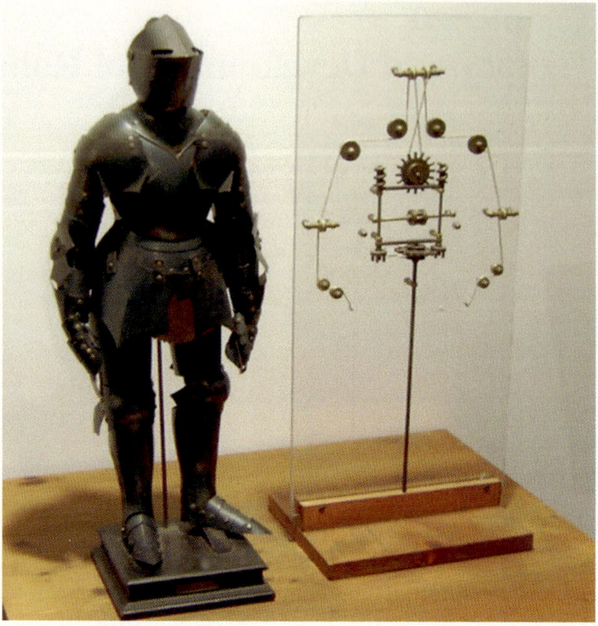

Fig. 20.1 Humanoid automaton, designed by Leonardo da Vinci, it is believed to be able to perform several human-like motions

"telepresence" surgical system to improve dexterity in microscopic hand surgery [4]. The focus then shifted from micro- surgical to macroscopic general surgical applications, largely driven by the demonstration of laparoscopic cholecystectomy in 1989 by Perissat and colleagues [5]. A revised telepresence system including a surgeon's console and remotely controlled tele-manipulators was developed with funding from the U.S. Department of Defense. These research projects eventually led to the da Vinci Surgical System (timeline summarized in Table 20.1).

Finally, we must make a clarification, the Oxford Dictionary of English defines robot as: "a machine capable of carrying out a complex series of actions automatically, especially one programmable by a computer," but this definition does exactly fit the so-called robotic surgical devices of today [6]. Most of the devices available to us are actually master-slave systems, where the surgeon (the master) has full control over the device (the slave), so fully articulating robotic arms mimic the movement of hands, allowing surgeons to have greater dexterity and control than is possible with conventional laparoscopic instruments.

Robotics in Surgery

The first time a robot was used in a surgical intervention was in 1985 in the Memorial Hospital of Los Angeles. The Unimation PUMA (Programmable Universal Manipulation Arm) 200 robot was used to hold a probe guide during a stereotactic brain biopsy. The robot was properly interfaced with a computerized tomographic (CT) scanner (Fig. 20.2). Once the target was identified on the CT imaging, a simple command

Table 20.1 Timeline of events in the history and development of robotics in urology

Date	Event
1495	Leonardo da Vinci designs the humanoid automaton, a robot knight that was able to stand, sit, raise its visor and independently maneuver its arms, and jaw.
1923	The word robot (Robota) is first coined by the Czech author Karel Capek in his science fiction book "Rossum's Universal robots".
1985	PUMA 200 was the first robot used in a surgical intervention during a stereotactic brain biopsy, in Los Angeles, USA.
1988	The PROBOT was used to perform transurethral surgery at imperial college (London, UK), this being the first application of robotics in urology.
1994	FDA approved AESOP®, the first robotic arm used to hold the camera during laparoscopy procedures.
1995	Intuitive surgical® in founded
2000	The FDA approved the da Vinci surgical system®. This year binder performed the first RALP in Frankfurt, Germany.
2000	First robotic nephrectomy in humans was performed by Guillonneau using a Zeus robotic surgical system.

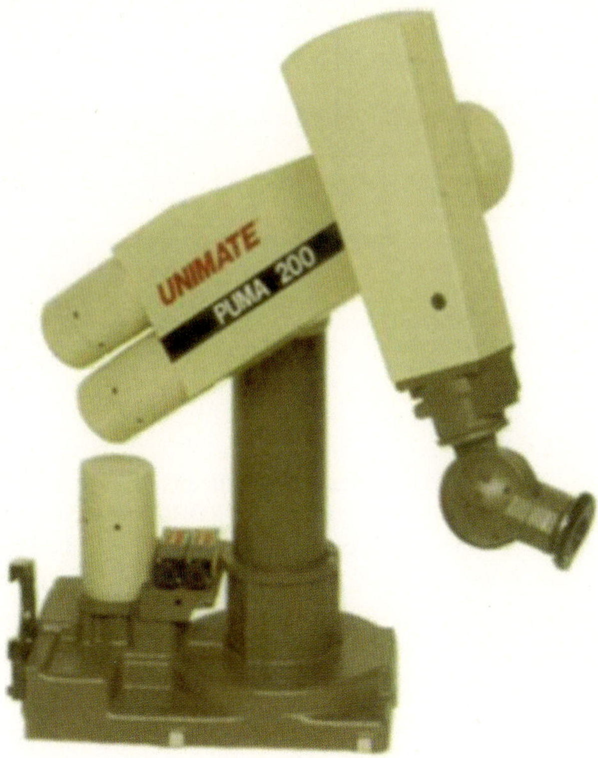

Fig. 20.2 Unimate PUMA 200 first robot used in a surgical intervention during a stereotactic brain biopsy

allowed the robot to move to a position such that the end-effector probe guided points toward the target. The main advantage of this technique was the improved accuracy that can be achieved by proper calibration of the robot [7]. This was followed by ROBODOC (Integrated Surgical Systems), a robotic system to aid orthopedic surgeons (Fig. 20.3).

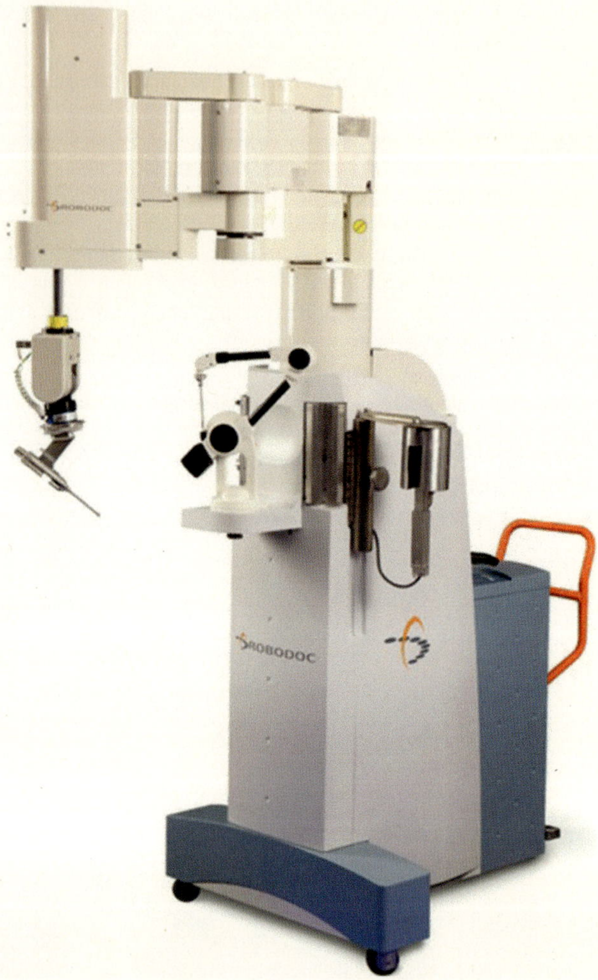

Fig. 20.3 ROBODOC used for the first time in 1988, during a total hip replacement

In 1988, ROBODOC was used for the first time to drill a hole in a patient's femur during a total hip replacement [8]. The ROBODOC System has assisted surgeons in more than 35,000 joint replacement procedures across the United States, Europe and Asia. Japan, Korea and India, and continues its role at the forefront of medical technology.

First Application of Robotics in Urology

In 1988 at Imperial College (London, UK) the PROBOT was used in clinical trials to perform transurethral surgery (Fig. 20.4). This prototype was able to execute a surgical task following a preoperatively established plan. First, the distance from the bladder neck to the verumontanum was measured. Then, an ultrasound probe was passed through the endoscope to scan the prostate in order to build a three dimensional image of the gland. Using this model the urologist designed the cavity

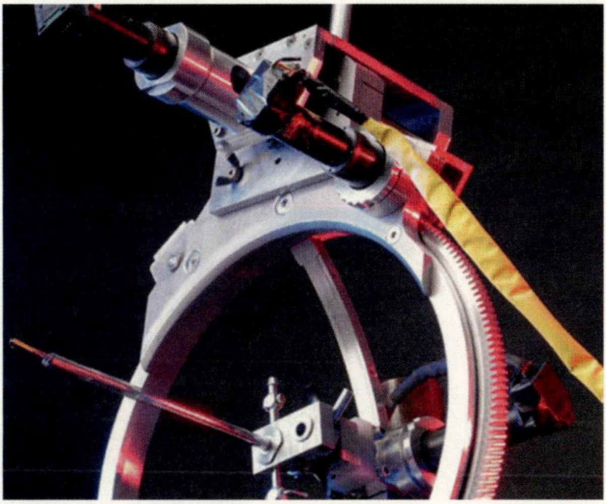

Fig. 20.4 The PROBOT was able to performed precise and repetitive cone shaped cuts of the prostate following a pre-establish plan

to be resected and the PROBOT was able to perform precise and repetitive cone shaped cuts from the verumontanum to the bladder neck [9]. The surgeon followed the progression of the procedure at the workstation and can adjust the cutting parameters or stop the robot at any time. In case of system failure, the surgeon can complete the operation manually.

Application of Robotics in Laparoscopy

In 1993, Computer Motion Inc. (Santa Barbara, California) released AESOP® (Automated Endoscope System for Optimal Positioning), a robotic arm designed to assist the surgeon in the era of laparoscopy by taking control of the laparoscopic camera (Fig. 20.5). This eliminates the need for an additional member of the surgical team, offering a steadier view and reducing instrument collisions. The system is composed of an articulated, electromechanical arm mounted to the operating room table. The arm provides 7 degrees of freedom (7-DOF) that are completely controlled by the surgeon. In 1994, AESOP® 1000 became the first robot to be approved by the U.S. Food and Drug Administration (FDA) [10]. When it was first introduced, it (AESOP® 1000) it was controlled via a foot pedal but future models (AESOP® 2000 in 1996 and AESOP® 3000 in 1998) were released with voice control.

AESOP® was followed by ZEUS® Robotic Surgical System (1998) which was also created by Computer Motion Inc. (Fig. 20.6). With ZEUS®, a master console allows the surgeon to control three independent articulated arms. This system combined an AESOP® robotic camera holder with two arms providing 6 degrees of freedom (6-DOF). Initially, this model was developed with a two-dimensional viewing system, however the final version was provided with a three-dimensional (3-D) view using glasses. The first procedure performed with this technology was a fallopian tube re-anastomosis in Cleveland, USA [11]. The ZEUS® Robotic Surgical

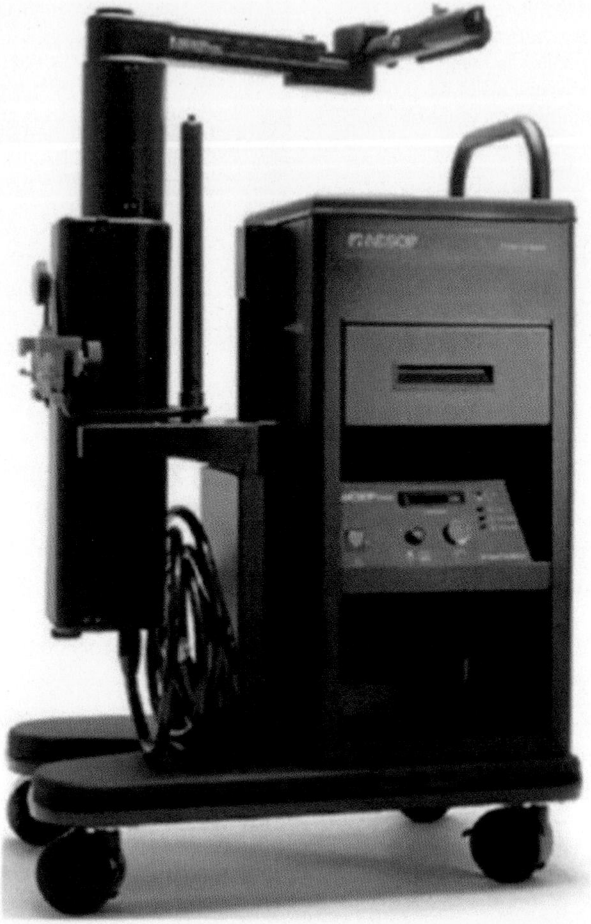

Fig. 20.5 AESOP® (Automated Endoscope System for Optimal Positioning), is a voice-activated robot used to hold the endoscope

System has the honor of being the first robotic system to be used in a transatlantic surgery. In 2001, Marescaux performed from New York, USA, an uneventful cholecystectomy on a female patient in Strasbourg, France, this procedure was also known as the "Lindbergh Operation" [12].

Modern Robotics Systems

In 1995, a group of scientists and medical entrepreneurs from Stanford Research Institute International (SRI International), Massachusetts Institute of Technology (MIT) and International Business Machines (IBM) founded Intuitive Surgical® with the idea of applying the principals of minimally invasive surgery to robotic-assisted surgery [13]. The company refined the SRI System into prototypes known originally as *Lenny* (used in animal trials) after the young Leonardo da Vinci, and *Mona*, for his masterwork the Mona Lisa. These prototypes were used in a human

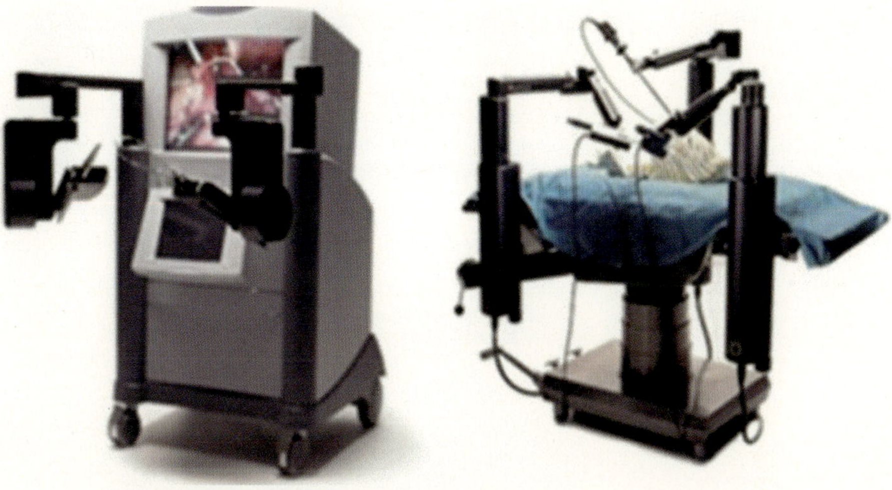

Fig. 20.6 The ZEUS Robotic Surgical System (ZRSS) was a medical robot designed to assist in surgery, originally produced by the American robotics company Computer Motion

cholecystectomy (Himpens and Cadiere) for the first time at the St. Blasius Hospital in Dendermonde, Belgium in 1997 [14].

Based on the initial experiences, the market ready version of the da Vinci robot had more advanced control and ergonomic features compared to the Mona Lisa, and final tests began in 1999. The robotic surgical system was based on three mechanisms: (1) a master-slave software driven system that provide intuitive control of the instruments with seven degrees of freedom; (2) a computerized binocular immersive vision system; (3) a safety system, with redundant sensors that checked instrument position every 750 μs.

The da Vinci Platform

In July of 2000, the FDA approved the Da Vinci® Surgical System (Fig. 20.7). The da Vinci is the most advanced master–slave system developed to date. The system has three components: (a) a surgeon console, (b) a patient-side cart and (c) an image- processing vision cart. The three-dimensional view from the endoscope is projected in the console at 10× magnification. The foot pedals allow control of the energy sources, camera and switching arms. Motion scaling enhances the elimination of tremor, allowing more smooth and precise movements. The robotic arms are mounted on the patient-side cart, one of which holds the high-resolution, three-dimensional endoscope. Specialized EndoWrist® (Intuitive Surgical, California, USA) instruments are mounted on the remaining arms. The vision cart includes the light source, video/image-processing equipment for the endoscope and the main electronic/software processing units. The vision cart also has a touch screen to view the endoscopic image and adjust system settings. The newest model (da-Vinci Xi) also has an integrated electrosurgical unit for activation of energy. The three-dimensional vision, enhanced magnification, motion

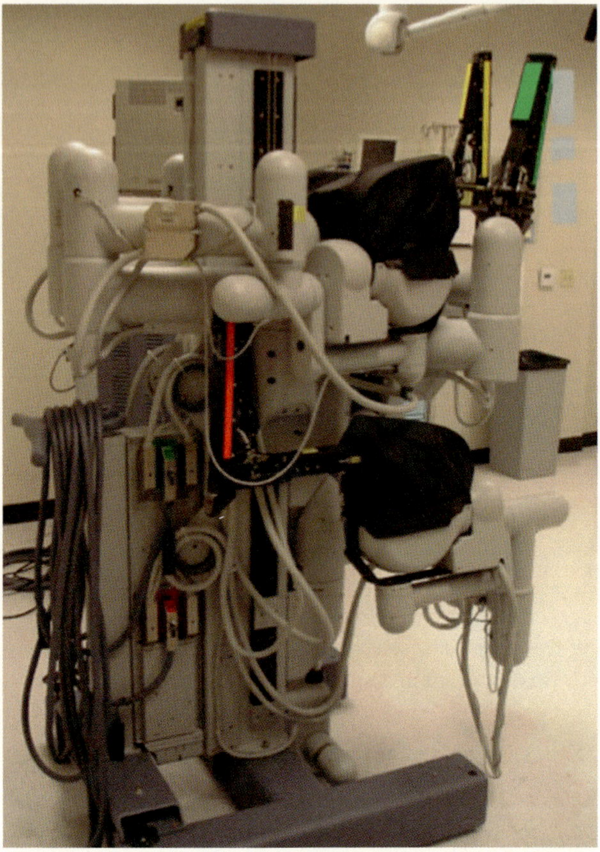

Fig. 20.7 da Vinci Standard System, model approved by the FDA in the year 2000

scaling and most importantly the EndoWrist® technology makes it easier for the operating surgeon to perform complex laparoscopic procedures.

Intuitive Surgical Systems has released four generations of the da Vinci® Surgical System so far. Starting with the "da Vinci" in 2000, that introduced the three-dimensional (3D) vision, the EndoWrist® instrumentation, the Intuitive® motion and later in 2003, the fourth arm. In 2006 the "da Vinci® S" was released with a high-definition, 3D endoscope (720p), streamlined setup, multi-quadrant access and visual inputs (TilePro) (Fig. 20.8). The "da Vinci® Si" was released in 2009 with a more ergonomic surgeon console, improvements in vision and the option of a dual console, as well as, the Firefly fluorescence imaging, this provides real-time, image-guided identification of key anatomical landmarks using near-infrared technology (Fig. 20.9). This enables two surgeons to collaborate during a procedure for *da Vinci*-enabled surgical assistance, exchange control of the instrument arms and endoscope and facilitate teaching comprehensively.

The da Vinci Xi is the newest model of the da Vinci Surgical System (Fig. 20.10). It is optimized for complex four-quadrant surgery featuring revolutionary anatomical access, crystal clear 3D-HD vision, and a platform designed to seamlessly integrate

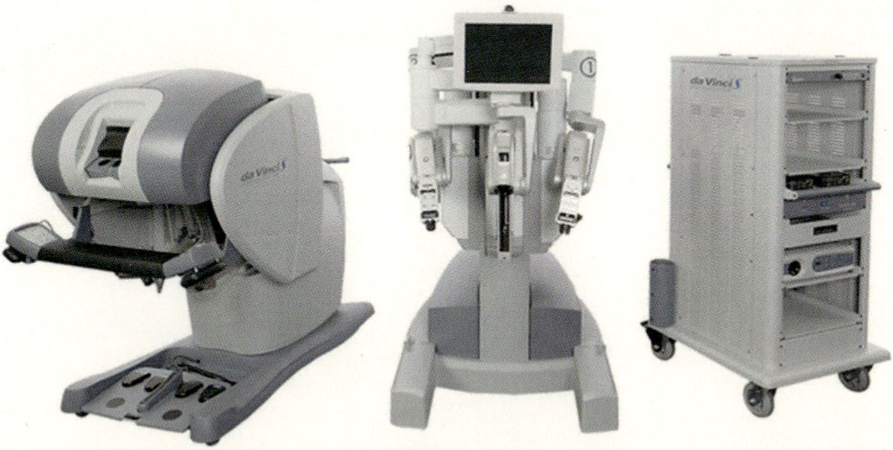

Fig. 20.8 The three components of the da-Vinci S (Intuitive Surgical, Sunnyvale, California), released in 2006: surgeon console, patient-side cart and the image- processing vision car

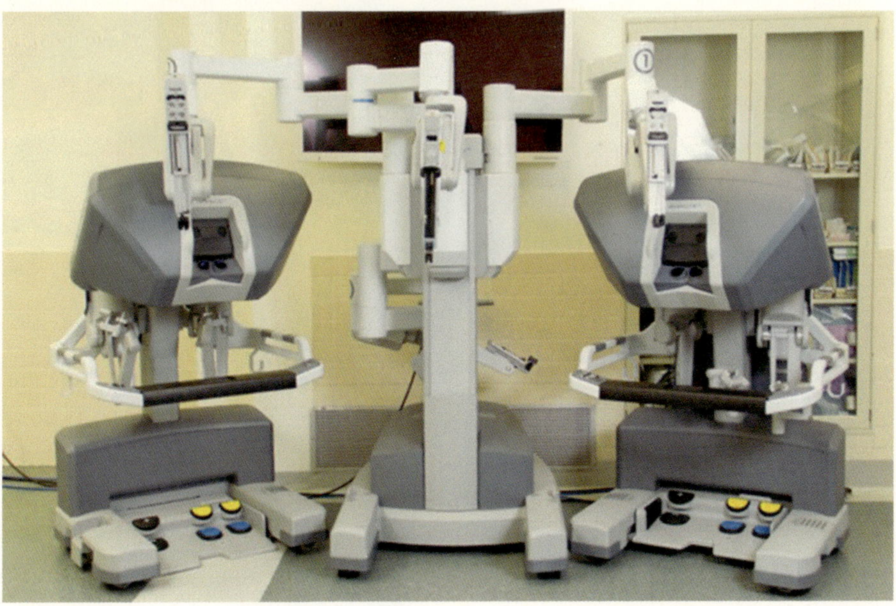

Fig. 20.9 The da Vinci Si dual console (Intuitive Surgical, Sunnyvale, California) allows a surgical mentor to teach with both the mentor and the trainee working at a surgeon console simultaneously

future innovations. Some of the new features are an overhead boom allowing the arms to rotate as a group, lighter arms, a laser target to facilitate the docking, an 8 mm endoscope which is lighter and easier to use with no draping and calibration required, and the instant toggling of the 30 degree endoscope with the touch of a button.

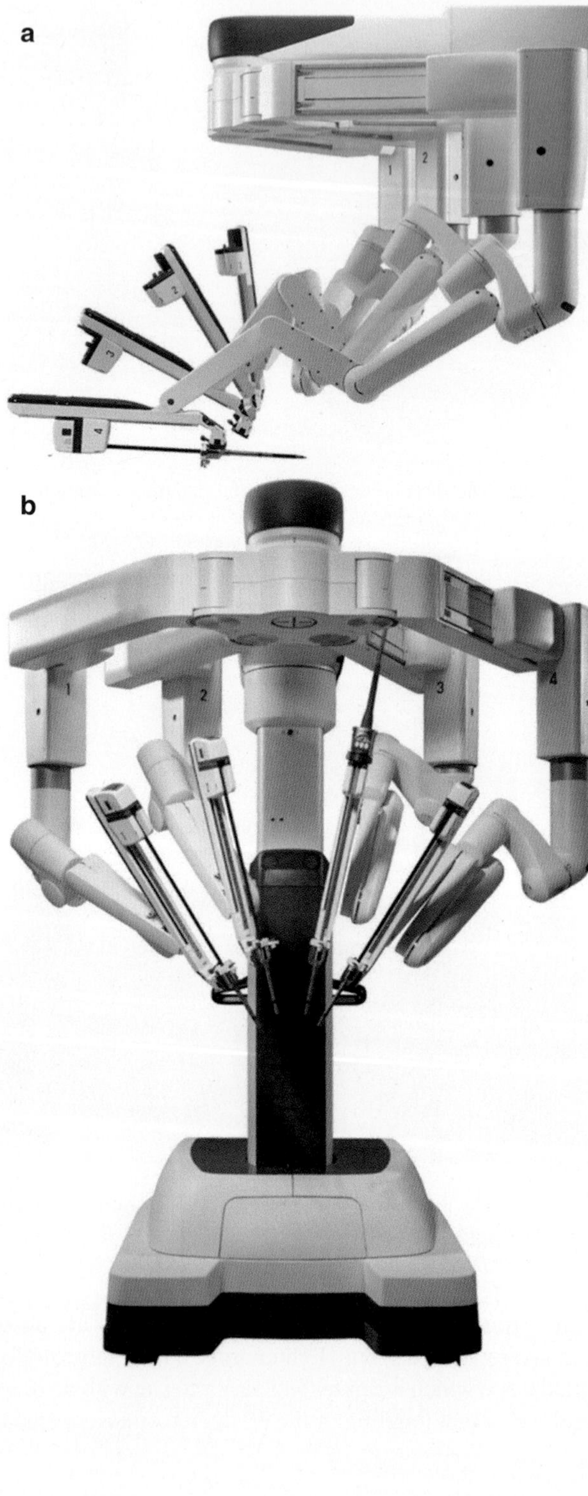

Fig. 20.10 da Vinci Surgical System Xi model released in 2014. (**a**) Overhead boom with lighter arms, the arms rotate as a group. (**b**) Laser target to facilitate the docking and the 8 mm endoscope

Beginning and Evolution of Robotic-Assisted Laparoscopic Prostatectomy

After a period of technical development and training on cadavers with the da Vinci Surgical System, Binder et al. performed the first Robotic-assisted Laparoscopic Prostatectomy (RALP) in May of 2000 in Frankfurt, Germany [15]. They were able to complete the RALP in nine out of the first ten patients with a median console time of 9 h. Despite the long operative surgical time their results were acceptable and highlighted the benefits of the da Vinci Surgical System over conventional laparoscopic surgery. These advantages included better visualization thanks to the three-dimensional vision, tenfold magnification, improved instrument handling facilitated by the EndoWrist technology and the fact that the surgery could be performed in a more ergonomic position at the surgical console. This was followed by Abbou (Paris, France), who described the technique for the first time, with a shorter operating time, catheterization time and hospital stay [16].

The same year, on the other side of the Atlantic Ocean, the first urologic robotic program in the world was built at the Vattikuti Urology Institute (Detroit, USA). Menon, who had no previous laparoscopic experience, but was mentored by Guillonneau and Vallancien, developed a standardized procedure to performed RALP, thus diminishing operative time, complications and cost [17]. Menon's experience is the origin of widespread use of robotics in radical prostatectomy worldwide.

Robotic Kidney Surgeries

The first simple robotic nephrectomy in humans was performed by Guillonneau in 2000 using a Zeus Robotic Surgical System [18]. The patient was a 77-year old woman with a nonfunctioning hydronephrotic right kidney due to ureteropelvic junction obstruction. Using a transperitoneal approach, the operative time for this first robotic nephrectomy was 200 min and the estimated blood loss was 100 mL. But it was not until November of 2002 that the first robotic-assisted partial nephrectomy (RAPN) was performed by Gettman et al. [19]. Later, they reported the outcomes of the first 13 patients that underwent RAPN using transperitoneal, as well as retroperitoneal approach, with tumor sizes ranging from 2 to 6 cm with encouraging results, such as 22 min of warm ischemia, 170 mL of estimated blood loss (EBL) and only one positive surgical margin.

In 2002, Horgan reported the series of ten consecutive cases of robotic-assisted laparoscopic living donor nephrectomies using the da Vinci platform. The nephrectomies were performed between January and May 2001. The mean operative time was 166 min and the mean hospital stay was 1.8 days. All kidneys were transplanted successfully [20].

Other Robotic Surgeries in Urology

Robotic Radical Cystectomy

Radical Cystectomy is one of the most complex procedures in urology. In 2003 Menon et al. published the first series of 17 patients who underwent Robotic-assisted Radical Cystoprostatectomy (RRCP) [21]. The first five patients experienced a surgical approach that mimicked the steps of open radical cystectomy. For the remaining of the patients the initial approach was performed through a transverse incision in the "cul de sac", dissecting out the ureter, the adnexal structures and developing the rectovesical plane. With more than acceptable mean operative time and blood loss during the RRCP, the urinary system was reconstructed by a second surgical team.

Robotic Pyeloplasty

The feasibility of pyeloplasty was proven in a porcine model in 1999. However, it was not until the following year when Guillonneau et al. performed the first robotic-assisted pyeloplasty in humans, using the dismembered technique describe by Anderson and Hynes in 1949 for the open approach [22]. The procedure highlighted the advantage of the robotic platform in reconstructive cases when one compared the ease of suturing compared to the laparoscopic approach.

Future

What is most remarkable about robotic surgery is what the future might hold. One development is long-distance operations and the creation of the tele-surgeons, where a surgeon could conceivably operate on a patient in another city, country or even a different continent. Practically, this would mean that surgical centers would be set up in different parts of the world and a doctor could go to a surgical center and sit in a control console while a patient in a different surgical center would be operated on by a robot controlled by that doctor. There is already a precedent for this as Marescaux performed the first transatlantic surgery [12].

Surgical instruments will also change. Although considerable progress has been achieved with robotic instrument design, great potential exists for further improvements. One change will be the development of the single-incision port, where a snake-like arm would be inserted through a single robotic trocar.

So far, we have seen only the beginning of robotics in surgery. Robotic surgery has proven its safety and feasibility, but what we have done so far only translates open surgical maneuvers into movement of the surgical arms. The future will include automation similar to what we see in the airline industry, however currently automated surgical robots are far from a reality due to subtle variations in human anatomy that demands human skills beyond the capabilities of an algorithm. Although not on the immediate horizon, automation may 1 day meet the safety challenges it faces and become a reality [23].

Microsurgery and further miniaturization will be another area that will be developed in the near future. Robots will be able to turn surgeons into microsurgeons, by translating large movements into minuscule ones, allowing the surgeon to solve specific problems [24]. But we are not only talking about smaller instruments and smaller cameras but also nanorobots, micron sized robots able to deliver targeted gene therapy or detect particular biologic pathogens [13].

Conclusion

Robotics have made a significant contribution to surgery in the past 30 years. This is especially evident in Urology where it has become the reference procedure in the radical surgery of the prostate and partial nephrectomy. Robotics is gaining more and more followers for other surgeries like: pyeloplasty, radical cystectomy and retroperitoneal lymph node dissection among others. Surgical robotics has seen a shift from early systems that assisted the surgeon to current teleoperator systems that can enhance surgical skills. Improvements in size, tactile sensation, instruments, and telesurgery are expected; there is no doubt that the future of surgical robotics is bright.

References

1. Moran ME. The da Vinci robot. J Endourol. 2006;20:986–90.
2. Capek K. Rossum's Universal Robots. [Playfair N, Selver P, trans]. In: Landes WA, editor. New York: Dobleday; 1923.
3. Devol G. U.S. Patent 2,988,237. Programmed article transfer. Filed December 10, 1954 and Issued June 13, 1961.
4. Hill JW, Holst PA, et al. Telepresence interface with applications to microsurgery and surgical simulation. Stud Health Technol Inform. 1998;50:96–102.
5. Perissat J, Collet DR, Belliard R. Gallstones: laprascopic treatment, intracorporeal lithotripsy followed by cholecystostomy or chole-cystectomy—a personal technique. Endoscopy. 1989;21:373–4.
6. Oxford English Dictionary. 2nd ed, vol. 20. Oxford: Oxford University Press; 1989.
7. Kwoh YS, Hou J, Jonckheere EA, Hayati S. A robot with improved absolute positioning accuracy for CT guided stereotactic brain surgery. IEEE Trans Biomed Eng. 1988;35:153–60.
8. Cowley G. Introducing 'Robodoc'. Robot finds his calling – in the operating room. Newsweek. 1992;120:86.
9. Harris SJ, Arambula-Cosio F, Mei Q, et al. The Probot – an active robot for prostate resection. Proc Inst Mech Eng H. 1997;211:317–25.
10. Unger SW, Unger HM, Bass RT. AESOP robotic arm. Surg Endosc. 1994;8:1131.

NOTES

The earliest documented attempt at abdominal surgery via a natural orifice was "ventroscopy" performed by Russian gynaecologist Dimitri Oskarovitch Ott. In 1901, he performed an examination of the pelvic and abdominal viscera via a posterior vaginal incision using a head lamp and a mirror [1]. However, as early as 1813, a technique for vaginal hysterectomy was described by Langenbeck, and is arguably the first instance of surgery performed via a natural orifice [2]. A lack of suitable instruments for visualisation and manipulation meant that these procedures were never widely adapted, and natural orifices were largely abandoned as access portals until the early twenty-first century.

In the era of modern surgery, the first documented human natural-orifice procedure was a pancreatic necrosectomy performed via the transgastric route in 2000 [3]. A transgastric appendectomy was reported in 2004, although never published [4]. Animal studies in 2005 and 2007 demonstrated that access via natural orifices to the peritoneal cavity was safe and viable, with reports of transgastric peritoneoscopy and oophorectomy as well as cholecystectomy via a combined transvesical and transgastric approach in porcine models [5, 6]. Nephrectomy, partial nephrectomy, cryoablation of renal lesions and partial cystectomy have also been demostrated via either the transgastric or transvaginal route [7].

Translating work on animal models to real-world clinical practice has proved challenging. Difficulties in dissection and retraction, as well reliable methods to achieve safe closure of the access portal have been highlighted [7]. There is also a lack of purpose-built instrumentation for access and intra-operative use, meaning that adaptation of existing instruments is required.

Despite these challenges, the range of procedures performed continues to grow with the transvaginal and transgastric routes emerging as the preferred methods of access. Nephrectomy, gastrectomy, cholecystectomy, appendectomy, splenectomy and hernia repairs have all been performed via the transvaginal route, while transgastric access has been used for cholecystectomy, appendectomy, partial gastrectomy and peritoneoscopy [8]. From a urological perspective, transvaginal extraction of a kidney after laparoscopic nephrectomy was described as early as 1993 with a subsequent series of ten cases in 2002 [9, 10]. Reports of pure NOTES transvaginal nephrectomy followed in 2009 and 2010 [11, 12]. Cadaveric radical prostatectomy via the transurethral route has been performed but limitations in extracting an intact specimen, difficulty in performing a secure vesico-urethral anastomosis and the impossibility of performing a lymph node dissection may preclude the progress of this procedure further [13] (Table 21.1).

One notable milestone in the inception and development of NOTES was the recognition that the adaptation of this novel surgical approach must be performed in a safe, structured and carefully monitored fashion. A summit was held in 2005 with members from the Society of American Gastrointestinal and Endoscopic Surgeons (SAGES) and the American Society for Gastrointestinal Endoscopy (ASGE) collaborating to determine the appropriate pathway for the safe and responsible

Table 21.1 Highlights of human NOTES procedures

Year	Procedure	Approach	References
2006	Appendectomy	Transgastric	Rao & Reddy [13]
2007	Cholecystectomy	Transvaginal	Zorron et al. [14]
2008	Colectomy	Transvaginal	Lacy et al. [15]
2008	Peritoneoscopy	Transgastric	Hazey et al. [16]
2008	Peritoneoscopy	Transvaginal	Zorron et al. [17]
2008	Appendectomy	Transvaginal	Palanivelu et al. [18]
2008	Gastrectomy	Transvaginal	Ramos et al. [19]
2009	Cholecystectomy	Transgastric	Auyang et al. [20]
2009	Nephrectomy	Transvaginal	Kaouk et al. [12]
2009	Splenectomy	Transvaginal	Targarona et al. [21]
2010	Gastric banding	Transvaginal	Michalik et al. [22]
2010	Incisional hernia repair	Transvaginal	Jacobsen et al. [23]
2011	Gastric mass resection	Transgastric	Willingham et al. [24]

development and evaluation of NOTES. This culminated in the publication of a white paper which set out the challenges and goals for NOTES, as well as a road-map for addressing them [25]. An organization called the Natural Orifice Surgery Consortium for Assessment and Research (NOSCAR) was formed to lead this effort, and to manage a registry of trials and human procedures in the field. A second white paper was published in 2011, reporting on progress made [26]. The uptake of NOTES has remained largely experimental, and numerous challenges continue to prevent widespread adoption of this surgical approach. It remains an exciting but challenging area for future development and progress.

LESS

While modern single-site laparoscopy is considered relatively new, the origins of laparoscopy were in fact in single-site procedures. In 1961 Platteborse described access to the abdominal cavity with a 12 mm trocar and a working channel [27], allowing biopsies of the liver and gall bladder. Around the same time Steptoe began gynaecological laparoscopic procedures [28], which would culminate in his collaboration with Edwards and the birth of in-vitro fertilisation. Using his technique of access, a series of 25 laparoscopic sterilisations was subsequently carried out at Johns Hopkins Hospital by Wheeless in 1969 [29].

As interest in laparoscopy grew it became apparent that multiple instruments and ports would be necessary to achieve the required retraction and triangulation in more complex procedures, as well as to reduce the potential for instrument clashes. The progression to multi-port laparoscopy enabled the technique to emerge as not only a viable alternative to traditional methods of open surgery, but eventually as the preferred surgical approach in many procedures today. There was still, however, interest in single-port surgery by some pioneers. Notably, the American gynaecologist Pelosi, who performed the first major extirpative single-site procedure in 1991—a hysterectomy with bilateral salpingo-oophrectomy via a single transumbilical port [30]. His group subsequently reported a supracervical hysterectomy and the earliest series of single-port appendectomies [31, 32]. In 1997 Navarra published his report of a single-port laparoscopic cholecystectomy [33]. Over the next decade, the indication and complexity of reported cases increased. Emergency procedures such as salpingectomy for ectopic pregnancy were carried out and described as "feasible and safe" by Ghezzi et al. in 2005 [34]. A series of paediatric procedures was reported by Cobellis et al. in 2006, where a single 10 mm transumbilical trocar was used to identify a Meckel's diverticulum and bring it to the skin, where the diverticulum was excised [35].

Single-port urological procedures were first described in the early twenty-first century. Hirano et al. reported a series of single-port adrenalectomies in 2005 [36]. These were performed using a large (4 cm) port inserted into the retroperitoneum, with no gas insufflation. However, significant complications were reported, including fulminant hepatitis, pulmonary embolism and death. The first successful laparo-endoscopic single-site urological procedure (a simple nephrectomy in a 36 year old man) was presented by Rane et al. at the World Congress of Endourology in 2007 [37]. A multichannel port (the R-port, Advanced Surgical Concepts, Wicklow, Ireland) was used via a single flank incision to insert a 5 mm telescope, two further 5 mm instruments and a 10 mm clip applier. The same group subsequently reported successful ureterolithotomy, orchidopexy and orchiectomy [37]. Raman et al. reported a series of nephrectomies in 2007, utilising multiple trocars and articulating instruments via a single umbilical incision [38]. These were performed for both benign as well as malignant disease. Radical nephrectomies as well as pyeloplasties were reported by Desai et al. in 2008, this time using custom-designed curved instruments and the R-port; a supplementary 2 mm needle port was also used [39].

The range and complexity of single-port urological procedures grew rapidly. Kaouk et al. reported laparoscopic renal cryoablation, wedge renal biopsy and sacrocolpopexy in 2008, and further experiences with LESS reconstructive procedures were reported including dismembered pyeloplasty, ureteral reimplantation with psoas hitch, ileal ureter construction and urteroneocystostomy [40, 41]. A series of live donor nephrectomies via a LESS approach was reported in 2008 by Gill et al., with no complications and excellent graft outcome [42]. This was followed by highly complex extirpative procedures successfully performed via a LESS approach, including radical prostatectomy and radical cystectomy with pelvic lymph node dissection [43, 44] (Table 21.2).

Despite the proven technical feasibility and safety of the LESS approach for a multitude of procedures, the wider uptake of this technique has not yet materialised. This can be attributed to a number of reasons. The approach is technically demanding and requires considerable practice and relearning of established laparoscopic skills, to learn the behaviour of crossed and articulating instruments. Working angles can be awkward and instrument clashes are common, despite advances in instrumentation and ports. Coupled with this, the incremental benefit that LESS

Table 21.2 Highlights of Laparoendoscopic Single-Site Surgery (LESS) procedures

Year	Procedure	Approach	References
1969	Tubal ligation	Single transumbilical trocar	Wheeless [29]
1991	Hysterectomy with bilateralsalpingo-oophorectomy	Single transumbilical trocar	Pelosi et al. [30]
1992	Supracervical hysterectomy with bilateral salpingo-oophorectomy	Single transumbilical trocar	Pelosi et al. [31]
1992	Appendectomy	Single transumbilical trocar	Pelosi et al. [32]
1997	Cholecystectomy	Single transumbilical trocar	Navarra et al. [33]
2001	Ovarian cystectomy	Single transumbilical trocar	Kosumi et al. [45]
2005	Salpingectomy for ectopic pregnancy	Single transumbilical trocar	Ghezzi et al. [34]
2005	Retroperitoneal adrenalectomy	Single retroperitoneal port. Noinsufflation used	Hirano et al. [36]
2006	Meckel's diverticulectomy	Single transumbilical trocar	Cobellis et al. [35]
2007	Simple nephrectomy, radical nephrectomy	Single transumbilical incision, multiple ports	Raman et al. [38]
2007	Simple nephrectomy	Single port through a flank incision	Rane et al. [37]
2008	Orchidectomy, orchidopexy, ureterolithotomy	Transumbilical R-port	Rane et al. [37]
2008	Simple nephrectomy	Single transumbilical port	Desai et al. [39]
2008	Pyeloplasty	Transumbilical port and 2 mm needle port	Desai et al. [39]
2008	Renal cryotherapy, radical nephrectomy, wedgekidney biopsy, sacrocolpopexy	Single transumbilical port	Kaouk et al. [40]
2008	Live donor nephrectomy	Transumbilical port and 2 mm needle port	Gill et al. [42]
2008	Paediatric varicocelectomy	Single transumbilical trocar	Kaouk et al. [46]
2008	Radical prostatectomy	Single transumbilical port	Kaouk et al. [43]
2008	Transvesical simple prostatectomy	Single port introduced percutaneously through the bladder	Desai et al. [47]
2008	Transvesical robotic radical prostatectomy (cadaveric)	Single port introduced percutaneously through the bladder	Desai et al. [48]
2008	Robotic single-port (RSP) surgery (radical prostatectomy, pyeloplasty, radical nephrectomy)	Single transumbilical port	Kaouk et al. [49]
2009	Ileal ureter, psoas hitch ureteroneocystostomy	Transumbilical port and 2 mm needle port	Desai et al. [41]

(continued)

Table 21.2 (continued)

Year	Procedure	Approach	References
2009	Transumbilical simple prostatectomy	Single transumbilical trocar	Sotelo et al. [50]
2009	Subtotal cystectomy and augmentation enterocystoplasty	Single transumbilical port	Noguera et al. [51]
2010	Radical cystectomy and pelvic lymph node dissection	Single transumbilical port	Kaouk et al. [52]
2010	Repair of retrocaval ureter	Single transumbilical port	Autorino et al. [44]

offers over traditional laparoscopic surgery may not be enough to overcome some of the difficulties mentioned. One potential game-changer, however, is the rise of robotic surgery. Initial experiences with robotic single-port surgery (RSP) have shown feasibility, initially in cadaveric models [53], with successful RSP radical prostatectomy, nephrectomy and pyeloplasty in live patients reported by Kaouk in 2009 [49]. Difficulties with clashing of robotic arms remain, but may be less of an issue using the newer Xi model of Da Vinci surgical robot. RSP also allows remapping of the right and left working arms to negate the effect of crossed instruments. A purpose-built RSP system with articulating instruments was initially reported in 2010 and is anticipated to become available in the near future [44]. This is likely to herald the wider uptake of LESS in the coming years.

References

1. Hatzinger M, Fesenko A, Büger L, Sohn M. Dimitrij Oscarovic Ott (1855–1929) "Die Ventroskopie": Sein Beitrag zur Entwicklung der Laparoskopie (Geschichte der Urologie). Urologe. 2013;52:1454–8.
2. Baskett TF. Hysterectomy: evolution and trends. Best Pract Res Clin Obstet Gynaecol. 2005;19:295–305.
3. Seifert H, Wehrmann T, Schmitt T, Zeuzem S, Caspary WF. Retroperitoneal endoscopic debridement for infected peripancreatic necrosis. Lancet. 2000;356:653–5.
4. Reddy N, Rao P. Per oral transgastric endoscopic appendectomy in human. Abstract presented at 45th Annual Conference of the Society of Gastrointestinal Endoscopy of India; 2004. pp. 28–29.
5. Wagh MS, Merrifield BF, Thompson CC. Endoscopic transgastric abdominal exploration and organ resection: initial experience in a porcine model. Clin Gastroenterol Hepatol. 2005;3:892–6.
6. Rolanda C, Lima E, Pêgo JM, Henriques-Coelho T, Silva D, Moreira I, Macedo G, Carvalho JL, Correia-Pinto J. Third-generation cholecystectomy by natural orifices: transgastric and transvesical combined approach (with video). Gastrointest Endosc. 2007;65:111–7.
7. Autorino R, Cadeddu JA, Desai MM, Gettman M, Gill IS, Kavoussi LR, Lima E, Montorsi F, Richstone L, Stolzenburg JU, Kaouk JH. Laparoendoscopic single-site and natural orifice transluminal endoscopic surgery in urology: a critical analysis of the literature. Eur Urol. 2011;59:26–45.
8. Clark MP, Qayed ES, Kooby DA, Maithel SK, Willingham FF. Natural orifice translumenal endoscopic surgery in humans: a review. Minim Invasive Surg. 2012;2012 doi:10.1155/2012/189296.

9. Breda G, Silvestre P, Giunta A, Xausa D, Tamai A, Gherardi L. Laparoscopic nephrectomy with vaginal delivery of the intact kidney. Eur Urol. 1992;24:116–7.
10. Gill IS, Cherullo EE, Meraney AM, Borsuk F, Murphy DP, Falcone T. Vaginal extraction of the intact specimen following laparoscopic radical nephrectomy. J Urol. 2002;167:238–41.
11. Sotelo R, de Andrade R, Fernandez G, Ramirez D, Di Grazia E, Carmona O, Moreira O, Berger A, Aron M, Desai MM, Gill IS. NOTES hybrid transvaginal radical nephrectomy for tumor: stepwise progression toward a first successful clinical case. Eur Urol. 2010;57:138–44.
12. Kaouk JH, White WM, Goel RK, Brethauer S, Crouzet S, Rackley RR, Moore C, Ingber MS, Haber GP. NOTES transvaginal nephrectomy: first human experience. Urology. 2009;74:5–8.
13. Rao GV, Reddy N. Transgastric appendectomy in humans. In: Proceedings of the American Gastrointestinal and Endoscopic Surgeons (SAGES) Conference. TX: Dallas; 2006.
14. Zorrón R, Filgueiras M, Maggioni LC, Pombo L, Carvalho GL, Oliveira AL. NOTES transvaginal cholecystectomy: report of the first case. Surg Innov. 2007;14:279–83.
15. Lacy AM, Delgado S, Rojas OA, Almenara R, Blasi A, Llach J. MA-NOS radical sigmoidectomy: report of a transvaginal resection in the human. Surg Endosc. 2008;22:1717–23.
16. Hazey JW, Narula VK, Renton DB, Reavis KM, Paul CM, Hinshaw KE, Muscarella P, Ellison EC, Melvin WS. Natural-orifice transgastric endoscopic peritoneoscopy in humans: initial clinical trial. Surg Endosc. 2008;22:16–20.
17. Zorrón R, Soldan M, Filgueiras M, Maggioni LC, Pombo L, Oliveira AL. NOTES: transvaginal for cancer diagnostic staging: preliminary clinical application. Surg Innov. 2008;15:161–5.
18. Palanivelu C, Rajan PS, Rangarajan M, Parthasarathi R, Senthilnathan P, Prasad M. Transvaginal endoscopic appendectomy in humans: a unique approach to NOTES—world's first report. Surg Endosc. 2008;22:1343–7.
19. Ramos AC, Zundel N, Neto MG, Maalouf M. Human hybrid NOTES transvaginal sleeve gastrectomy: initial experience. Surg Obes Relat Dis. 2008;4:660–3.
20. Auyang ED, Hungness ES, Vaziri K, Martin JA, Soper NJ. Human NOTES cholecystectomy: transgastric hybrid technique. J Gastrointest Surg. 2009;13:1149–50.
21. Targarona EM, Gomez C, Rovira R, Pernas JC, Balague C, Guarner-Argente C, Sainz S, Trias M. NOTES-assisted transvaginal splenectomy: the next step in the minimally invasive approach to the spleen. Surg Innov. 2009;16:218–22.
22. Michalik M, Orlowski M, Bobowicz M, Frask A, Trybull A. The first report on hybrid NOTES adjustable gastric banding in human. Obes Surg. 2011;21:524–7.
23. Jacobsen GR, Thompson K, Spivack A, Fischer L, Wong B, Cullen J, Bosia J, Whitcomb E, Lucas E, Talamini M, Horgan S. Initial experience with transvaginal incisional hernia repair. Hernia. 2010;14:89–91.
24. Willingham FF, Garud SS, Davis SS, Lewis MM, Maithel SK, Kooby DA. Human hybrid endoscopic and laparoscopic management of mass lesions of the foregut (with video). Gastrointest Endosc. 2012;75:905–12.
25. Rattner D, Kalloo A. ASGE/SAGES working group on natural orifice translumenal endoscopic surgery. Surg Endosc. 2006;20:329–33.
26. Rattner DW, Hawes R, Schwaitzberg S, Kochman M, Swanstrom L. The second SAGES/ASGE white paper on natural orifice transluminal endoscopic surgery: 5 years of progress. Surg Endosc. 2011;25:2441–8.
27. Platteborse R. Laparoscopy, laparophotography, punch biopsy of the liver, gallbladder punch biopsy and collection of specimens of the peritoneal organs through a single trocar. Acta Gastro-Enterol Belg. 1961;24:696.
28. Litynski GS, Patrick C. Steptoe: laparoscopy, sterilization, the test-tube baby, and mass media. JSLS. 1998;2:99.
29. Wheeless CR Jr. A rapid inexpensive and effective method of surgical sterilization by laparoscopy. J Reprod Med. 1969;3:65–9.
30. Pelosi MA, Pelosi MA 3rd. Laparoscopic hysterectomy with bilateral salpingo-oophorectomy using a single umbilical puncture. N J Med. 1991;88:721–6.
31. Pelosi MA, Pelosi MA 3rd. Laparoscopic supracervical hysterectomy using a single-umbilical puncture (mini-laparoscopy). J Reprod Med. 1992;37:777–84.

32. Pelosi MA, Pelosi MA 3rd. Laparoscopic appendectomy using a single umbilical puncture (minilaparoscopy). J Reprod Med. 1992;37:588.
33. Navarra G, Pozza E, Occhionorelli S, Carcoforo P, Donini I. One-wound laparoscopic cholecystectomy. Br J Surg. 1997;84:695.
34. Ghezzi F, Cromi A, Fasola M, Bolis P. One-trocar salpingectomy for the treatment of tubal pregnancy: a 'marionette-like' technique. BJOG. 2005;112:1417–9.
35. Cobellis G, Cruccetti A, Mastroianni L, Amici G, Martino A. One-trocar transumbilical laparoscopic-assisted management of Meckel's diverticulum in children. J Laparoendosc Adv Surg Tech A. 2007;17:238–41.
36. Hirano D, Minei S, Yamaguchi K, Yoshikawa T, Hachiya T, Yoshida T, Ishida H, Takimoto Y, Saitoh T, Kiyotaki S, Okada K. Retroperitoneoscopic adrenalectomy for adrenal tumors via a single large port. J Endourol. 2005;19:788–92.
37. Desai MM, Rao PP, Aron M, Pascal-Haber G, Desai MR, Mishra S, Kaouk JH, Gill IS. Scarless single port transumbilical nephrectomy and pyeloplasty: first clinical report. BJU Int. 2008;101:83–8.
38. Rané A, Rao P, Rao P. Single-port-access nephrectomy and other laparoscopic urologic procedures using a novel laparoscopic port (R-port). Urology. 2008;72:260–3.
39. Kaouk JH, Haber GP, Goel RK, Desai MM, Aron M, Rackley RR, Moore C, Gill IS. Single-port laparoscopic surgery in urology: initial experience. Urology. 2008;71:3–6.
40. Gill IS, Canes D, Aron M, Haber GP, Goldfarb DA, Flechner S, Desai MR, Kaouk JH, Desai MM. Single port transumbilical (E-NOTES) donor nephrectomy. J Urol. 2008;180:637–41.
41. Sotelo RJ, Astigueta JC, Desai MM, Canes D, Carmona O, De Andrade RJ, Moreira O, Lopez R, Velásquez A, Gill IS. Laparoendoscopic single-site surgery simple prostatectomy: initial report. Urology. 2009;74:626–30.
42. Kaouk JH, Palmer JS. Single-port laparoscopic surgery: initial experience in children for varicocelectomy. BJU Int. 2008;102:97–9.
43. Desai MM, Aron M, Canes D, Fareed K, Carmona O, Haber GP, Crouzet S, Astigueta JC, Lopez R, de Andrade R, Stein RJ. Single-port transvesical simple prostatectomy: initial clinical report. Urology. 2008;72:960–5.
44. Haber GP, White MA, Autorino R, Escobar PF, Kroh MD, Chalikonda S, Khanna R, Forest S, Yang B, Altunrende F, Stein RJ. Novel robotic da Vinci instruments for laparoendoscopic single-site surgery. Urology. 2010;76:1279–82.
45. Kosumi T, Kubota A, Usui N, Yamauchi K, Yamasaki M, Oyanagi H. Laparoscopic ovarian cystectomy using a single umbilical puncture method. Surg Laparosc Endosc Percutan Tech. 2001;11:63–5.
46. Kaouk JH, Goel RK, Haber GP, Crouzet S, Desai MM, Gill IS. Single-port laparoscopic radical prostatectomy. Urology. 2008;72:1190–3.
47. Desai MM, Aron M, Berger A, Canes D, Stein RJ, Kamoi K, Crouzet S, Brandina R, Irwin BH, Goel RK, White WM. Transvesical robotic radical prostatectomy. J Urol. 2009;181(4):335.
48. Kaouk JH, Goel RK, Haber GP, Crouzet S, Stein RJ. Robotic single-port transumbilical surgery in humans: initial report. BJU Int. 2009;103:366–9.
49. Desai MM, Stein R, Rao P, Canes D, Aron M, Rao PP, Haber GP, Fergany A, Kaouk J, Gill IS. Embryonic natural orifice transumbilical endoscopic surgery (E-NOTES) for advanced reconstruction: initial experience. Urology. 2009;73:182–7.
50. Noguera RJS, Astigueta JC, Carmona O, De Andrade RJ, Luis S, Cuomo B, Manrique J, Gill IS, Desai MM. Laparoscopic augmentation enterocystoplasty through a single trocar. Urology. 2009;73:1371–4.
51. Kaouk JH, Goel RK, White MA, White WM, Autorino R, Haber GP, Campbell SC. Laparoendoscopic single-site radical cystectomy and pelvic lymph node dissection: initial experience and 2-year follow-up. Urology. 2010;76:857–61.
52. Autorino R, Khanna R, White MA, Haber GP, Shah G, Kaouk JH, Stein RJ. Laparoendoscopic single-site repair of retrocaval ureter: first case report. Urology. 2010;76:1501–5.
53. Humphreys MR, Krambeck AE, Andrews PE, Castle EP, Lingeman JE. Natural orifice translumenal endoscopic surgical radical prostatectomy: proof of concept. J Endourol. 2009;23:669–75.

Chapter 22
The History of Focused Ultrasound Therapy in Urology

Albert Gelet, Sebastien Crouzet, Olivier Rouviere, Emmanuel Blanc, and Jean-Yves Chapelon

Principle of High Intensity Focused Ultrasound (HIFU)

The first description of HIFU was made in 1942 and it was first used to destroy tissue in 1944 [1]. HIFU is a non-ionizing and non-surgical physical therapy that produces biological effects by thermal and mechanical means. Heating tissue denatures proteins and leads to cell death, whereas mechanical effects disrupt cells by the collapse of micro bubbles generated by cavitation, in both cases, regardless of

---

The authors have published some materials of this book chapter in 2012 in Chapter 6 of "Management of Prostate, A Multidisciplinary Approach". Springer, Bolla, Michel, van Poppel, Hendrik (Eds.), 2012, pp. 191–212 and in 2016 in Chapter 2 of Therapeutic Ultrasound, Advances in Experimental Medicine and Biology, Springer, J.-M. Escoffre, A. Bouakaz (eds.), Vol. 880, 2016, pp. 22–41.

A. Gelet (✉) • S. Crouzet
Department of Urology, Edouard Herriot Hospital, Lyon, France

Laboratory of Therapeutic Applications of Ultrasound (LabTAU), Inserm, Lyon, France

University of Lyon, Lyon F-69003, France
e-mail: albert.gelet@gmail.com

O. Rouviere

Laboratory of Therapeutic Applications of Ultrasound (LabTAU), Inserm, Lyon, France

Université de Lyon, Lyon F-69003, France

Department of Radiology, Edouard Herriot Hospital, Lyon, France

E. Blanc
Edap-TMS, Vaulx en Velin, France

J.-Y. Chapelon
Laboratory of Therapeutic Applications of Ultrasound (LabTAU), Inserm, Lyon, France

University of Lyon, Lyon F-69003, France

S.R. Patel et al. (eds.), *The History of Technologic Advancements in Urology*,
DOI 10.1007/978-3-319-61691-9_22

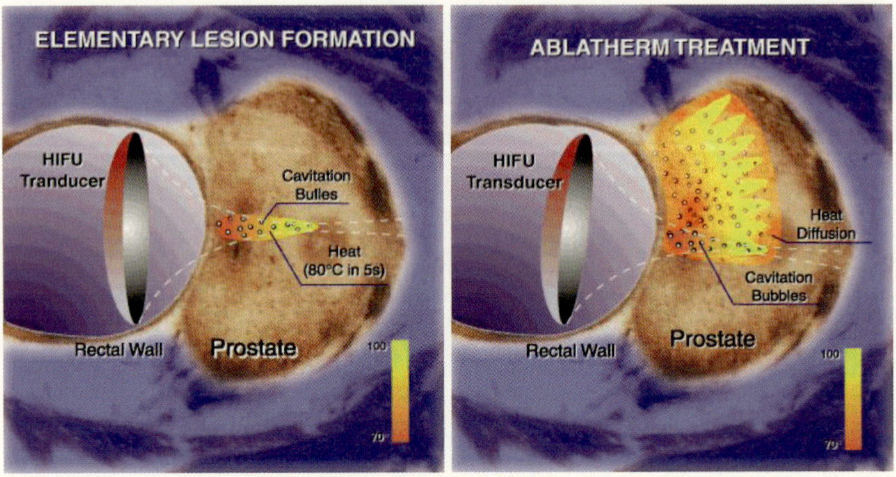

Fig. 22.1 (**a**, **b**) Principle of HIFU for prostate treatment: Prostate treatment is performed by the repetition and juxtaposition of several elementary lesions

whether they are normal or abnormal. In most applications, spherically shaped power transducers are used to focus the ultrasound energy onto a target point deep within the body. This results in thermal tissue coagulation necrosis, cavitation and heat shock. Each sonication heats only a small focal target, creating an elementary lesion with extreme precision and accuracy. Subsequently, multiple sonications (lesions), side-by-side and layer after layer, are necessary to cover large volumes of tissue targeted for ablation (Fig. 22.1). The main sonication parameters are acoustic intensity, duration of exposure, on/off duty cycle, the distance between two elementary lesions and the displacement path when multiple lesions are made.

HIFU in Animal Models

In 1989 a multidisciplinary "task force" was created in Lyon, France for use HIFU in the treatment of cancer in urology. This team consisted of scientists, engineers, radiologist and urologists. The main goal was to provide minimally invasive therapies for urological cancers, especially to patients with localized prostate cancer who were not suitable candidates for radical surgery.

In 1991, Chapelon et al. established the ultrasound parameters required to induce irreversible tissue lesions in animals [2]. In 1992, Chapelon et al. demonstrated in rats (R 3327 AT2 Dunning tumor) that HIFU could be used to ablate tumors and cure cancer without causing metastasis [3]. A complete tumor necrosis occurred in 24 out of 25 animals (96%) receiving high-intensity ultrasound therapy (Fig. 22.2a). A local regrowth of tumor from the periphery was identified in seven animals (28%). Sixteen rats were still alive after treatment without any pathological evidence of tumor regrowth or metastasis (64%). There was a significant difference ($P < 0.0001$) in survival curves between the two groups (Fig. 22.2b). All rats in the control group died of progressive tumor growth. Of these, seven developed lymph node metastasis (28%).

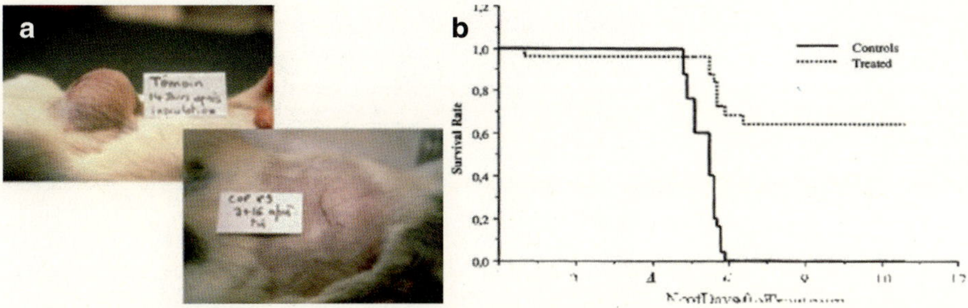

Fig. 22.2 Dunning tumor study. (**a**) Complete tumor necrosis occurred in animals receiving high-intensity ultrasound therapy (**b**) Survival curves for 50 rats with AT2 subline R 3327

Fig. 22.3 Experimental trial in canine prostates (**a**) Prototype probe used for canine prostate ablation (**b**) Lesions in canine prostate

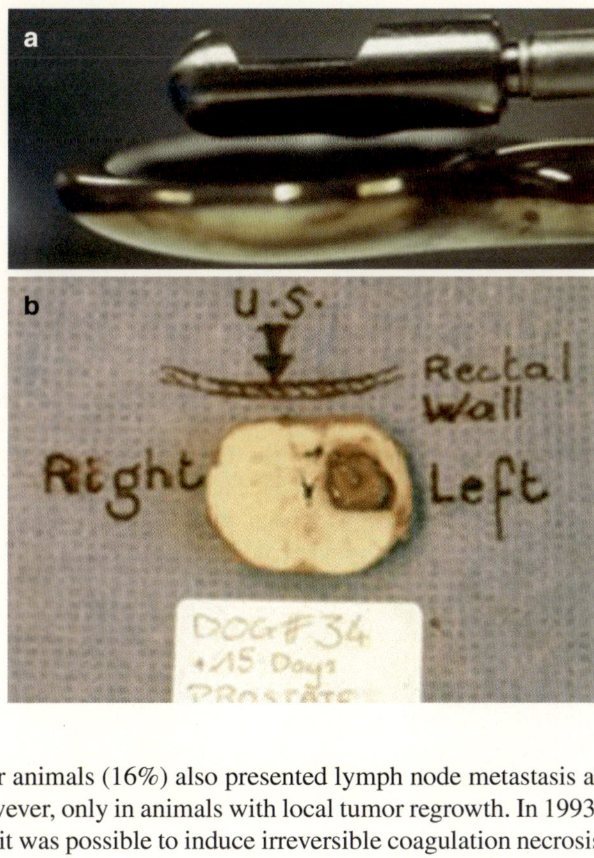

In the treatment group, four animals (16%) also presented lymph node metastasis at autopsy. This occurred, however, only in animals with local tumor regrowth. In 1993, Gelet et al. established that it was possible to induce irreversible coagulation necrosis lesions in dog prostates using a transrectal route without damaging the rectal wall [4]. The experimental probe combined a firing transducer (working at 2.25 MHz) and a rotating imaging system B&K (Fig. 22.3a). Thirty-seven dogs were treated. Lesions in the prostate gland occurred with a combination of moderate acoustic intensity (720 W/cm^2) and longer shot duration (4 s). The temperature reached at the focal point of the transducer was 85 °C. The study confirmed the possibility of creating irreversible lesions in the prostatic tissue through the rectal wall (Fig. 22.3b).

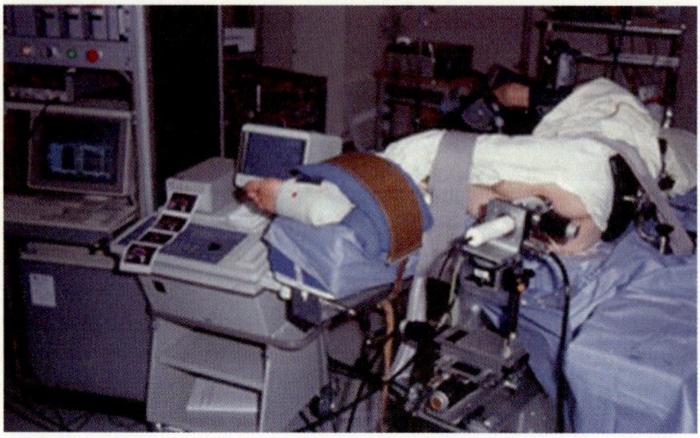

Fig. 22.4 HIFU Prototype used for the first prostate ablation trials in human

First Human Trials in Lyon

The next goal was to find appropriate acoustic parameters able to induce irreversible coagulation necrosis lesions in human prostate via the transrectal route without damaging the rectal wall. The first trial was conducted in 1992: HIFU was carried out with the first prototype in human prostatic adenoma [5] (Fig. 22.4). The device used to produce the HIFU combined a firing system (homemade power amplifier and therapy transducer) and an imaging system (Kretz ultrasound scanner). Nine patients were treated under epidural anesthesia with an ultrasound intensity similar to or higher than the acoustic intensity used in the experiments on canine prostates. Open surgical ablation of adenoma was performed 1 week after the HIFU session. Irreversible necrosis lesions were obtained in the prostate adenoma without any damage to the rectal wall. These lesions were also histologically determined to be coagulation necrosis with a complete destruction of the glandular tissue. The second trial was a pilot study conducted with the same prototype in 1993, in 14 patients with prostate cancer who were not candidates for surgery [6]. Control biopsies demonstrated coagulative necrotic lesions of the treated prostate zones with secondary development into fibrosis. A satisfactory local control with negative control biopsies was achieved in 50% of the cases in this pilot study.

First Trials in Europe: 1995–2009

The first commercial HIFU prototype was the Ablatherm® from Edap-TMS company which was completed in 1995 and introduced to five centers in Europe (Lyon, Paris, Munich, Regensburg, Nijmegen) (Fig. 22.5). The device combined a 2.25-MHz therapy transducer and a 7.5-MHz trans-rectal biplane ultrasound scanner probe. Phase one of the study was performed in Nijmegen [7]. The HIFU treatments were performed 1 week before radical prostatectomy, and meticulous histopathologic examination of the prostate specimens were performed: complete necrosis was seen in the treated region in all cases. Following phase one of the study, almost

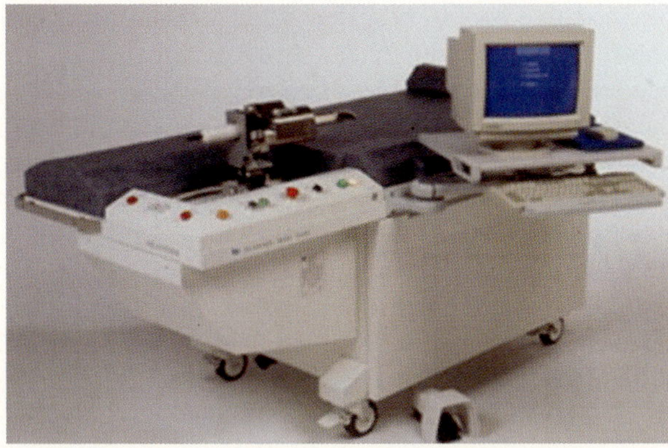

Fig. 22.5 First prototype of the Ablatherm used for the multiple center study (1995–2000)

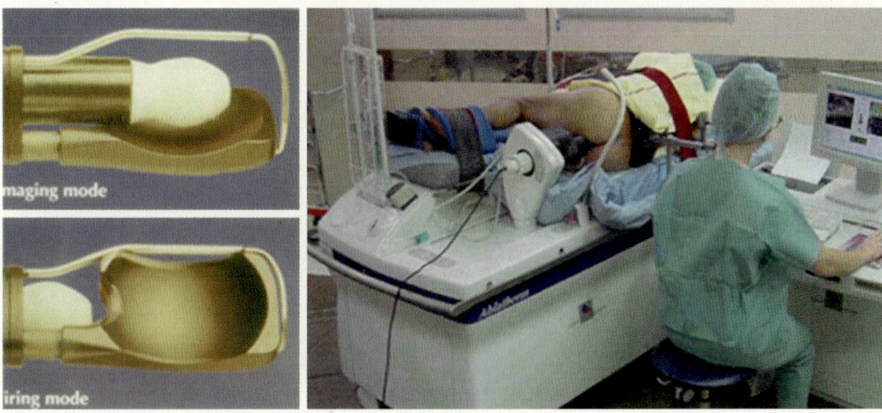

Fig. 22.6 Ablatherm Maxis, Probe and device (2000–2005)

500 patients were successfully treated between 1995 and 1999 in France and Germany. Middle term results of these patient treatments were published in 1996 and 1999 [8]. After this study, the company Edap obtained the CE mark for the Ablatherm Maxis® that was used commercially in Europe from 2000 to 2005.

Development of HIFU Devices Dedicated to Localized PCa (2000–2010)

The first commercially available device from Edap-TMS combined two separate probes: a bi-plane imaging probe (Kretz) and a therapy probe working at 3 MHz with a mono-element piezo-composite transducer (Fig. 22.6). Results achieved in 227 consecutive patients treated with the Ablatherm Maxis were published in 2006 in European Urology [9]. Histological results showed 81.8% of the patients had negative control biopsies. Their median nadir prostate-specific antigen (PSA) was 0.16 ng/mL, with 72.7% of the patients having a nadir PSA $\leq$ 0.5 ng/mL. The actuarial 5-year disease free rate which combined the histological and the biochemical outcomes was 63% for the overall population, ranging from 78% in the low-risk subgroup to 47% in the high-risk subgroup. The Ablatherm II® (Integrated Imaging) was completed in 2005 this device used a new endo-rectal probe. The therapy probe (working at 3 MHZ) had a 45-mm focal length with a 61-mm aperture where the imaging transducer (working at 7.5 MHZ) was placed in the center of the probe (Fig. 22.7). At the same time, another HIFU device for prostate treatment was developed in the USA, the Sonablate (SonaCare Medical LLC, Charlotte, NC, USA) [10]. This device used double-sided and dual-mode transducers for imaging (6.3 MHz) and treatment (4 MHz) (Fig. 22.8a). The probes were available with two focal lengths (from 30 to 40 mm). The probes were capable of creating an elementary lesion 10–12 mm in length and 3 mm in diameter. The Sonablate procedure was conducted with the patient in a supine position on a regular operating table

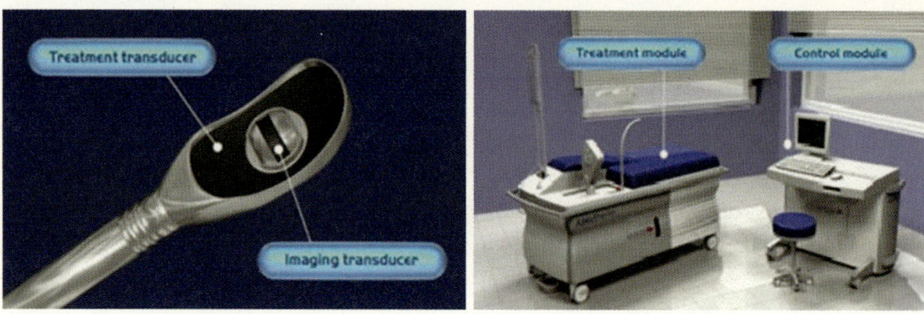

Fig. 22.7 Ablatherm II, probe and device (2006–2013)

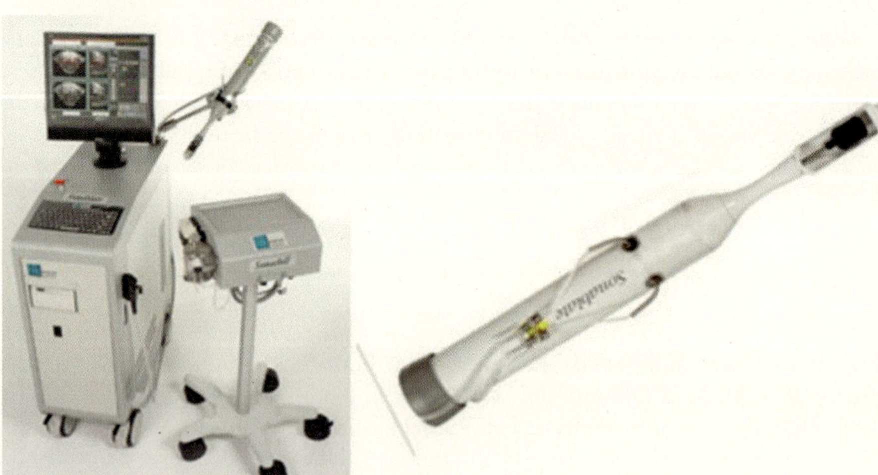

Fig. 22.8 Sonablate: Probe and device

(Fig. 22.8b). The Sonablate used a single treatment protocol in which the power had to be adapted manually by the operator. The probe chosen depended on the prostate size, with larger glands requiring longer focal length probes.

Results of Whole Gland Ablation as Primary Care Treatment of Localized PCa

Using HIFU as a primary treatment for prostate cancer is usually recommended for patients with localized prostate cancer (clinical stage T1-T2, NX/0 MX/0) for whom radical prostatectomies are not an option for one the following reasons: age > 70 year old, life expectancy ≤10 years, major co-morbidities which preclude surgery, or the simple refusal on the part of the patient to undergo one. The five most recent studies reported outcomes of at least 500 patients [11–15]. Articles published from three European urology departments confirmed the long-term efficacy (mean follow-up of 76–97 months) of HIFU treatment with the Ablatherm device [11–13]. Crouzet et al. reported results of 1002 patients treated for localized PCa from 1997 to 2009 [11]. At 10 years, the PCa-specific survival rates (PCSSR) and metastasis-free survival rates (MFSR) were 97% and 94%, respectively. Salvage therapies included external beam radiation therapy (EBRT) (13.8%), EBRT + androgen deprivation (ADT) (9.7%), and ADT alone (12.1%). Thuroff et al. published outcomes of 709 patients with primary localized prostate cancer [12]. Mean follow-up was 5.3 years. Cancer specific survival was 99%, metastasis-free survival was 95%, and 10-year salvage treatment-free rates were 98% in low risk, 72% in intermediate risk and 68% in high risk patients. Ganzer et al. reported results of a prospective study on 538 consecutive patients who underwent primary HIFU for clinically localized PCa [13]. The mean follow-up was 8.1 years. Metastatic disease was reported in 0.4%, 5.7% and 15.4% of low, intermediate and high-risk patients, respectively. The salvage treatment rate was 18%. PCa-specific death was registered in 18 (3.3%) patients. Two recent articles confirmed the efficacy of whole gland HIFU treatment with the Sonablate device. The study performed by Uchida et al. included 918 patients treated with Sonablate™ devices during 1999–2012 [14]. The 10-year overall and cancer-specific survival rates were 89.6% and 97.4%, respectively. The 5-year biochemical disease-free survival rates in the different versions of the Sonablate device's tissue change monitor groups were 48.3%, 62.3%, and 82.0% respectively ($p < 0.0001$). Dickinson et al. reported outcomes in 569 men receiving primary whole-gland HIFU [15]. One hundred and sixty three (29%) of the 569 patients required the HIFU procedures to be redone. Median follow-up was 46 months. Failure-free survival, at 5 years after first HIFU, was 70%, it was 87%, 63% and 58% for low, intermediate and high-risk groups, respectively. Complication rates were low: Urethro-rectal fistula occurred in 0.23–0.7% in the large studies treated with Ablatherm device [11–13]. Erectile Dysfunction (ED) occurred in 35–45% of previous potent patients and bladder outlet obstruction in 24–28% (66–67). Incontinence rates reported in recent studies were: 4–5.5% grade I and 1.5–3.1%

grade II/III. In the largest study published in [11], severe incontinence and bladder outlet obstruction (BOO) decreased from 5.7% and 10.2% to 3.1% and 5.9%, respectively, thanks to refinement in technology.

Results of Whole Gland Ablation as Salvage Treatment of Locally Recurrent PCa After Radiation Therapy

The rate of positive biopsy after External Beam Radio Therapy (ERBT) for prostate cancer in the literature is between 25 and 32%. Patients with a locally proven recurrence after external-beam radiation therapy and no metastasis are usually treated with androgen deprivation. Since 1995 the Ablatherm device has been used as a salvage treatment in patients with local recurrence after EBRT without metastasis. The first study was published in 2004 [16, 17]. Crouzet et al. examined the outcomes of salvage HIFU in 290 consecutive patients with biopsy-confirmed locally radio recurrent PCa, without evidence of metastasis [18]. Progression was defined using Phoenix biochemical failure criteria or the introduction of androgen deprivation (AD). Local cancer control with negative biopsy results were obtained in 169 patients out of 208 who underwent post-HIFU biopsies (81%). The median PSA nadir was 0.14 ng/mL. The cancer-specific and metastasis free survival rates at 7 years were 80% and 79.6%, respectively. The Progression Free Survival Rate (PFSR) was significantly influenced by three factors: the pre-HIFU PSA level, the Gleason score and a previous AD treatment. With the use of dedicated acoustic parameters, the rate of severe side effects decreased significantly from standard parameters: recto urethral fistula (0.4%), grade II/III incontinence (19.5%), and bladder outlet obstruction (14%). Rouvière et al. demonstrated in [19] that the MRI localization of cancer recurrence anterior to the urethra is an independent significant predictor of salvage HIFU failure after EBRT. Therefore, MRI may be useful for patient selection before post-EBRT salvage HIFU ablation. Two articles reported outcomes of salvage HIFU performed with the Sonablate [20, 21], showing the biochemical survival rate was 71% at 9 months and 52% at 5 years. Nevertheless, the risk–benefit ratio of salvage HIFU compares favorably with those of the other available techniques and with less morbidity and similar oncological outcomes. In this context, HIFU appears to be an effective curative treatment option for local recurrence after radiation failure.

Accurate Mapping of Prostate Cancer with MRI Plus Guided Biopsies and Evaluation of the Destruction of the Target Volume: The Keys for Focal Therapy

For a long time, it has been considered that prostate cancer could not be reliably detected by imaging methods. As a result, even today, it is diagnosed by means of systematically-distributed prostate biopsies. However, current 12-core systematic biopsy schemes can miss prostate cancer in up to 20% of patients. They also may underestimate prostate cancer volume and aggressiveness. The localization value of positive samples is also limited [22, 23]. Extensive research has been performed since the 1990s to develop an imaging method that can accurately show the position and volume of the different prostate cancer foci within the gland. This would dramatically improve the assessment of the tumor volume and aggressiveness by improving the sampling of the suspicious areas. As a result, it would also improve patient management, by selecting the appropriate treatment on more precise data. It is also a necessary condition for any focal treatment [23]. Despite recent improvements, ultrasound-based methods cannot currently provide an accurate mapping of intraprostatic cancer foci [24]. T2-weighted MRI has long been used as a staging method for prostate cancer as it provides a favorable contrast between the hyperintense normal peripheral zone and the hypointense cancer tissue. Unfortunately, it only achieves a 25–60% sensitivity in localizing prostate cancer foci [25–27]. Hydrogen MR spectroscopy can provide molecular information, but its added value to T2-weighted imaging has been disappointing [28]. The use of dynamic contrast-enhanced (DCE) imaging at the turn of the 2000s dramatically improved the sensitivity of MRI [27] and started to show good results in predicting biopsy results [29]. The advent of diffusion-weighted imaging a few years later further improved the diagnostic performance of MRI [30] which became the so-called multiparametric MRI (mpMRI), associating T2-weighted imaging with DCE, diffusion-weighted and/or spectroscopic imaging [31]. mpMRI has shown excellent results in detecting aggressive cancers with detection rates of 56–63% and 88–92% for Gleason 7 cancers of less and greater than 0.5 cc, respectively, and of 96% for Gleason ≥8 cancers [32]. Biopsies guided by mpMRI findings can also outperform systematic biopsies in detecting aggressive cancer [33, 34]. Because of these good results, mpMRI has currently become the cornerstone of focal treatment planning. However, mpMRI has two limitations. First, many benign conditions may mimic prostate cancer when using mpMRI. As a result, 40–75% of focal lesions seen at mpMRI are benign [32, 35]. It is therefore mandatory to biopsy all focal lesions before selecting patients for focal treatment. These so-called targeted biopsies have first been performed using cognitive guidance. The operator uses anatomical landmarks to target under transrectal ultrasound guidance the prostate area that was abnormal on mpMRI. However, there is potential for error in the extrapolation from MR to transrectal ultrasound images, because MR and ultrasound images are not acquired along the same plane. Sophisticated techniques of US/MRI fusion have been developed over the last 10 years to help the biopsy operator target the right area [36]. Some researchers have also proposed direct in-bore MR guidance [37]. This later technique is potentially very accurate but is limited by its cost and the need for dedicated scanning time. mpMRI is also limited by the fact that it underestimates the histological tumor volume [38, 39]. There is currently no reliable estimation of the safety margin that should be applied around malignant focal lesions seen on mpMRI to have a reasonable chance of destroying the entire histological tumor. This will probably be the topic of intensive research in the near future. Some US/MR fusion systems can register the position of the biopsy cores within the prostate. By retrospectively indicating which cores are positive, it is possible to define a target volume for focal treatment. These so-called 3D biopsies can be performed either transrectally or using a transperineal template. The precision of the tumor localization depends on the co-registration accuracy of the biopsy cores and on the number of cores. Although there is no large series of focal treatment using these 3D co-registered biopsies for treatment planning, this method could be interesting in addition to the tumor mapping provided by mpMRI.

In addition to a precise preoperative mapping of prostate cancer foci, there is also a need for an imaging method that can evaluate the destruction of the target volume. The ablated prostate volume appears on gadolinium-enhanced MRI as a devascularized zone that persists for 1–3 months postoperatively [40]. However, MRI is usually performed a few days following the treatment. It has recently been shown that contrast-enhanced ultrasound (CEUS) using Sonovue (Bracco, Milan, Italy) as a contrast medium showed similar findings as the postoperative gadolinium-enhanced MRI and could predict the presence of residual living tissue at postoperative biopsy [41]. On CEUS images, destroyed tissue appears as devascularized within minutes following the treatment [41]. It is therefore possible to immediately retreat the patient in case of unsatisfactory results.

Development of FocalOne: HIFU Device Dedicated to Focal Therapy of Localized PCa (CE Mark 2014)

The FocalOne was developed to overcome the limitations of devices which use a transducer with a fixed focus. FocalOne is a new device specifically designed for focal therapy of Prostate Cancer, combining the necessary tools to visualize, target, treat and validate the focal treatment (Fig. 22.9). MR images are imported through the hospital's network or USB drive. The operator defines the contours of the

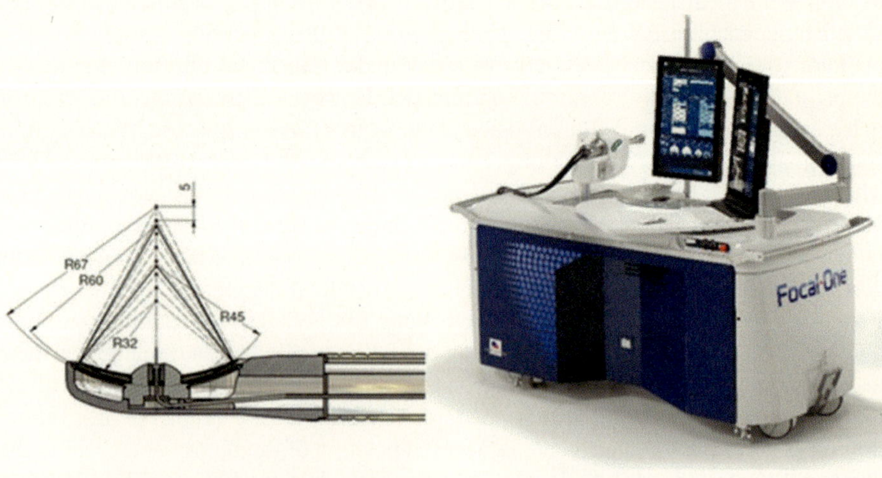

Fig. 22.9 Focal One, Probe and device

prostate and the regions of interests that have been confirmed as prostate tumors. The same contouring of the prostate is performed on the live ultrasound volume acquired by the transrectal probe. The software proceeds to create an "elastic fusion": the live ultrasound volume is considered as the reference volume and the MR volume is smoothly deformed so the 3D contour of the prostate on the MR volume matches perfectly the contours of the prostate on the Ultrasound Volume. The same 3D elastic transformation is applied to the ROIs initially indicated on the MR image (Fig. 22.10a, b). They thus appear at the correct position on the real-time ultrasound images guiding the planning process (Fig. 22.10c). FocalOne is equipped with a new generation of HIFU probe that is able to electronically vary the focal point along the acoustic axis using a HIFU multi-element transducer (Fig. 22.9a).

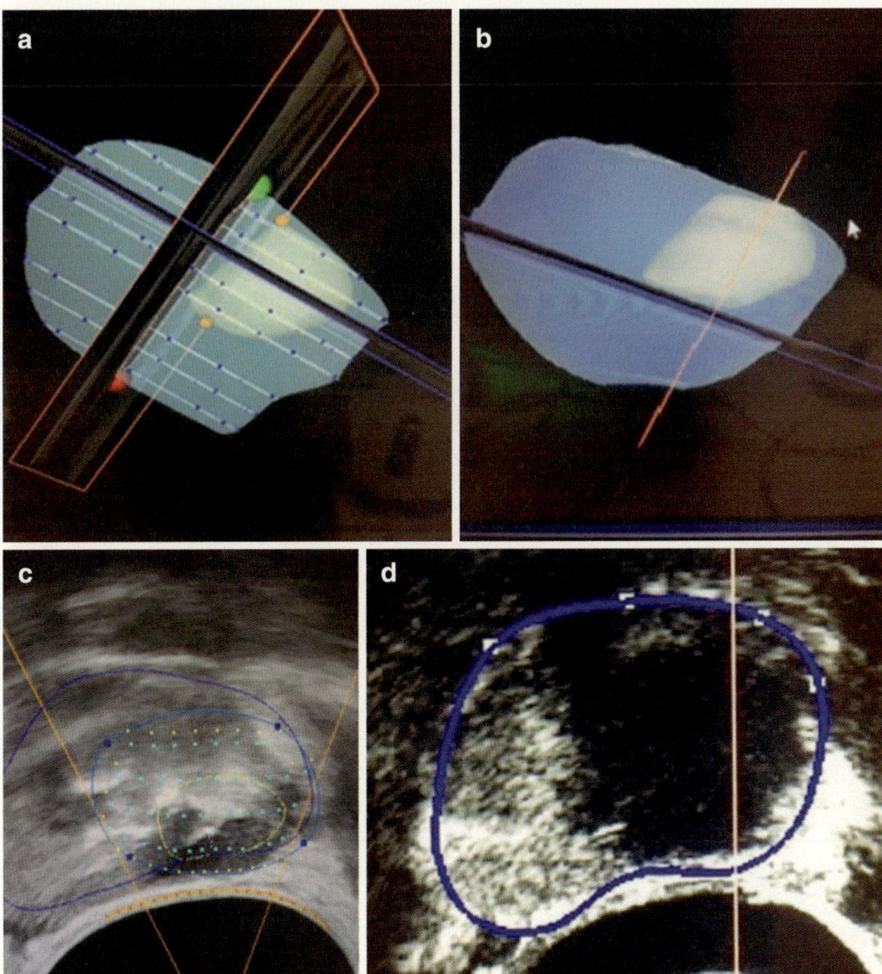

Fig. 22.10 (**a**) Imported MR Image with ROIs (**b**) Image fusion after elastic transformation (**c**) Focal one treatment planning (**d**) contrast-enhanced ultrasound (CEUS) of the treated area

The Dynamic Focusing transducer is made of 16 confocal rings that allow electronic steering of the focal point to a maximum of eight different points at 32–67 mm from the transducer. The Dynamic Focusing treatment consists of stacking several unitary HIFU lesions. The elementary HIFU lesion height is 5 mm and stacking two to eight unitary lesions leads to necrotic lesion of 10–40 mm height. The shooting process is a 1 s fire at each foci with no OFF between different foci. When compared to a fixed focusing treatment, dynamic focusing allows the treatment of bigger prostates with maximum lesion height of 40 mm instead of 26 mm. The wide range of lesion heights (10–40 mm) allows obtaining a better contouring of the prostate. HIFU treatment of the prostate cancer should be faster due to the shooting process with no time OFF between firings. Several studies were conducted in animals (rabbit and pigs) to determine effective acoustic parameters. Another advantage of dynamic focusing HIFU treatment is a more homogeneous necrotic zone due to a better energy distribution. During the HIFU energy delivery process, the operator sees a live ultrasound image of what is being treated and, if necessary, can readjust the treatment in real-time. At the end of the treatment process, a Contrast-enhanced Ultrasound volume is acquired showing the de-vascularized area (Fig. 22.10d). This CEUS volume can be fused with the treatment planning as well as the initial MR image showing immediate concordance between targeted and treated areas.

Preliminary Results of HIFU Focal Treatment of Localized PCa

HIFU focal therapy is another pathway that is being explored due to the increased accuracy and reliability of PCa mapping techniques. HIFU would be particularly suitable for such a therapy since it is clear that HIFU results and toxicity are relative to treated prostate volume.

Focal Therapy as Primary Care Treatment

Active surveillance has been adopted as an option for men who have low risk prostate cancer. The advantages of active surveillance must be weighed against the very real possibility of missing the "window" to cure the cancer because of delayed treatment. Focal therapy is emerging as an alternative in the management of low to intermediate risk patients. Mouraviev et al. identified unilateral cancers in 19.2% of 1184 radical prostatectomy specimens [42]. This study suggests, without taking into account cancer significance, that almost a fifth of the patients who are candidates for radical surgery could be amenable to hemi-ablation using thermal therapy targeting one lobe of prostate. Some evidence exists which shows the largest tumor (the index tumor) is the main driver of progression, outcome and prognosis; small secondary cancers might be clinically irrelevant [43, 44]. Focal therapy is currently only being considered for use in carefully selected patient populations for future prospective trials (Gleason 6 or Gleason 7 (3 + 4), small solitary cancer foci). The concept of the index tumor potentially allows for the use of focal therapy on patients with bilateral tumors. HIFU might be one of the best techniques for focal therapy because it is performed under real-time control using ultrasound or MRI. An immediate control of the boundaries of the necrosis area is possible using contrast agents (either with ultrasound and/or MRI). HIFU procedures can also be repeated if necessary. Finally, salvage standard curative therapies are feasible after HIFU (EBRT, surgery or cryo-ablation).

In 2008, Muto et al. reported the outcomes of 29 patients treated with Sonablate™ device [45]. In selected patients whose cancer was confined to only one lobe by multi regional biopsies, the total peripheral zone and a half portion of the transitional zone were ablated: 17 patients underwent control biopsies 12 months after the procedure: A residual cancer foci was found in four patients (23.5%). No significant change was found on IPSS score and Maximal Flow Rate before and 12 months after the procedure.

The first study (20 patients) of prostate hemi ablation with HIFU was published in 2011 [46]. Inclusion criteria were men with low to moderate risk (Gleason − 7, PSA = 15 μg/mL), unilateral PCa on TRUS biopsy underwent MRI and 5 mm-spaced transperineal template biopsies to localize disease. Of the patients, 25% had low risk and 75% intermediate risk cancer, their mean PSA pre HIFU was 7.3 ng/mL. Their mean PSA decreased to 1.5 ng/mL ± 1.3 at 12 months. A total of 89% of the patients had no histological evidence of any cancer. An erection sufficient for penetrative sex occurred in 95% of the patients and 95% of patients were pad free. Ahmed et al. reported in 2015, the outcomes of 56 patients with multifocal localized prostate cancer treated with HIFU Focal Ablation targeting the Index Lesion [47]. The median PSA was 7.4 ng/mL. The median PSA nadir was 2.4 ng/mL at 12 months. 80.8% of the patients had histological absence of clinically significant cancer (Gleason <7, <2 positive cores and no cancer core length > 3 mm regardless of grade) and 85.7% had no measurable prostate cancer (biopsy and/or mpMRI). Two (3.6%) patients had clinically significant disease in untreated areas not detected at baseline. Pad-free and leak-free continence was preserved in 92.3% and 92.0% of patients, respectively. Erections sufficient for intercourse were preserved in 76.9% of patients. The French Urological Association (AFU) has started a multi-institutional study to evaluate hemi ablation with HIFU as a primary treatment for patients >50 years, T1C or T2A, PSA < 10 ng/mL, Gleason 6 or 7 (3 + 4), in no more than one lobe after MRI, random and targeted biopsies. Only one prostatic lobe is treated. So far, the primary outcome has been the absence of clinically significant cancer (CSC) on control biopsy (Gleason <7, <2 positive cores and no cancer core length > 3 mm regardless of grade). Secondary outcomes have been the presence of any cancer on biopsy, biochemical response, radical treatment free survival (RTFS). A total of 111 patients have been treated. On control biopsy, 12 patients (11.9%) had a CSC (5 ipsilateral; 7 contralateral). Secondary treatments were technically uneventful and the radical treatment free survival rate at 2 years was 89%. Their mean PSA decrease at 2 years was 62.8% compared with initial PSA pre-treatment value.

At 12 months urinary and erectile functions were preserved in 97.2% and 78.4% of patients. Similar results after HIFU hemi ablation were reported by Cordeiro Feijoo et al. in [48]. Van Velthoven published the first long term results of a prospective clinical trial of HIFU hemi ablation for clinically localized prostate cancer [49]. Hemi ablation HIFU was primarily performed in 50 selected patients with biopsy-proven clinically localized unilateral, low-intermediate risk prostate cancer in complete concordance with the prostate cancer lesions identified by magnetic resonance. The median follow-up was 39.5 months. Their mean nadir PSA value was 1.6 ng/mL, which represents 72% reduction compared with initial PSA pre-treatment value ($P < 0.001$). Biochemical recurrence, according to Phoenix definition, occurred in 28% of patients. The 5-year actuarial metastases-free survival, cancer-specific survival and overall survival rates were 93%, 100% and 87%, respectively. Out of the eight patients undergoing biopsy, six patients had a positive biopsy for cancer occurring in the untreated contralateral ($n = 3$), treated ipsilateral lobe ($n = 1$) or bilaterally ($n = 2$). Complete continence (no pads) and erection sufficient for intercourse were documented in 94% and 80% of patients, respectively. After Hemi-ablation with HIFU, the rate of clinically significant disease was low and associated with low morbidity and preservation of quality of life. This treatment strategy does not preclude future definitive therapies. New devices (i.e. FocalOne) will make HIFU an even more precise treatment option for focal therapy. Preliminary results compare favorably with those of hemi ablation studies [50].

Focal Therapy as Salvage Treatment (Focal Salvage HIFU)

Early identification of a local relapse after radiation therapy failure is feasible using MRI and targeted biopsies performed soon after the biochemical failure (Phoenix criteria). Focal Salvage HIFU is a new therapeutic option. The aim of Focal Salvage HIFU (FSH) is to destroy the recurrent cancer with a minimal risk of severe side effects. The study of Ahmed et al. demonstrated that, focal therapy with HIFU can achieve a local control of the disease with minimal morbidity in patients with unilateral relapse after EBRT [51]. Baco and Gelet reported outcomes of 48 men with unilateral radio recurrent prostate cancer treated with Hemi salvage HIFU (HSH) [52]. After HSH the mean PSA nadir was 0.69 ng/mL at a median follow-up of 16.3 months. Progression-free survival rates at 12, 18, and 24 months were 83%, 64%, and 52%, respectively. Severe incontinence occurred in 8% of the 48 patients, 17% required one pad a day, and 75% were pad-free.

Conclusion

After 25 years of clinical research, HIFU is now used to treat PCa in clinical practice and in different clinical situations. The outcomes achieved for primary care patients seem close to those obtained by standard definitive therapies. On the other hand, HIFU has a considerable potential for local recurrence after radiation failure. HIFU is an evolving technology perfectly adapted for focal treatment. Sophisticated techniques of US/MRI fusion have been developed over the last 10 years allowing better targeting of the index tumor. Some early experiences on focal therapy suggest that HIFU provides an excellent opportunity to achieve local control of the disease in low to intermediate risk prostate cancer and in early identified local relapse after EBRT. Therefore, focal HIFU should find its place between active surveillance and radical therapies.

References

1. Lynn JG, Putnam TJ. Histology of cerebral lesions produced by focused ultrasound. Am J Pathol. 1944;20(3):637–49.
2. Chapelon JY, Margonari J, Theillère Y et al. Effects of high energy focused ultrasound on kidney tissue in the rate and the dog. Eur. Urol.1992;22:147–152.
3. Chapelon JY, Margonari J, Vernier F, Gorry F, Ecochard R, Gelet A. In vivo effects of high-intensity ultrasound on prostatic adenocarcinoma Dunning R3327. Cancer Res. 1992;52(22):6353–7.
4. Gelet A, Chapelon JY, Margonari J, Theillere Y, Gorry F, Cathignol D, et al. Prostatic tissue destruction by high-intensity focused ultrasound: experimentation on canine prostate. J Endourol. 1993;7(3):249–53.
5. Gelet A, Chapelon JY, Margonari J, Theillere Y, Gorry F, Souchon R, et al. High-intensity focused ultrasound experimentation on human benign prostatic hypertrophy. Eur Urol. 1993;23(Suppl 1):44–7.
6. Gelet A, Chapelon JY, Bouvier R, Souchon R, Pangaud C, Abdelrahim AF, et al. Treatment of prostate cancer with transrectal focused ultrasound: early clinical experience. Eur Urol. 1996;29(2):174–83.
7. Beerlage HP, van Leenders GJ, Oosterhof GO, Witjes JA, Ruijter ET, van de Kaa CA, et al. High-intensity focused ultrasound (HIFU) followed after one to two weeks by radical retropubic prostatectomy: results of a prospective study. Prostate. 1999;39(1):41–6.
8. Gelet A, Chapelon JY, Bouvier R, Pangaud C, Lasne Y. Local control of prostate cancer by transrectal high intensity focused ultrasound therapy: preliminary results. J Urol. 1999;161(1):156–62.
9. Poissonnier L, Chapelon JY, Rouviere O, Curiel L, Bouvier R, Martin X, et al. Control of prostate cancer by transrectal HIFU in 227 patients. Eur Urol. 2007;51(2):381–7.
10. Koch MO, Gardner T, Cheng L, Fedewa RJ, Seip R, Sanghvi NT. Phase I/II trial of high intensity focused ultrasound for the treatment of previously untreated localized prostate cancer. J Urol. 2007;178:2366–70. discussion 70–71
11. Crouzet S, Chapelon JY, Rouvière O, Mege-Lechevallier F, Colombel M, Tonoli- Catez H, Martin X, Gelet A. Whole-gland ablation of localized prostate cancer with high-intensity focused ultrasound: oncologic outcomes and morbidity in 1002 patients. Eur Urol. 2014;65(5):907–1464.
12. Thüroff S, Chaussy C. Evolution and outcomes of 3 MHz high intensity focused ultrasound therapy for localized prostate cancer during 15 years. J Urol. 2013;190(2):702–10.
13. Ganzer R, Fritsche HM, Brandtner A, Bründl J, Koch D, Wieland WF, Blana A. Fourteen-year oncological and functional outcomes of high-intensity focused ultrasound in localized prostate cancer. BJU Int. 2013;112(3):322–9.
14. Uchida T, Tomonaga T, Kim H, Nakano M, Shoji S, Nagata Y, Terachi T. Improved outcomes with advancements in high intensity focused ultrasound devices for the treatment of localized prostate cancer. J Urol. 2015;193(1):103–10.
15. Dickinson L, Arya M, Afzal N, Cathcart P, Charman SC, Cornaby A, Hindley RG, Lewi H, McCartan N, Moore CM, Nathan S, Ogden C, Persad R, van der Meulen J, Weir S, Emberton

35. Rouvière O, Papillard M, Girouin N, et al. Is it possible to model the risk of malignancy of focal abnormalities found at prostate multiparametric MRI? Eur Radiol. 2012;22(5):1149–57.
36. Costa DN, Pedrosa I, Donato F Jr, Roehrborn CG, Rofsky NM. MR imaging-transrectal US fusion for targeted prostate biopsies: implications for diagnosis and clinical management. Radiographics. 2015;35(3):696–708.
37. Hambrock T, Hoeks C, Hulsbergen-van de Kaa C, et al. Prospective assessment of prostate cancer aggressiveness using 3-T diffusion-weighted magnetic resonance imaging-guided biopsies versus a systematic 10-core transrectal ultrasound prostate biopsy cohort. Eur Urol. 2012;61(1):177–84.
38. Bratan F, Melodelima C, Souchon R, et al. How accurate is multiparametric MR imaging in evaluation of prostate cancer volume? Radiology. 2015;275(1):144–54.
39. Le Nobin J, Orczyk C, Deng FM, et al. Prostate tumour volumes: evaluation of the agreement between magnetic resonance imaging and histology using novel co-registration software. BJU Int. 2014;114(6b):E105–12.
40. Rouvière O, Lyonnet D, Raudrant A, et al. MRI appearance of prostate following transrectal HIFU ablation of localized cancer. Eur Urol. 2001;40(3):265–74.
41. Rouvière O, Glas L, Girouin N, et al. Transrectal HIFU ablation of prostate cancer: assessment of tissue destruction with contrast-enhanced ultrasound. Radiology.
42. Mouraviev V, Mayes JM, Sun L, Madden JF, Moul JW, Polascik TJ. Prostate cancer laterality as a rationale of focal ablative therapy for the treatment of clinically localized prostate cancer. Cancer. 2007;110(4):906–10.
43. Wise AM, Stamey TA, McNeal JE, Clayton JL. Morphologic and clinical significance of multifocal prostate cancers in radical prostatectomy specimens. Urology.
44. Noguchi M, Stamey TA, McNeal JE, Nolley R. Prognostic factors for multifocal prostate cancer in radical prostatectomy specimens: lack of significance of secondary cancers. J Urol. 2003;170(2 Pt 1):459–63.
45. Muto S, Yoshii T, Saito K, Kamiyama Y, Ide H, Horie S. Focal therapy with high-intensity-focused ultrasound in the treatment of localized prostate cancer. Jpn J Clin Oncol.
47. Ahmed HU, Dickinson L, Charman S, Weir S, McCartan N, Hindley RG, Freeman A, Kirkham AP, Sahu M, Scott R, Allen C, Van der Meulen J, Emberton M. Focal ablation targeted to the index lesion in multifocal localised prostate cancer: a prospective development study. Eur Urol. 2015;68(6):927–36.
48. Feijoo ER, Sivaraman A, Barret E, Sanchez-Salas R, Galiano M, Rozet F, Prapotnich D, Cathala N, Mombet A, Cathelineau X. Focal high-intensity focused ultrasound targeted hemiablation for unilateral prostate cancer: a prospective evaluation of oncologic and functional outcomes. Eur Urol. 2016;69(2):214–20.
49. Van Velthoven R, Aoun F, Marcelis Q, Albisinni S, Zanaty M, Lemort M, Peltier A, Limani K. A prospective clinical trial of HIFU hemiablation for clinically localized prostate cancer. Prostate Cancer Prostatic Dis. 2016;19(1):79–83.
50. Gelet A, Crouzet S, Rouvière O, Bratan F, Chapelon JY. Focal treatment of prostate cancer using focal one device: pilot study results. J Ther Ultrasound. 2015;3(Suppl 1):O6–4.
51. Ahmed HU, Cathcart P, McCartan N, Kirkham A, Allen C, Freeman A, Emberton M. Focal salvage therapy for localized prostate cancer recurrence after external beam radiotherapy: a pilot study. Cancer. 2012;118(17):4148–55.
52. Baco E, Gelet A, Crouzet S, Rud E, Rouvière O, Tanougast-Debbeche H, Berge V, Chapelon JY, Eggesbø HB. Hemi salvage high-intensity focused ultrasound (HIFU) in unilateral radiorecurrent prostate cancer: a prospective two-centre study. BJU Int. 2014;114(4):532–40.

Chapter 23
Development and Application of Histotripsy

William W. Roberts

Scientific Background

Histotripsy was defined as the application of high-intensity acoustic pulses of short duration (<50 μs) to induce controlled cavitation. When a sufficiently negative pressure is applied to fluid or tissue, microbubbles can form as fluid vaporizes and dissolved gas is released [1]. This phenomenon is called cavitation. Once the microbubbles have formed, they oscillate, coalesce, and collapse with release of substantial localized energy that produces mechanical disruption of cells and architectural features of tissues [2]. The low duty cycle (generally <1%) ensures predominance of mechanical rather than thermal tissue bioeffects [3].

To experimentally assess the process of cumulative tissue disruption, varying numbers of histotripsy pulses were applied transcutaneously to kidneys in an *in-vivo* rabbit model [4]. Scattered focal zones of hemorrhage and some cellular debris were produced with application of only ten histotripsy pulses. With application of increasing numbers of pulses, these focal zones of disruption enlarged and ultimately merged with adjacent disruption zones to create a larger homogenous zone of tissue disruption contained by a smooth margin of undamaged tissue [4, 5]. Application of greater than 1000 pulses, did not expand the zone of disruption, suggesting a self-limited process [4].

Tissue treated with histotripsy appears grossly and microscopically different than tissue after thermal ablation. To better understand the source of this distinction, thermocouples were placed in an *ex-vivo* porcine kidney model, at target

W.W. Roberts, M.D.
University of Michigan, 3879 Taubman Center, 1500 East Medical Center Drive, Ann Arbor, MI 48109-5330, USA
e-mail: willrobe@umich.edu

S.R. Patel et al. (eds.), *The History of Technologic Advancements in Urology*,
DOI 10.1007/978-3-319-61691-9_23

points which were treated with focus ultrasound parameter sets spanning the range from HIFU to histotripsy [6]. Lesions were characterized based on gross appearance. Disrupted lesions (where liquefied material spilled out of a cavity after sectioning) corresponded to application of high amplitude, short pulse acoustic parameters where tissue temperature increase was less than 27 °C. Desiccated lesions were produced by acoustic parameters of moderate amplitude but much longer pulse width and higher duty cycle and were associated with tissue temperature increases of 40 °C or greater. These results confirmed that with histotripsy acoustic pulse sequences, it is possible to induce cavitational mechanical effects while minimizing thermal tissue deposition [6]. This effect has also been validated with a similar acoustic pulsing strategy known as "boiling histotripsy" [7, 8].

The microbubbles that are produced with controlled cavitation and cause tissue disruption also happen to reflect ultrasound energy very well and hence provide real-time feedback of the histotripsy process. When monitoring histotripsy with conventional US imaging, the microbubble cloud appears as hyperechoic (bright) [3, 4]. This effect allows direct localization of the bubble cloud with US imaging and has proven very useful for target co-localization. Additionally, during treatment as the tissue is progressively disrupted, the appearance of the cloud evolves and the US signature of the tissue changes as well. Fractionated tissue appears hypoechoic as many of the structures that would have reflected US energy have disintegrated [4, 9]. Analysis of US backscatter data and assessment with shear wave imaging have also been evaluated as methods to more finely follow the progressive disruption of tissue with histotripsy acoustic pulses [10, 11].

Histotripsy can be applied with high precision as tissue disruption will only occur when negative pressure exceeds the cavitational threshold. The applied pressure field is tightly controlled based on the geometry of the histotripsy transducer. Using a phantom model composed of red blood cells and agar, histotripsy was applied in specific geometric patterns. Tissue disruption in this model was indicated by a color change resulting from lyses of the red blood cells (Fig. 23.1) [12]. The millimeter precision that can be achieved with histotripsy is apparent from the straight line and right angle corner boundaries of the disrupted regions. A further increase in precision is also possible by removing residual bubble nuclei with specialized acoustic pulses to reduce reflection and energy scatter before delivery of histotripsy pulses [13].

Earlier, the distinction between the acute appearance of histotripsy and thermal ablation lesions was discussed. Similarly, the biological response to tissue treated with histotripsy is also different than the response to thermal tissue coagulation. Histotripsy was applied to kidneys in an *in-vivo* rabbit model. The kidneys were harvested from 1 to 60 days later [14]. The debris within the disrupted lesions was resorbed quickly with little evidence of a residual lesion at 45–60 days and minimal fibrotic tissue deposition [14]. In subsequent canine prostate studies, the liquefied consistency of the disrupted prostate tissue following histotripsy treatment allowed drainage of this debris via the urethra, producing a TURP-like cavity within the prostate [9, 15, 16].

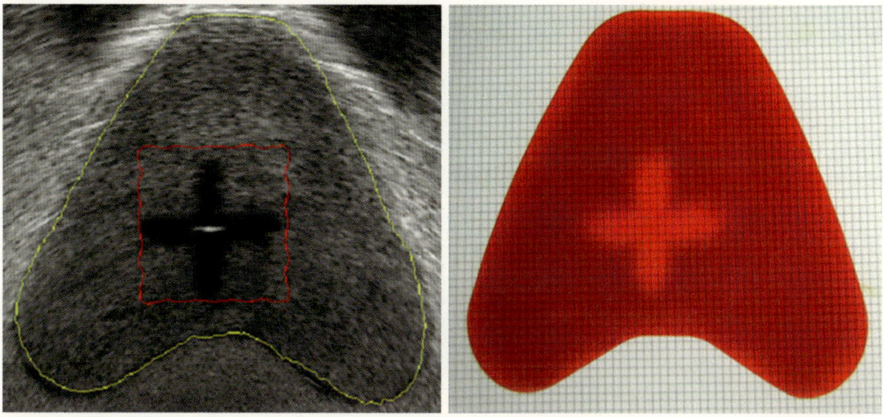

Fig. 23.1 A transverse section of a red blood cell prostate phantom (*left*) treated with histotripsy in a "plus" pattern. Lysis of the red blood cells (*lighter region*) is a marker of histotripsy tissue effect. Ultrasound imaging of the prostate phantom prior to sectioning (*right*) demonstrates the same pattern of tissue disruption

Translation to Clinical Application

Potential advantages of using histotripsy to treat BPH include extracorporeal application of energy, feedback with real-time US, rapid tissue disintegration, and reduction of debris to a liquefied state passable via the urethra. To capitalize on these features, A stepwise research approach was followed, building on initial feasibility studies, to characterize the number of acoustic pulses needed to disrupt each of the tissues within the prostate (glandular, stromal, periurethral) and to assess safety. Specifically, studies were performed to characterize the lack of substantial bleeding with histotripsy treatment, to quantify pain and assess tolerability, and to understand the consequence of inadvertently applying histotripsy to critical structures adjacent to the prostate. In all of these studies, intact older male canines were used as the model that was anatomically most similar to the human prostate. Histotripsy was applied transabdominally in anesthetized supine canine subjects with a water bolus positioned over the suprapubic region. The histotripsy transducer was placed in the water bolus and its focal volume co-localized within the prostate (Fig. 23.2). High resolution US images of the prostate and bubble cloud were obtained from A 10 MHz TRUS probe. The bubble cloud was translocated through the treatment region either by following a prescribed pattern or manually with joystick controls to produce volume ablation.

The feasibility of prostate histotripsy was first established in acute studies [9]. Based on initial observations of variability in tissue disruption, additional studies were conducted demonstrating that glandular tissue was more easily disrupted than periurethral prostatic tissue (28,000 pulses/cm^3 vs. 270,000 pulses/cm^3) [15]. In cases where the prostatic urethra was not completely treated, the endoscopic appearance after histotripsy correlated with the probability of prostatic urethral

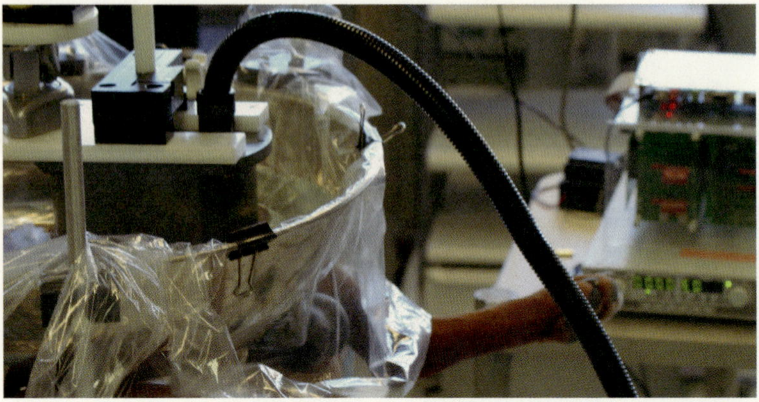

Fig. 23.2 The histotripsy transducer is positioned over the lower abdomen of a canine subject positioned supine. The focal volume of the transducer is co-localized within the prostate. A transrectal ultrasound probe is inserted in the rectum to provide imaging of the prostate and bubble cloud during treatment. The power supply and driving electronics are seen in the background

disintegration by 14 days. This was a desired outcome in order to permit disintegrated material in the treatment cavity to drain via the urethra [17]. An alternative urethral-sparing treatment strategy was evaluated, where only a modest 1–2 cm^3 volume of glandular tissue was disrupted and the periurethral tissue spared. This strategy resulted in pools of liquefied debris within the prostate that resorbed over an 8 week period. Residual treatment sites contained simple fluid and prostate volume decreased by 12% without evidence of abscess or increased chronic inflammation [18].

Limited hematuria and little hemorrhage were observed in previous studies. This prompted further exploration in nine canine subjects that were anticoagulated with warfarin (international normalized ratio ranged from 1.2 to 11.3) and then underwent large-volume histotripsy treatment of the prostate producing TURP-like defects [19]. Serial assessment of serum hemoglobin did not reveal a decrease and only mild hematuria without clots was noted in the first 48 h after treatment, before clearing. This suggested that histotripsy tissue treatment exhibits a hemostatic effect even in anticoagulated subjects.

In order to move towards human translation of this technology, it was important to characterize local and systemic effects of histotripsy. Eighteen canine subjects underwent histotripsy treatment to produce at least a 4 cm^3 volume treatment cavity. Upon harvest (between 0 and 56 days after treatment) a vacuous treatment cavity was confirmed. Validated pain scoring revealed mild post-treatment discomfort that resolved with catheter removal. On several occasions, the treatment volume inadvertently included a portion of rectum, which resulted in a prostatorectal fistula in one case. In all other subjects, minimal hematuria and only transient abnormalities in blood tests were noted which resolved after several days [16]. The treatment cavity in each case exhibited only minimal residual debris and was covered with new urothelium 28 days after treatment (Fig. 23.3).

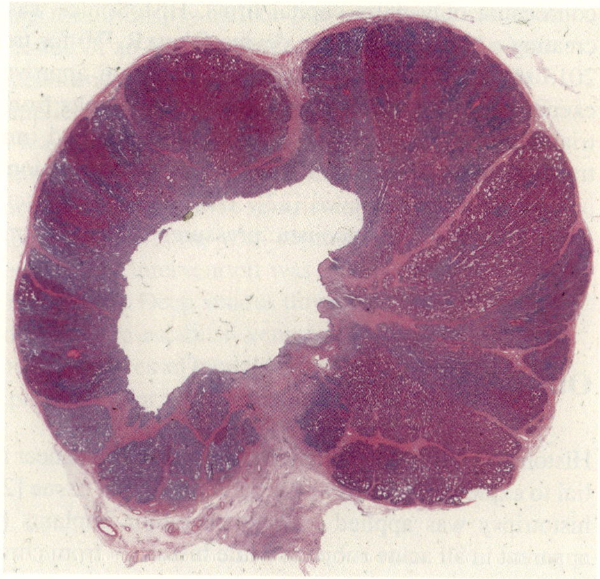

Fig. 23.3 Four weeks after transcutaneous in-vivo histotripsy treatment in a canine model, the prostate was harvested sectioned and stained with hematoxylin and eosin. The roughly *rectangular* empty cavity encompassing both glandular and prostatic urethral tissue elements represents a section of the rectangular treatment cavity

The prostate is surrounded by critical structures which must be spared of injury during prostate treatment. Although histotripsy is precise, targeting errors or patient motion may result in inadvertent treatment of these structures. It was apparent from earlier studies that damage thresholds from histotripsy vary based on tissue type [15, 20]. Studies were conducted to establish the damage thresholds of critical periprostatic structures by applying 1000, 10,000, or 100,000 histotripsy pulses directly on the urinary sphincter, neurovascular bundle, rectum, and 750,000 pulses to the bladder trigone, and ureteral orifices [21, 22]. After 10,000 pulses, the rectum exhibited moderate collagen disruption and focal mucosal disruption. The other structures however were more resilient. After 100,000 pulses the urinary sphincter was structurally intact and exhibited minimal histologic muscle fiber disruption. Arteries, veins, and nerves within the neurovascular bundles appeared intact, though extensive destruction of surrounding loose connective tissue was observed [21]. Cystoscopy, after histotripsy was applied to the bladder trigone, revealed moderate edema, though all ureteral orifices were preserved and patent [22].

Commercialization Efforts

After 5 years of successful research funded by National Institutes of Health and several foundations, our research group realized that additional resources would be needed to move further along the translational pathway towards human application. After evaluation of the options, it became clear that we needed to create a start-up company. HistoSonics, Inc. was formed in December 2009 and financed by a

References

1. Maxwell AD, Wang T, Cain CA, et al. Cavitation clouds created by shock scattering from bubbles during histotripsy. J Acoust Soc Am. 2011;130:1888–98.
2. Xu Z, Raghavan M, Hall TL, et al. Evolution of bubble clouds induced by pulsed cavitational ultrasound therapy – histotripsy. IEEE Trans Ultrason Ferroelectr Freq Control. 2008;55:1122–32.
3. Parsons JE, Cain CA, Abrams GD, Fowlkes JB. Pulsed cavitational ultrasound therapy for controlled tissue homogenization. Ultrasound Med Biol. 2006;32:115–29.
4. Roberts WW, Hall TL, Ives K, et al. Pulsed cavitational ultrasound: a noninvasive technology for controlled tissue ablation (histotripsy) in the rabbit kidney. J Urol. 2006;175:734–8.
5. Winterroth F, Xu Z, Wang T, et al. Examining and analyzing subcellular morphology of renal tissue treated by histotripsy. Ultrasound Med Biol. 2011;37:78–86.
6. Kieran K, Hall TL, Parsons JE, et al. Refining histotripsy: defining the parameter space for the creation of non-thermal lesions with high intensity pulsed ultrasound in the in vitro kidney. J Urol. 2007;178:672–6.
7. Wang Y, Khokhlova T, Bailey M, et al. Histological and biochemical analysis of mechanical and thermal bioeffects in boiling histotripsy lesions induced by high intensity focused ultrasound. Ultrasound Med Biol. 2013;39:424–38.
8. Simon JC, Sapozhnikov OA, Khokhlova VA, et al. Ultrasonic atomization of tissue and its role in tissue fractionation by high intensity focused ultrasound. Phys Med Biol. 2012;57:8061–78.
9. Lake AM, Hall TL, Kieran K, et al. Histotripsy: minimally invasive technology for prostatic tissue ablation in an in vivo canine model. Urology. 2008;72:682–6.
10. Wang T, Xu Z, Winterroth F, et al. Quantitative ultrasound backscatter for pulsed cavitational ultrasound therapy – histotripsy. IEEE Trans Ultrason Ferroelectr Freq Control. 2009;56:995–1005.
11. Wang T, Hall TL, Xu Z, et al. Imaging feedback of histotripsy treatments using ultrasound shear wave elastography. IEEE Trans Ultrason Ferroelectr Freq Control. 2012;59:1167–81.
12. Maxwell AD, Wang T, Yuan L, et al. A tissue phantom for visualization and measurement of ultrasound-induced cavitation damage. Ultrasound Med Biol. 2010;36:2132–43.
13. Wang T, Xu Z, Hall TL, et al. Active focal zone sharpening for high-precision treatment using histotripsy. IEEE Trans Ultrason Ferroelectr Freq Control. 2011;58:305–15.
14. Hall TL, Kieran K, Ives K, et al. Histotripsy of rabbit renal tissue in vivo: temporal histologic trends. J Endourol. 2007;21:1159–66.
15. Hall TL, Hempel CR, Wojno K, et al. Histotripsy of the prostate: dose effects in a chronic canine model. Urology. 2009;74:932–7.
16. Hempel CR, Hall TL, Cain CA, et al. Histotripsy fractionation of prostate tissue: local effects and systemic response in a canine model. J Urol. 2011;185:1484–9.
17. Schade GR, Styn NR, Hall TL, Roberts WW. Endoscopic assessment and prediction of prostate urethral disintegration after histotripsy treatment in a canine model. J Endourol. 2012;26:183–9.
18. Schade GR, Hall TL, Roberts WW. Urethral-sparing histotripsy of the prostate in a canine model. Urology. 2012;80:730–5.
19. Wheat JC, Hall TL, Hempel CR, et al. Prostate histotripsy in an anticoagulated model. Urology. 2010;75:207–11.
20. Lake AM, Xu Z, Cain CA, et al. Renal ablation by histotripsy: does it spare collecting system? J Urol. 2008;179:1150–4.
21. Styn N, Hall TL, Fowlkes JB, et al. Histotripsy homogenization of the prostate: thresholds for cavitation damage of periprostatic structures. J Endourol. 2011;25:1531–5.
22. Allam C, Wilkinson JE, Cheng X, et al. Histotripsy effects on the bladder trigone: functional and histologic consequences in the canine model. J Endourol. 2013;27:1267–71.
23. Wei JT, Schuster TG, Hendlin K, et al. Histotripsy for treatment of benign prostatic hyperplasia using the Vortx Rx: safety and initial efficacy results. J Endourol. 2015;29(Suppl. 1):A195.

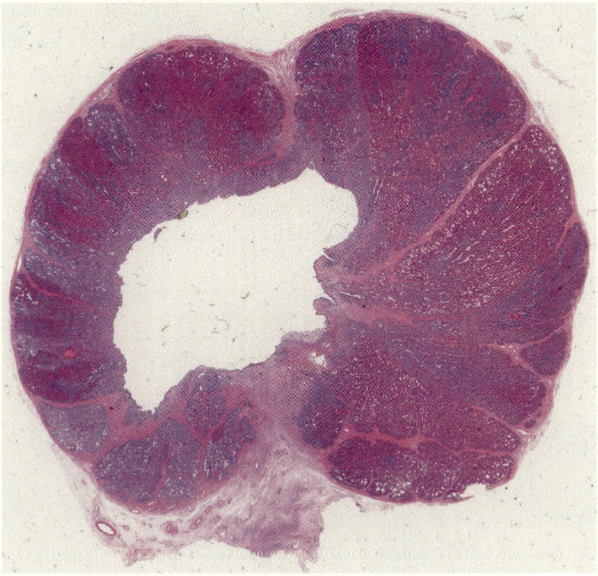

Fig. 23.3 Four weeks after transcutaneous in-vivo histotripsy treatment in a canine model, the prostate was harvested sectioned and stained with hematoxylin and eosin. The roughly *rectangular* empty cavity encompassing both glandular and prostatic urethral tissue elements represents a section of the rectangular treatment cavity

The prostate is surrounded by critical structures which must be spared of injury during prostate treatment. Although histotripsy is precise, targeting errors or patient motion may result in inadvertent treatment of these structures. It was apparent from earlier studies that damage thresholds from histotripsy vary based on tissue type [15, 20]. Studies were conducted to establish the damage thresholds of critical periprostatic structures by applying 1000, 10,000, or 100,000 histotripsy pulses directly on the urinary sphincter, neurovascular bundle, rectum, and 750,000 pulses to the bladder trigone, and ureteral orifices [21, 22]. After 10,000 pulses, the rectum exhibited moderate collagen disruption and focal mucosal disruption. The other structures however were more resilient. After 100,000 pulses the urinary sphincter was structurally intact and exhibited minimal histologic muscle fiber disruption. Arteries, veins, and nerves within the neurovascular bundles appeared intact, though extensive destruction of surrounding loose connective tissue was observed [21]. Cystoscopy, after histotripsy was applied to the bladder trigone, revealed moderate edema, though all ureteral orifices were preserved and patent [22].

Commercialization Efforts

After 5 years of successful research funded by National Institutes of Health and several foundations, our research group realized that additional resources would be needed to move further along the translational pathway towards human application. After evaluation of the options, it became clear that we needed to create a start-up company. HistoSonics, Inc. was formed in December 2009 and financed by a consortium of venture capital firms. HistoSonics was subsequently successful at creating a human prototype device (VortxR$_X$™) for treatment of BPH and in May 2013 the US Food and Drug Administration approved an investigational device exemption to conduct a human pilot trial. Results from this 25 patient first-in-man trial demonstrated an excellent safety profile and improvement in lower urinary tract symptoms, however TURP-like tissue destruction as seen in the canine model has not yet been achieved [23]. The histotripsy system will need to be refined in order to enhance the acoustic pressures needed for more effective cavitation and tissue disruption.

Other Applications

Histotripsy has been applied in a canine ACE-1 cancer model with metastatic potential to explore histotripsy effects on malignant tissue [24]. In seven canine subjects, histotripsy was applied to prostate tumor implants [25]. Tumor disruption was apparent in all acute subjects while histology from chronic subjects revealed necrosis and hemorrhage. Metastases were apparent in all three tumor implanted controls, while none of the histotripsy treated chronic subjects exhibited metastases [25].

A similar study in rabbits with subcapsular renal implants of VX-2 tumor demonstrated pools of homogenized tumor, while kidneys harvested at 24 h after treatment also exhibited an acute inflammatory response [26]. This study confirmed malignant tissue in the kidney could be homogenized with histotripsy and led to a subsequent study to measure the metastatic burden after histotripsy [27]. Thirteen days after tumor implantation in the kidney, histotripsy was applied, followed by nephrectomy 1 day later and necropsy 7 days later. There was no statistical difference in total lung metastases or density of metastases when comparing histotripsy treated and control rabbits [27]. Similar results have been reported in a murine model treated with mechanical HIFU, a focused ultrasound therapy that combines cavitational and thermal effects [28]. These studies, though not definitive, do suggest that histotripsy may have a direct or indirect effect that impedes tumor metastases. Further studies are needed to verify these findings.

Induction and control of cavitation is the fundamental concept that underlies histotripsy. SWL treatment of urinary stones is also, at least partially, dependent on cavitation. Histotripsy was used to erode Ultracal-30 model stones and produced particles no larger than 100 μm [29, 30]. While SWL breaks down stone by progressive subdivision, histotripsy uses cavitation to produce surface erosion. Understanding this mechanistic difference led to the hypothesis that SWL and histotripsy could be used synergistically to improve treatment of urinary stones. When both histotripsy and SWL acoustic pulses were applied to model stones, stone comminution was more efficient and the distribution of stone fragments was shifted to smaller sizes than seen with SWL alone [31].

Additional urologic applications for histotripsy include non-invasive fenestration of ureteroceles which has been tested in an *ex-vivo* tissue model [32] and *in-vitro* histotripsy treatment of urinary stents and catheters to destroy Escherichia Coli biofilms [33]. Histotripsy has application for non-urologic diseases as well. Transcutaneous liver ablation is feasible in an in-vivo porcine model and could be applied as treatment for hepatocellular carcinoma and liver metastases [34]. Histotripsy has been used to puncture the intracardiac ventricular septum in porcine models. This has utility for temporizing newborns with sever cardiac defects [35]. Intrauterine histotripsy for potential fetal intervention was successful in ablating liver and renal tissue in a sheep model [36]. Deep venous thrombi can also be disintegrated with non-invasive histotripsy to re-establish venous flow as demonstrated in porcine models [37]. In phantom blood vessel models it has been possible to create an acoustic embolus trap to prevent larger particles from escaping during histotripsy thrombolysis [38].

Conclusion

Histotripsy, based upon control of acoustic cavitation, is effective at disrupting tissue and eroding urinary stones. It is distinct from other ablative modalities as it is non-thermal and image-guided with real-time feedback which enhances targeting and monitoring of treatment effects. Histotripsy, originally conceived and pioneered at the University of Michigan, has been disseminated with active research efforts now established at other academic institutions. A pilot human clinical trial has been conducted for treatment of BPH and other pre-clinical exploration is ongoing for other urologic and non-urologic diseases.

Timeline

- Feb 2006 Histotripsy first defined in the literature [4].
- Oct 2007 First histotripsy survival pre-clinical animal study published [14].
- Dec 2009 HistoSonics, Inc. founded to develop human prototype for histotripsy treatment of BPH.
- May 2013 Investigational Device Exemption approved by FDA allowing first-in-man human trial.
- Oct 2015 First-in-man histotripsy human pilot study results reported [23].

Acknowledgements Conflicts of Interest: WWR has equity, royalty, and consulting interests in HistoSonics, Inc. He is the principal investigator on a sponsored research grant from HistoSonics, Inc.

References

1. Maxwell AD, Wang T, Cain CA, et al. Cavitation clouds created by shock scattering from bubbles during histotripsy. J Acoust Soc Am. 2011;130:1888–98.
2. Xu Z, Raghavan M, Hall TL, et al. Evolution of bubble clouds induced by pulsed cavitational ultrasound therapy – histotripsy. IEEE Trans Ultrason Ferroelectr Freq Control. 2008;55:1122–32.
3. Parsons JE, Cain CA, Abrams GD, Fowlkes JB. Pulsed cavitational ultrasound therapy for controlled tissue homogenization. Ultrasound Med Biol. 2006;32:115–29.
4. Roberts WW, Hall TL, Ives K, et al. Pulsed cavitational ultrasound: a noninvasive technology for controlled tissue ablation (histotripsy) in the rabbit kidney. J Urol. 2006;175:734–8.
5. Winterroth F, Xu Z, Wang T, et al. Examining and analyzing subcellular morphology of renal tissue treated by histotripsy. Ultrasound Med Biol. 2011;37:78–86.
6. Kieran K, Hall TL, Parsons JE, et al. Refining histotripsy: defining the parameter space for the creation of non-thermal lesions with high intensity pulsed ultrasound in the in vitro kidney. J Urol. 2007;178:672–6.
7. Wang Y, Khokhlova T, Bailey M, et al. Histological and biochemical analysis of mechanical and thermal bioeffects in boiling histotripsy lesions induced by high intensity focused ultrasound. Ultrasound Med Biol. 2013;39:424–38.
8. Simon JC, Sapozhnikov OA, Khokhlova VA, et al. Ultrasonic atomization of tissue and its role in tissue fractionation by high intensity focused ultrasound. Phys Med Biol. 2012;57:8061–78.
9. Lake AM, Hall TL, Kieran K, et al. Histotripsy: minimally invasive technology for prostatic tissue ablation in an in vivo canine model. Urology. 2008;72:682–6.
10. Wang T, Xu Z, Winterroth F, et al. Quantitative ultrasound backscatter for pulsed cavitational ultrasound therapy – histotripsy. IEEE Trans Ultrason Ferroelectr Freq Control. 2009;56:995–1005.
11. Wang T, Hall TL, Xu Z, et al. Imaging feedback of histotripsy treatments using ultrasound shear wave elastography. IEEE Trans Ultrason Ferroelectr Freq Control. 2012;59:1167–81.
12. Maxwell AD, Wang T, Yuan L, et al. A tissue phantom for visualization and measurement of ultrasound-induced cavitation damage. Ultrasound Med Biol. 2010;36:2132–43.
13. Wang T, Xu Z, Hall TL, et al. Active focal zone sharpening for high-precision treatment using histotripsy. IEEE Trans Ultrason Ferroelectr Freq Control. 2011;58:305–15.
14. Hall TL, Kieran K, Ives K, et al. Histotripsy of rabbit renal tissue in vivo: temporal histologic trends. J Endourol. 2007;21:1159–66.
15. Hall TL, Hempel CR, Wojno K, et al. Histotripsy of the prostate: dose effects in a chronic canine model. Urology. 2009;74:932–7.
16. Hempel CR, Hall TL, Cain CA, et al. Histotripsy fractionation of prostate tissue: local effects and systemic response in a canine model. J Urol. 2011;185:1484–9.
17. Schade GR, Styn NR, Hall TL, Roberts WW. Endoscopic assessment and prediction of prostate urethral disintegration after histotripsy treatment in a canine model. J Endourol. 2012;26:183–9.
18. Schade GR, Hall TL, Roberts WW. Urethral-sparing histotripsy of the prostate in a canine model. Urology. 2012;80:730–5.
19. Wheat JC, Hall TL, Hempel CR, et al. Prostate histotripsy in an anticoagulated model. Urology. 2010;75:207–11.
20. Lake AM, Xu Z, Cain CA, et al. Renal ablation by histotripsy: does it spare collecting system? J Urol. 2008;179:1150–4.
21. Styn N, Hall TL, Fowlkes JB, et al. Histotripsy homogenization of the prostate: thresholds for cavitation damage of periprostatic structures. J Endourol. 2011;25:1531–5.
22. Allam C, Wilkinson JE, Cheng X, et al. Histotripsy effects on the bladder trigone: functional and histologic consequences in the canine model. J Endourol. 2013;27:1267–71.
23. Wei JT, Schuster TG, Hendlin K, et al. Histotripsy for treatment of benign prostatic hyperplasia using the Vortx Rx: safety and initial efficacy results. J Endourol. 2015;29(Suppl. 1):A195.

24. Keller JM, Schade GR, Ives K, et al. A novel canine model for prostate cancer. Prostate. 2013;73(9):952.
25. Schade GR, Keller J, Ives K, et al. Histotripsy focal ablation of implanted prostate tumor in an ACE-1 canine cancer model. J Urol. 2012;188:1957–64.
26. Styn NR, Wheat JC, Hall TL, Roberts WW. Histotripsy of VX-2 tumor implanted in a renal rabbit model. J Endourol. 2010;24:1145–50.
27. Styn NR, Hall TL, Fowlkes JB, et al. Histotripsy of renal implanted VX-2 tumor in a rabbit model: investigation of metastases. Urology. 2012;80:724–9.
28. Xing Y, Lu X, Pua EC, Zhong P. The effect of high intensity focused ultrasound treatment on metastases in a murine melanoma model. Biochem Biophys Res Commun. 2008;31:645–50.
29. Duryea AP, Hall TL, Maxwell AD, et al. Histotripsy erosion of model urinary calculi. J Endourol. 2011;25:341–4.
30. Duryea A, Maxwell A, Roberts W, et al. In vitro comminution of model renal calculi using histotripsy. IEEE Trans Ultrason Ferroelectr Freq Control. 2011;58:971–80.
31. Duryea AP, Roberts WW, Cain CA, Hall TL. Controlled cavitation to augment SWL stone comminution: mechanistic insights *in-vitro*. IEEE Trans Ultrason Ferroelectr Freq Control. 2013;60:301–9.
32. Maxwell AD, His RS, Bailey MR, et al. Pulsed focused ultrasound as a method for noninvasive treatment of ureteroceles. Abstract, Engineering & Urology Society Annual Meeting. 2013.
33. Bigelow TA, Northagen T, Hill TM, Sailer FC. Ultrasound histotripsy and the destruction of *Escherichia Coli* biofilms. Conf Proc IEEE Eng Med Biol Soc. 2008;2008:4467–70.
34. Vlaisavljevich E, Kim Y, Allen S, et al. Image-guided non-invasive ultrasound liver ablation using histotripsy: feasibility study in an *in vivo* porcine model. Ultrasound Med Biol. 2013;39:1398–409.
35. Owens GE, Miller RE, Owens ST, et al. Intermediate-term effects of intracardiac communications created noninvasively by therapeutic ultrasound (histotripsy) in a porcine model. Pediatr Cardiol. 2012;33:83–9.
36. Kim Y, Fifer CG, Gelehrter SK, et al. Developmental impact and lesion maturation of histotripsy-mediated non-invasive tissue ablation in a fetal sheep model. Ultrasound Med Biol. 2013;39:1047–55.
37. Maxwell AD, Owens G, Gurm HS, et al. Noninvasive treatment of deep venous thrombosis using pulsed ultrasound cavitation therapy (histotripsy) in a porcine model. J Vasc Interv Radiol. 2011;22:369–77.
38. Park S, Maxwell AD, Owens GE, et al. Non-invasive embolus trap using histotripsy – an acoustic parameter study. Ultrasound Med Biol. 2013;39:611–9.

Chapter 24
Nanotechnology in Urology: History of Development and Applications in Urology

James Liu and Benjamin R. Lee

Introduction

In 1959, future Nobel Laureate (1965) Dr. Richard Feynman presented a landmark lecture entitled "There's Plenty of Room at the Bottom" to the American Physical Society where he postulated the miniaturization of science and challenged the audience: "How small can you make machinery?" Dr. Feynman's early visions and conceptual thoughts of shrinking down our understanding of the physical realm and examining the elemental parts on a small scale was the earliest invitation for our exploration into the realm of nanotechnology [1].

Nanotechnology, a term coined by Professor Norio Taniguichi from the University of Tokyo in 1974, refers to the study, creation, and manipulation of materials on the scale of 1–1000 nm (10^{-9} M) [2] (Fig. 24.1). Today, it is a rapidly expanding new field with pervasive applications across many disciplines. Within medicine, nanotechnology has provided groundbreaking solutions to the detection, characterization, and treatment of disease through unique pathways. Nanoparticles, due to their small size, have high surface area- to- volume ratio and versatile construction allowing for maximum manipulation. In the field of urology nanotechnology has already proven to be incredibly innovative [3, 4]. Particles like liposomes and polymers like poly lactic-co glycolic acid (PLGA) have already become mainstay research vectors for the study of drug delivery and gene therapy [3]. Other particles like carbon nanotubes and gold nanoshells are actively being explored in the use of more precise thermal ablation of tissue with both prostate cancer as well as renal cell carcinoma [4]. Finally, particles like magnetic iron oxide cover the gamut of use from improved metastatic cancer imaging to magnetic hyperthermia ablation modalities [3]. This

J. Liu, M.D.
Tulane University School of Medicine, New Orleans, LA, USA

B.R. Lee, M.D. (✉)
University of Arizona College of Medicine, Tucson, AZ, USA
e-mail: brlee@surgery.arizona.edu

S.R. Patel et al. (eds.), *The History of Technologic Advancements in Urology*,
DOI 10.1007/978-3-319-61691-9_24

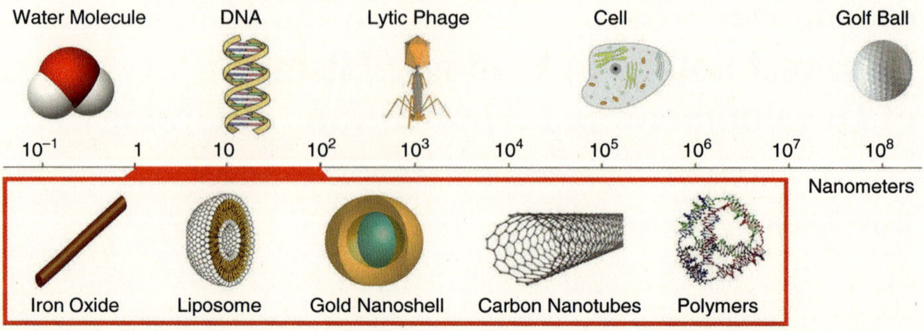

Fig. 24.1 The most investigated nanoparticles include Iron Oxide, Liposomes, Gold nanoshells, and carbon nanotubes

chapter aims to summarize the development and application of nanotechnology in urology in the specific modalities of imaging, gene therapy, drug delivery, thermal ablation, and tissue engineering.

Imaging

Contemporary imaging like MRI and CT has already improved our ability to detect anatomical and oncologic abnormalities. However, there are still limitations restricting the sensitivity and specificity of our modern technology [5]. Nanoparticles provide an interesting solution by utilizing high surface area; these nanoparticles allow extensive space for attachment of imaging agents and tumor-targeted ligands. Likewise, due to their specific size, nanoparticles undergo a process called enhanced permeability and retention (EPR) allowing them to escape renal clearance, while being small enough to extravasate and concentrate in the leaky vascular and lymphatic drains of developing tumors [3].

The first landmark paper on urological imaging was published in 2003. Dr. Harinsghani's group at Massachusetts General Hospital demonstrated the use of superparamagnetic nanoparticles in detection of occult metastatic prostate cancer. In a study of 80 prostate cancer patients of whom 33 had positive lymph nodes the authors reported that superparamagnetic particles via MRI were able to identify 100% of those patients preoperatively. This improvement was compared to a 45.4% detection based on standard MRI size criteria. By gaining access to interstitial lymphatic fluid these particles were able to enhance high-resolution MRI to detect clinically occult lymph node metastasis [6]. Feldman et al. applied the same technology in the lymph node metastasis detection in prostate, bladder, penile, and testicular cancers and found significant improvements in the sensitivity, specificity, and accuracy compared to conventional imaging [7].

As nanoparticle innovation continues to improve, further investigation has achieved targeted imaging enhancement. Recently, Mirzaei et al. has synthesized a nanodendrimer conjugated with a monoclonal antibody against prostate cancer and further chelating the particle with the imaging contrast agent, gadolinium. The group's early research with a complex nanoprobes demonstrates the capability to develop highly sensitive, specific, and targeted imaging augmentations [8].

Another promising vector for nanotechnology in imaging is the exploration of quantum dots. These are nano sized fluorescence-based optical probes with long half-lives, strong luminescence, and narrow emission range which can be tuned to near infrared light, allowing unmatched sensitivity in deeper penetrating [9]. Several *in vivo* and *in vitro* trials have shown potential for quantum dots. However, debate exists about the relative toxicity and low clearance of these particles [3]. Researchers like Ma et al. have developed potential solutions. The authors created a novel chitosan coated quantum dot that has increased sensitivity to zinc, a compound found in high concentrations in prostate cancer, while the coating also reduces any potential toxicity leak [10]. Quantum dots continue to provide promise in the diagnosis of urologic cancers.

Gene Therapy

Gene therapy has been a heavily researched field due to the promise of overcoming genetic illness with the introduction or ectopic expression of healthy genes. Nanoparticles have been implemented as non-viral vectors as a result of good biocompatibility, unlimited DNA carrying capacity, and specific cell targeting [11]. Early research has focused on cationic lipids such as liposomes in the delivery of genes. Larchian and his group from The Cleveland Clinic, in 2000, developed a liposome-mediated immune gene therapy using interleukin-2 and B71 in a murine bladder cancer model. The authors found that their regiment significantly improved tumor-free survival and was a safer and more effective compared to retroviral systems [12]. Other researchers like Hattori and Maitani developed nanoparticles with the addition of novel folate-link ligands for more specific delivery to prostate cancer. Their research was the first to selectively deliver DNA to prostate cancer *in vitro* that then enhanced gene expression [13]. Moffatt et al. from MD Anderson Cancer Center as well as Mukherjee from Johns Hopkins have been able to pair nanoparticles with prostate specific membrane antigen (PSMA) [14, 15]. Moffatt et al. using a targeted DNA molecular vector was also able to demonstrate a 20-fold increase in gene delivery over control in a mouse model [14]. These early studies illustrate the ability to create effective non-viral gene carriers while also improving uptake via surface markers and specific ligands.

Drug Delivery

Nanotechnology as a vector for drug delivery is perhaps the most studied platform for this new technology. Nanoparticles can effectively package drugs and thereby protect them from the *in vivo* microenvironment while also decreasing and minimizing systematic toxicity. Likewise, particles can be tagged with targeted ligands and markers and due to the EPR effect; particles have increased drug half-life, circulation, and enhanced bioavailability [16]. The earliest milestone for nanotechnology in drug delivery was the FDA approval of Doxil, a liposomal-based doxorubicin formulation, in 1995. This decision opened the floodgates for research to encapsulate other drugs for nanoparticle delivery [17].

In 1994 Okada et al. successfully loaded PLGA particles with leuprorelin for the treatment of prostate cancer. The group was able to use the stability of PLGA particles to create a 3-month depot injectable with linearly sustained drug release over 13 weeks [18]. Other groups like Sahoo et al. were also able to formulate paclitaxel-loaded PLGA particle with the addition of transferrin conjugation thereby selectively targeting prostate cancer. The authors were able to show in a murine prostate model that particles with transferrin and paclitaxel selectively killed tumor greater than drug or drug and particle alone [19].

In a phase II clinical trial of 34 patients with unresectable transitional cell carcinoma Winquist et al. investigated an IV pegylated-liposomal doxorubicin. The authors showed that six patients had partial response while seven had stable disease. Likewise, the authors noticed no clinical cardiotoxicity in the cohort, a typical dose-limiting factor in free drug regiments. Therefore, the authors demonstrated that nanoparticle formulations could alter toxicity profiles and improve response rate [20].

In the treatment of renal cell carcinoma (RCC) Sumitomo et al. in 2008 explored the use of an SN38 releasing nanodevice in disease progression. The authors found the nanoparticle was able to significantly decrease the number of pulmonary metastasis in a murine model versus control or drug alone [21]. In 2014 Liu et al. from Tulane University was able to successfully encapsulate the tyrosine kinase inhibitor Sorafenib one of the front line medications for the treatment of RCC, demonstrating that the class of tyrosine kinase inhibitor drugs and their hydrophobic interactions could be overcome [22].

Nanotechnology is also being used in the treatment of bladder cancer. Early research by Kiyokawa et al. in 1999 showed that injected liposomal doxorubicin in canines demonstrated 15–100 times greater concentration in regional lymph nodes and 70–930 times greater in whole bladder wall [23]. Lu et al. showed similar improvements with their formulation of paclitaxel loaded gelatin nanoparticles. The authors showed a 2.6 times greater concentration of drug dose in canine bladder model versus commercial free drug formulation while also demonstrating rapidly releasing drug with good cell kill [24]. Research in drug delivery has also branched out to incorporate other forms of nanoparticles. The group Chen et al. was able to develop a pirarubicin-loaded carbon nanotube. The authors found significant tumor depression both in vitro and in a rat bladder cancer model compared to drug alone. Interestingly the authors also noted that in contrast to free drug groups the rats treated with nanoparticles did not exhibit any significant side effects and no changes to both hepatic and renal function [25].

Finally, McKiernan from Columbia University demonstrated in a Phase II trial of intravesical nanoparticle albumin bound paclitaxel, an increased response rate of 35.7% in treatment of nonmuscle invasive bladder cancer following bacillus Calmette-Guerin treatment failure. The intravesicle nanoparticle paclitaxel had minimal toxicity with complete response rate remaining durable at 1 year follow-up [26].

Thermal Ablation

Thermal ablation to treat urological maladies has significant clinical precedent. High intensity focused ultrasound, cryotherapy, and radiofrequency ablation are surgical ablation modalities used worldwide. Combination of thermal treatment with nanocarriers is an interesting new concept that allows synergistic targeted effect while sparing unaffected tissue [3]. Stern et al. from University of Texas Southwestern Medical Center explored gold nanoshells in the ablation of prostate cancer cells *in vitro*. The group found that laser combined with nanoshells could eradicate all cells, while laser or shells alone had no influence on viability [27]. The same group applied their platform to a mouse model and showed a 93% tumor necrosis and regression after harvest in the treatment arm. Likewise, when paired the laser and gold had a mean temperature change of 28.9 versus 13.8 °C in just laser and saline [28]. In a similar animal study done by Lee et al. a dual gold nanorod and tyrosine kinase inhibitor albumin particle was formulated. The authors reported that when activated by laser there was synergistic response in both thermal ablation and drug release that could more effectively eradicate tumor [29].

Another model commonly used in ablation is magnetic iron oxide. Kawai et al. used magnetic cationic liposomes to ablate prostate cancer in a mouse model using an alternating magnetic field. The authors were able to reach core tumor temperatures of 45 °C with negligible body temperature change in the rest of the mouse. Likewise, measuring heat shock proteins, they found a significant immune response along with noticeable cellular necrosis [30]. The exploration of magnetic hyperthermia will be an interesting platform for nanotechnology since it can successfully ablate tumors based on image guidance, in addition, avoids the potential of skin burns experienced with some of the ablation modalities [31].

Carbon nanotubes, first discovered in 1991 by physicist Sumio Iijima, have also been heavily studied in thermal ablation [3]. Fisher et al. demonstrated in both murine renal cancer and in vitro prostate cancer cell lines that multi wall carbon nanotubes (MWCNT) incubated in cell lines and activated with 5 min of laser could lead to temperature increase of 43 °C and 100% cell death [32]. Likewise the group Burke et al. used MWCNT in the ablation of RCC in nude mice. Despite using short treatment times with low laser settings the authors were able to achieve greater than 3.5-month remission in 80% of the mice treated [33].

Tissue Engineering

The development of tissue engineering is of particular interest since its success would be able to effectively improve treatment and potentially cure a number of urological maladies. As early as 2000 Hume et al. have started to develop an implantable bioartifical kidney. Using nanoporous silica filtration membrane cultured with renal tubule progenitor cells the authors created a device that mimics the function of filtration and reclamation as well as the metabolic activity of the natural kidney [34]. Similarly, Nissenson et al. have developed an artificial nephron system that mimics both the function of the glomerulus and renal tubules thereby providing a potential treatment for renal failure. Other urological organs are also being studied [35]. In 2005 Pattison et al. developed a three-dimensional porous PLGA and polyether urethane scaffold that allows cell adhesion and growth of implanted human bladder smooth muscle cells to form viable replacement material for bladder wall [36]. Other research is applying nanoparticles to enable bladder tissue growth by delivery substrates and factors, ultimately altering the growth microenvironment [37]. In effect nanotechnology is playing a substantial role in tissue engineering and the promise of being able to replace vital organs.

Conclusion

Since its conception in 1959 nanotechnology has grown in leaps and bounds (Fig. 24.2). Exciting advances, especially in the field of urology, are laying the foundation to revolutionize diagnosis and treatment. Early research in the fields of imaging, gene therapy, drug delivery, thermal ablation, and tissue engineering are but a glimpse of the full potential nanotechnology can have (Table 24.1). In the near future we will begin to see these promising basic research studies translate to significantly impact clinical urological practice.

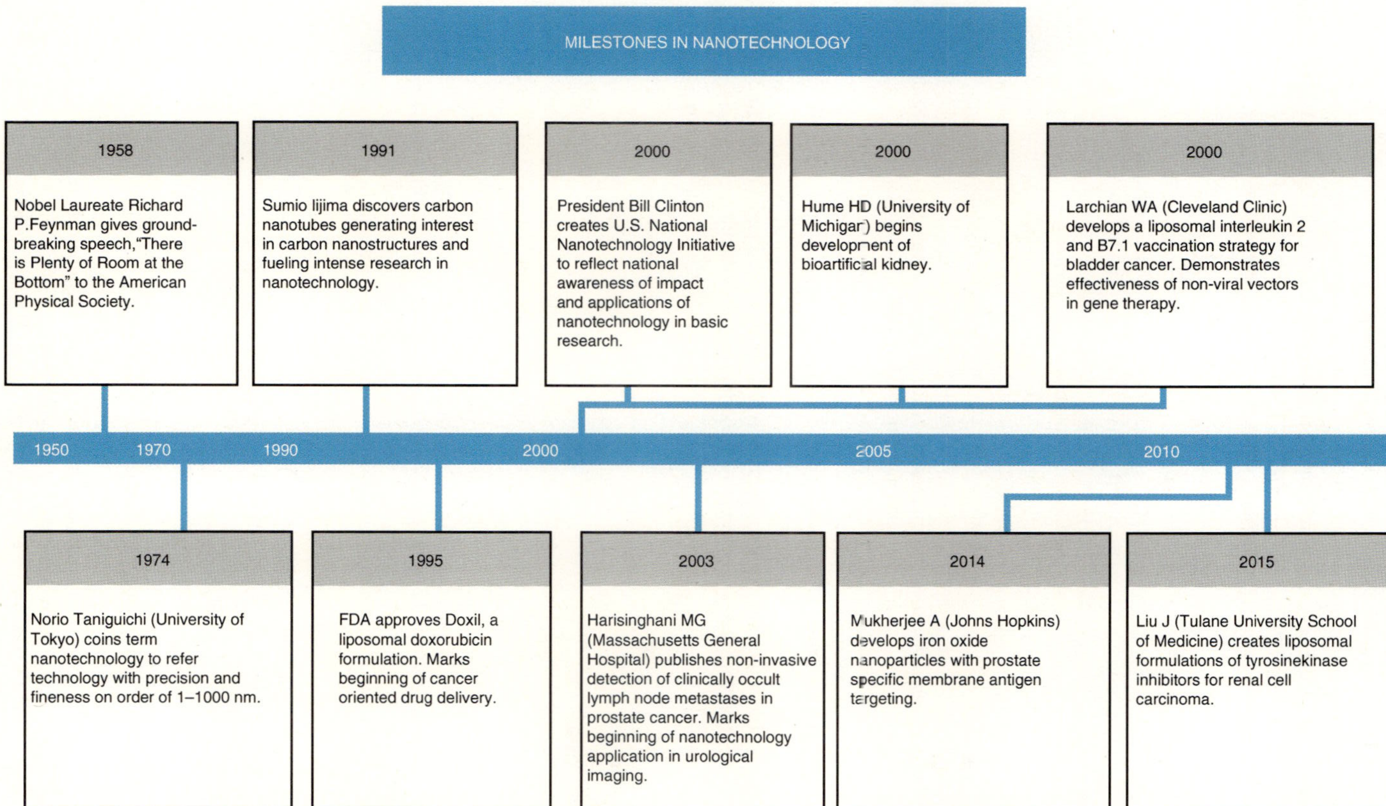

Fig. 24.2 Milestones in nanotechnology

Table 24.1 Summary of current nanotechnology development advantages and limitations

Summary of current nanotechnology development/limitations				
Particles	Applications	Developments	Limitations	Shape/size
Liposome/ Albumin	Drug delivery and ablation vector	Viable and flexible organic model that increases uptake efficacy, low systemic toxicity, and circumvent resistance	Drug release determined by cell uptake	Hollow sphere 100–170 nm
PLGA	Drug delivery and ablation vector	Viable and flexible polymer model that improves uptake efficacy, lowers systemic toxicity and circumvents resistance	Drug release independent of cell uptake	Solid sphere 150–200 nm
Gold	Laser thermal ablation	Excitation by NIR laser creates hyperthermia and destroys local cancer. Flexible construction	Potential toxicity with CTAB binder	Rod 40 × 10 nm
Iron Oxide	Laser thermal ablation, magnetic hyperthermia, and imaging	Excitation by NIR laser or electromagnetic field creates hyperthermia and destroys local cancer. Particles enhance imaging modalities	Limited efficacy with laser ablation, potential toxicity	Rod 3–10 nm
Carbon	Laser thermal ablation	Excitation by NIR laser creates hyperthermia and destroys local cancer	Size variability, difficulty solubilizing particle, particle toxicity	Rod 200–2000 nm

References

1. Feynman RP. There's plenty of room at the bottom (data storage). J Microelectromech Syst. 1992;1(1):60–6.
2. Taniguchi N. On the basic concept of 'Nano Technology'. Proceedings of the International Conference on Production Engineering, Tokyo, Part II (Japan Society of Precision Engineering). 1974.
3. Maddox MM, Liu J, Mandava SH, et al. Nanotechnology applications in urology: a review. Br J Urol. 2014;114:653–60.
4. Gommersall L, Shergill IS, Ahmed HU, et al. Nanotechnology and its relevance to the urologist. Eur Urol. 2007;52:368–75.
5. Chow EK, Ho D. Cancer nanomedicine: from drug delivery to imaging. Sci Transl Med. 2013;5:216.
6. Harisinghani MG, Barentsz J, Hahn PF, et al. Noninvasive detection of clinically occult lymph-node metastases in prostate cancer. N Engl J Med. 2003;348:2491–9.
7. Feldman AS, McDougal WS, Harisinghani MG. The potential of nanoparticle-enhanced imaging. Urol Oncol. 2008;26:65–73.
8. Mirzaei M, Mehravi B, Ardestani MS, et al. In vitro evaluation of Gd(3+)–anionic linear globular dendrimer-monoclonal antibody: potential magnetic resonance imaging contrast agents for prostate cancer cell imaging. Mol Imaging Biol. 2015;17(6):770.
9. Shi C, Zhu Y, Cerwinka WH, et al. Quantum dots: emerging applications in urologic oncology. Urol Oncol. 2008;26:86–92.

10. Ma Q, Lin ZH, Yang N, et al. A novel carboxymethyl chitosan-quantum dot-based intracellular probe for ZN (2+) ion sensing in prostate cancer cells. Acta Biomater. 2014;10:868–74.
11. Fortier C, Dorucher Y, De Crecenzo G. Surface modification of nonviral nanocarriers for enhanced gene delivery. Nanomedicine. 2014;1:135–51.
12. Larchian WA, Horiguchi Y, Nair SK, et al. Effectiveness of combined interleukin 2 and B7.1 vaccination strategy is dependent on the sequence and order: a liposome-mediated gene therapy treatment for bladder cancer. Clin Can Res. 2000;6:2913–20.
13. Hattori Y, Maitani Y. Enhanced in vitro DNA transfection efficiency by novel folate-linked nanoparticles in human prostate cancer and oral cancer. J Control Release. 2004;97:173–83.
14. Mofatt S, Papasakelariou C, et al. Successful in vivo tumor targeting of prostate-specific membrane antigen with a highly efficient J591/PEI/DNA molecular conjugate. Gene Ther. 2006;13:761–72.
15. Mukherjee A, Darlington T, Baldwin R, et al. Development and screening of a series of antibody-conjugated and silica-coated iron oxide nanoparticles for targeting the prostate-specific membrane antigen. ChemMedChem. 2014;19:1356–60.
16. Haley B, Frenkel E. Nanoparticles for drug delivery in cancer treatment. Urol Oncol. 2008;26:57–64.
17. Barenholz Y. Doxil- the first FDA approved nano-drug: lessons learned. J Control Release. 2012;160:117–34.
18. Okada H, Doken Y, Ogawa Y, et al. Preparation of three-month depot injectable microspheres of leuprorelin acetate using biodegradable polymers. Pharm Res. 1994;11:1143–7.
19. Sahoo SK, Ma W, Labhasetwar V. Efficacy of transferrin-conjugated paclitaxel-loaded nanoparticles in a murine model of prostate cancer. Int J Cancer. 2004;112:335–40.
20. Winquist E, Ernst DS, Jonker D, et al. Phase II trial of pegylated-liposomal doxorubicin in the treatment of advanced unresectable or metastatic transitional cell carcinoma of the urothelial tract. Eur J Cancer. 2003;39:1866–71.
21. Sumitomo M, Koizumi F, Asano T, et al. Novel SN-38-incorporated polymeric micelle, NK012, strongly suppresses renal cancer progression. Cancer Res. 2008;68:1631–5.
22. Liu J, Boonkaew B, Arora J, et al. Comparison of Sorafenib-loaded poly (lactic/glycolic) acid and DPPC liposome nanoparticle in the in vitro treatment of renal cell carcinoma. J Pharm Sci. 2014;104:1187–96.
23. Kiyokawa H, Igawa Y, Mursahi O, et al. Distribution of doxorubicin in the bladder wall and regional lymph nodes after bladder submucosal injection of liposome doxorubicin in the dog. Urology. 1999;161:665–7.
24. Lu Z, Yeh TK, Tsai M, et al. Paclitaxel-loaded gelatin nanoparticles for intravesical bladder cancer therapy. Clin Can Res. 2004;10:7677–84.
25. Chen G, He Y, Wu X, et al. In vitro and in vivo studies of pirarubicin-loaded SWNT for the treatment of bladder cancer. Braz J Med Biol Res. 2012;45:771–6.
26. McKiernan JM, Holder DD, Ghandour RA, et al. Phase II trial of intravesical nanoparticle albumin bound paclitaxel for the treatment of nonmuscle invasive urothelial carcinoma of the bladder after bacillus Calmette-Guerin treatment failure. J Urol. 2014;192:1633–8.
27. Stern JM, Stanfield J, Lotan Y, et al. Efficacy of laser-activated gold nanoshells in ablating prostate cancer cells in vitro. J Endourol. 2007;8:939–43.
28. Stern JM, Stanfield J, Kabbani W, et al. Selective prostate cancer thermal ablation with laser activated gold nanoshells. J Urol. 2008;179:748–53.
29. Lee BR, Callaghan C, Mandava SH, et al. Nanotechnology combination therapy for renal cell carcinoma: gold nanorods bound with tyrosine kinase inhibitor produce synergistic treatment response when combined with laser thermal ablation in a renal cell carcinoma animal model. MP1–5, J Endo. 2015.
30. Kawai N, Ito A, Nakahara Y, et al. Anticancer effect of hyperthermia on prostate cancer mediated by magnetite cationic liposomes and immune-response induction in transplanted syngeneic rats. Prostate. 2005;64:373–81.
31. Patil US, Adireddy S, Jaiswal A, et al. In vitro/in vivo toxicity evaluation and quantification of iron oxide nanoparticles. Int J Mol Sci. 2015;16:24417–50.

32. Fisher JW, Sarkar S, Buchanan CF, et al. Photothermal response of human and murine cancer cells to multiwalled carbon nanotubes after laser irradiation. Cancer Res. 2010;70:9855.
33. Burke A, Ding X, Singh R, et al. Long-term survival following a single treatment of kidney tumors with multiwalled carbon nanotubes and near-infrared radiation. Proc Natl Acad Sci U S A. 2009;106:12897.
34. Humes HD. Bioartificial kidney for full renal replacement therapy. Semin Nephrol. 2000;20:71–82.
35. Nissenson AR, Ronco C, Pergamit G, et al. Continuously functioning artificial nephron system: the promise of nanotechnology. Hemodial Int. 2005;9:210–7.
36. Pattison MA, Wurster S, Webster TJ, et al. Three-dimensional, nanostructured PLGA scaffolds for bladder tissue replacement applications. Biomaterials. 2005;26:2491–500.
37. Roth CC. Urologic tissue engineering in pediatrics: from nanostructures to bladders. Pediatr Res. 2010;67:509–13.

Chapter 25
History and Development of Regenerative Medicine and Tissue Engineering in Urology

Michael B. Rothberg and Anthony Atala

Over the course of the past half-century, the field of urology has born witness to the translation of a multitude of tissue engineering and regenerative medicine technologies from the laboratory to the bedside. While early advancements involved the use of synthetic materials for structural replacement along the genitourinary tract, further development of cell and tissue culturing techniques, along with breakthroughs in the disciplines of cellular and molecular biology, gave rise to the field of tissue engineering, which combined this newfound understanding of cell and tissue growth with material science and engineering. Along with the biotechnology of cell transplantation and nuclear transfer, the field of tissue engineering sought to regenerate living tissues and organs, hence giving birth to the concept of regenerative medicine. Major discoveries in the field of genitourinary regenerative medicine over the past 30 years have progressed from injectable biomaterials to synthetic polymer and naturally-derived scaffolds seeded with cellular material and subsequently implanted. Over time, these scaffolds have advanced from simple onlay grafts to tubularized structures, hollow organs, and organs with highly complex stromal and vascular architectures.

M.B. Rothberg, M.D.
Department of Urology, Wake Forest School of Medicine, Winston-Salem, NC, USA

A. Atala, M.D. (✉)
Department of Urology, Wake Forest School of Medicine, Winston-Salem, NC, USA

Wake Forest Institute for Regenerative Medicine, Winston-Salem, NC, USA
e-mail: aatala@wakehealth.edu

S.R. Patel et al. (eds.), *The History of Technologic Advancements in Urology*,
DOI 10.1007/978-3-319-61691-9_25

Injectable Therapies for Vesicoureteral Reflux and Urinary Incontinence

Vesicoureteral reflux is most commonly observed in the pediatric patient population, with the goal of contemporary first-line therapies, namely observation or antibiotic prophylaxis, to prevent sequelae such as reflux nephropathy and subsequent renal scarring. Prior to the development of injectable materials and the advent of endoscopic technology for their delivery, the earliest surgical interventions for these patients were highly invasive and involved either intravesical or extravesical approaches for reimplantation of the distal ureter into the bladder mucosa [1, 2]. Urinary incontinence is more prevalent in women and increases in incidence directly with age, but also occurs in males, most commonly in a post-radical pelvic surgery setting [3]. For female patients with stress urinary incontinence, endoscopic urethral bulking is a viable option following failure of first-line therapies. In the setting of both reflux and urinary incontinence, the properties of ideal injectable materials have been identified throughout the literature as those which are non-migratory, non-tumorigenic, non-antigenic, biocompatible, and will conserve their volume long-term following injection in order to maintain functionality. In an attempt to identify materials that demonstrate these properties, a spectrum of novel agents have been evaluated in the laboratory and clinical settings over the past century, ranging from non-autologous, synthetic materials and evolving over time towards patient-derived autologous therapies and stem cell-derived therapies.

Non-autologous, Synthetic Biomaterials

The earliest materials evaluated for use as injectable therapies date back to the early twentieth century when Gersuny performed urethral injections with paraffin as a sclerosing agent to treat urinary incontinence [4]. Over the next 70 years a variety of injectable sclerosing agents were evaluated clinically, but were unable to demonstrate long-term efficacy and were discredited by reports of local tissue sloughing and pulmonary emboli, eventually resulting in their abandonment as therapeutic options for incontinence [5–7]. The next generation of biomaterials to be used as injectable bulking therapies was ushered in by Berg, who in 1973 first utilized polytetrafluoroethylene (Teflon) paste for the treatment of urinary incontinence [8]. Teflon injections for periurethral bulking became more widespread in the mid-1970s, as Politano reported good functional outcomes in treating urinary incontinence, and became rapidly adopted to treat reflux as an endoscopically-delivered subureteral bulking agent, as first reported by Matouschek in 1981 [9, 10]. Throughout the 1970s and 1980s, Teflon was the primary injectable bulking agent utilized to treat thousands of ureters for reflux, yielding resolution at rates of upwards of 76–82% following a single injection in patients with long-term follow-up [11, 12]. However, the use of Teflon was mostly discontinued, as several reports surfaced over concerns of particle migration and systemic granuloma formation, with an 80 μm particle size proposed as the threshold to prevent the migration of injectables [13, 14]. As this major disadvantage to Teflon usage became realized, the search for a safer, but equally efficacious, bulking agent as a therapy for both reflux and urinary incontinence ensued. In the early 1990s, a variety of new injectable biomaterials were developed and evaluated in animal models, including polyvinyl alcohol, silicone microparticles in hydrogel, and injectable bioglass [15–17]. Unfortunately, these biomaterials were plagued by complications, with reports of distant particle migration, potential tumorigenesis, and diminished implant volume over time. As a result, these biomaterials did not gain substantial traction within the urologic community.

From the initial reports of its clinical application for the treatment of urinary incontinence in 1989 and reflux in 1991, glutaraldehyde cross-linked bovine collagen (GAX35; bovine collagen, containing at least 95% type I collagen and up to 5% type III collagen, cross-linked with glutaraldehyde at 35 mg/mL) has been widely utilized as an endoscopic injectable therapy [18, 19]. Intermediate-term outcomes for treatment of urinary incontinence have varied widely, with reported rates of symptom improvement as low as 57% and as high as 94% at 2-years of follow-up [20, 21]. Moreover, a relatively poor durability of cure of urinary incontinence upon completion of the last injection therapy was observed, with only a 45% cure rate at 3 years [22]. Although GAX collagen is cross-linked to prevent degradation by collagenases, several studies evaluating its use as an injectable therapy have reported decreasing implant volume over time and high rates of failure following a single injection therapy necessitating retreatment [23–25]. Up until its production was discontinued in 2010, GAX collagen was the most commonly used and extensively studied injectable biomaterial for these applications.

Additional biomaterials have been clinically evaluated as injectable therapies and are still currently in use today for the treatment of reflux and urinary incontinence. Dextranomer/hyaluronic acid (HA) microspheres (Deflux) were first described for the treatment of reflux in 1995, with reported success rates for correction of reflux between 72 and 86% following a single treatment with up to 1-year follow-up [26–28]. Use of dextranomer/HA for treatment of urinary incontinence has also been reported with an initial improvement of incontinence symptoms of 85% and a sustained response of 69% at 5-years follow-up [29]. Although a 23% loss of implant volume at 3 months following treatment has been reported, dextranomer/HA is touted for its ease of delivery and generally favorable durability; it is widely regarded as the contemporary standard for endoscopic injectable treatment of reflux [26].

Polydimethylsiloxane (Macroplastique) was first described for the treatment of reflux, but has been primarily used in the setting of urinary incontinence, with a systematic review and meta-analysis reporting a long-term (>18 months) cure rate of 36%, symptom improvement rate of 64%, and a 30% median reinjection rate to achieve these long-term outcomes [30–32]. Moreover, a large meta-analysis compiling data on over 8000 renal units that received endoscopic injectable therapy for reflux reported reflux resolution rates after a single course of treatment as 76.5% for polydimethylsiloxane, 68.7% for dextranomer/HA, and 56.9% for bovine cross-linked collagen [33].

Carbon-coated zirconium beads (Durasphere) were first described for treatment of urinary incontinence in a multi-center, double-blind trial, where patients were randomized to receive endoscopic injections of either Durasphere or cross-linked bovine collagen [34]. At 1-year of follow-up, a higher rate of patients receiving Durasphere reported at least one grade of continence improvement versus patients receiving bovine collagen (80.3% vs. 69.1%, respectively, $p = 0.16$). Moreover, the required injection volume for patients receiving Durasphere was significantly lower than the reported injection volumes for bovine collagen (4.83 vs. 6.23 mL, respectively, $p < 0.001$). Of note, this investigation experienced a 45% loss to follow-up from initial enrollment to the 1-year time point. The same group later reported their long-term follow-up experience with Durasphere as an injectable therapy for urinary incontinence in 2004, where patients treated with Durasphere were age-matched to patients treated with bovine collagen [35]. At 2- and 3-years follow-up, Durasphere produced cure rates of 33% and 21%, while bovine collagen produced cure rates of 19% and 9%, respectively. The authors note neither Durasphere nor bovine collagen provided patients with durable improvement in incontinence. To date, no investigations have demonstrated favorability of outcomes for Durasphere over bovine collagen.

Calcium hydroxyapatite (Coaptite) was first described for the treatment of reflux in 2006 in a 2-year, multi-center trial in which 155 ureters received endoscopic injections [36]. Resolution of reflux was achieved in 46% of ureters at 1-year and 40% of ureters at 2-years follow-up, with good safety and durability of treatment reported. Additionally, calcium hydroxyapatite was described for the endoscopic treatment of urinary incontinence in 2007 in a 1-year, prospective, randomized trial versus glutaraldehyde cross-linked collagen, where patients could receive no more than five treatments in the first 6 months of the injectable therapy to which they were randomized [37]. At 1-year, although there was not a significant difference in improvement of patient-reported Stamey grade, patients receiving calcium hydroxyapatite injections were more likely to receive only a single therapy with a lower average injected volume when compared to bovine collagen.

Tissue and Cell-Based Therapies

Recognizing the limitations of the synthetic biomaterials, several groups sought to develop and investigate new injectable therapies for reflux and urinary incontinence with improved safety, efficacy, and durability profiles. The use of autologous adipose tissue was first reported for the treatment of urinary incontinence in 1989 with 15 women and 5 men undergoing abdominal wall liposuction and endoscopic periurethral injection, yet only 23% of patients reported improvement of symptoms [38]. Intermediate-term outcomes (median 18 months follow-up) for autologous adipose as an injectable therapy for urinary incontinence were reported in 21 patients who underwent a similar abdominal wall harvest and periurethral injection, but improvement of symptoms in a subset of female patients were only achieved after one to four injections (mean 2.4 injections) [39]. After a randomized, controlled, double-blind trial comparing periurethral injections of autologous adipose to saline demonstrated poor rates of improvement at 3 months of 22.2% and 20.7%, respectively, and no difference in treating urinary incontinence compared to placebo, autologous adipose was abandoned as an injectable therapy [40].

The first use of tissue derived cells as an injectable therapy was proposed in the early 1990s with the concept of suspending chondrocytes in a biodegradable alginate polymer. Subcutaneous injections in a mouse model demonstrated several important characteristics, namely the suspensions were non-migratory, conserved their implant volume, were non-immunogenic, and enabled progressive replacement of polymer gels with cartilage [41]. Further studies demonstrated the feasibility of endoscopic subureteral injections of chondrocyte-alginate gel suspensions to resolve reflux in a porcine model of reflux via replacement of the polymer gel with growth of cartilage [42]. This technology found its way to the bedside in 1999 when 29 children with reflux underwent ear cartilage biopsy, expansion of cells in culture, and endoscopic subureteral injection of chondrocytes [43]. Overall, reflux was corrected in 83% of treated ureters following one or two treatments at the 3-month time point. At 1-year follow-up for this cohort of patients, resolution of reflux was maintained in 70% of ureters [44]. Autologous chondrocyte-alginate gel suspensions were also used for periurethral bulking in the setting of urinary incontinence, with 81.3% of patients reporting improved continence following a single treatment and patients reporting significant improvements in quality of life scores [45].

In a similar fashion to chondrocytes, use of smooth muscle cells suspended in a biodegradable alginate polymer as an injectable therapy was proven feasible by demonstrating progressive replacement of the implanted polymer gel with muscle cells in a mouse model [46]. Follow-up studies for this technology were also performed using a porcine model of reflux, where muscle cells were harvested, expanded in culture, complexed with the alginate polymer, and injected for subureteral bulking of a refluxing ureter [47]. Reflux was corrected in all ureters receiving injections and histologic examination of the injection site demonstrated the implants were biocompatible, non-migratory, and non-immunogenic.

Other muscle cell therapies have also been evaluated as an injectable therapy. First described in 2000 using a rat model, cultured cells from a myoblast cell line were injected periurethrally and resulted in formation of myotubes and myofibers on histologic evaluation 3–4 days following injection [48]. The same group advanced this technology by harvesting and injecting autologous muscle-derived cells into the urethral and bladder wall of a rat model, reporting cell survival and gene transfer in this setting [49]. When injected periurethrally in a stress urinary incontinence rat model, muscle-derived cells were superior in improving urethral contraction and leak point pressures (LPP), without causing urinary retention, when compared to fibroblasts [50].

Injectable autologous myoblasts and fibroblasts were eventually evaluated in patients with stress urinary incontinence in a randomized, controlled clinical trial, where patients were assigned to receive either transurethral injections of autologous myoblasts and fibroblasts or injections of collagen [51]. Although the rates of continence were promising for patients receiving injections of autologous cells, concerns over irregularities in conducting the trial ultimately led to retraction of the manuscript. In the pediatric setting, injectable autologous myoblasts were evaluated in a series of patients with bladder exstrophy and urinary incontinence [52]. Following staged repairs and bladder neck reconstruction, patients underwent a regimen of pelvic floor electrical stimulation and pelvic floor exercises for 1 year prior to injection therapy, resulting in 88% of patients socially continent, defined as dryness during the daytime for more than 3 h. In another clinical trial, eight women received transurethral injections of muscle-derived stem cells (MDSC) for stress urinary incontinence [53]. Investigators reported an improvement of symptoms in five of eight patients, with the onset of symptom improvement between 3 and 8 months and a duration of improvement for a median 10 months following therapy.

Functional electrical stimulation has also been used post-operatively following ultrasound-guided transurethral injection of autologous myoblasts in an attempt to accelerate myoblast integration and promote early tissue functionality [54]. Patients continued electrical stimulation at home for 5 weeks post-operatively. At 6-month follow-up, 24% of patients considered their urinary incontinence cured, while 53% of patients reported improvement of symptoms. In an attempt to determine the appropriate concentration of MDSCs to yield optimal improvement of urinary incontinence, 1-year outcomes of two pooled phase II trials were reported [55]. Following harvesting biopsies and preparation in culture, patients received injections ranging in concentration from 10 to 200×10^6 autologous MDSCs. Those receiving higher concentrations of autologous MDSCs were more likely to have reported at least a 50% reduction in stress leaks and pad weights, while all patients reported significantly improved UDI-6 and IIQ-7 scores at 1-year follow-up. Other groups have sought to circumvent the necessity to prepare cells in culture, with the objective of decreasing time and cost, by harvesting and mincing autologous striated muscle at the time of injection [56]. At 1-year follow-up, 25% and 63% of patients with uncomplicated stress urinary incontinence, along with 7% and 57% of patients with complicated stress urinary incontinence, reported cure and improvement of symptoms, respectively.

Adipose-derived stem cells (ADSC) have been suggested as an alternative source of tissue engineered smooth muscle for the lower genitourinary tract. Lipoaspirate was harvested from female patients, processed in culture to induce pleuripotency, and injected into the urethra and bladder wall of both a rat and mouse model [57]. As early as 8 weeks following injection, the processed lipoaspirate (PLA) demonstrated markers of smooth muscle differentiation; up to 12 weeks following implantation, the injected PLA maintained viability *in vivo*. In another investigation, ADSCs were harvested from rats, induced towards myoblastic differentiation in culture, and injected into the urethra and bladder neck of a rat model of stress urinary incontinence [58]. Urodynamics and histological analyses performed at 1- and 3-months post-injection revealed significant increases in LPP and increased number of myoblasts and large longitudinal muscle bundles compared to controls, respectively. This technology was further developed with a report of combining autologous ADSCs with nerve growth factor (NGF) encapsulated in PLGA microspheres for injection into a rat model of stress urinary incontinence, allowing for controlled-release of NGF and resulting in improved ADSC viability [59].

In the first therapeutic application of ADSCs for urinary incontinence in humans, three male patients with stress urinary incontinence secondary to prior prostate surgery underwent harvesting of abdominal adipose, isolation of ADSCs, and transurethral injection [60]. Continence outcomes were reported to have improved as early as 2 weeks following injections, with patients experiencing decreased frequency and volume of incontinence at 6 months. Functionally, increases in both functional profile length and maximum urethral closing pressure were identified on urodynamics studies. In another clinical investigation, five female patients with stress urinary incontinence underwent harvesting of subcutaneous adipose, expansion of cells in culture, and transurethral injection of a mixture of ADSCs and bovine collagen gel [61]. Investigators identified the cough test as the primary outcome for this study, and at 1-year follow-up, three patients had a negative test.

Biomaterials Scaffolds for Urethral Tissue Regeneration

A variety of clinically challenging urologic conditions may necessitate reconstruction of the urethra to restore functionality and ideally improve a patient's overall quality of life. Most commonly, urethral stricture disease, urogenital trauma, congenital abnormalities, such as hypospadias in the pediatric population, or genitourinary malignancies are the conditions requiring such a complex reconstructive procedure. Historically, when the urethral defect is substantial or the quantity or quality of urethral tissue available is inadequate, making an excision and reanastamosis urethroplasty unfeasible, reconstruction with autologous tissues has been the clinical standard. Typically, buccal mucosa, bladder epithelium, or epidermal grafts have been the principle source of autologous tissue for urethral repair; however, use of these tissues not only requires patients undergo an additional harvesting procedure, but has also been associated with complications, primarily bladder mucosal glandular protrusion and diverticula, hair growth, and stricture formation with skin grafts [62–64]. Autologous tissue grafts must also be adequately vascularized and received by the native tissue bed. In seeking potential substitutes for autologous tissues, several challenges in designing scaffolds must be overcome; specifically, vascularization of new tissue, promotion of cellular localization, adhesion, and interaction, and creation of a biomaterial that mimics the physical properties of surrounding natural tissues [65].

Either naturally derived or synthetic acellular scaffolds have long been used in regenerative medicine, having become popularized for their biodegradability. Acellular polyglactin (PGA) fiber mesh tubes coated with polyhydroxybutyric aci were used to repair urethral defects in a canine model [66]. PGA was bioabsorbable and at 12 months following grafting demonstrated substantial urothelial regeneration and viable surrounding tissues without evidence of stricture. Investigators also have explored the feasibility of collagen-based, xenogenic tissues for urethral regeneration. Segments of harvested acellular porcine small intestinal submucosa (SIS), initially used experimentally for vascular grafts in the 1980s, were used as a graft for urethral tissue regeneration in an animal model [67]. The acellular patch grafts proved successful in promoting tissue neovascularization, along with urothelial and smooth muscle regeneration while remaining non-immunogenic. The first use of acellular matrices in patients for organ regeneration in the field of regenerative medicine occurred in 1996 through the use of acellular bladder submucosal collagen matrices for urethral patch grafting for failed previous hypospadias repairs or for urethral stricture disease, showing good results long term [68, 69].

Additional studies were performed, and when randomized to either buccal mucosal or acellular bladder collagen matrix grafts for patch graft repair of urethral defects, patients with healthy, uncomplicated native tissue beds demonstrated patent urethras over the length of follow-up regardless of the source of their graft, whereas patients with either unhealthy native tissue beds or multiple prior interventions who received acellular bladder submucosa matrix grafts demonstrated higher failure rates compared to those who received buccal mucosal grafts [70]. From this trial arose a juxtaposition between these two grafting options for urethral regeneration: while buccal mucosa provides superior reconstructive outcomes, it carries several risks, including prolonged operative times and increased morbidity associated with tissue harvesting, unrelated to the use of acellular collagen matrices.

Other clinical experiences with acellular matrices have been reported. Acellular tubularized SIS was evaluated for repair of bulbar and membranous urethral strictures in human patients, but the investigation was terminated early due to high rates of post-graft stricture development [71]. Clinical evaluation of acellular SIS grafts for patch bulbar urethroplasty was initially reported in 2007, with results after a median follow-up of 71 months detailing a 76% overall success rate, but 100% failure rate for urethral defects greater than 4.0 cm in length [72, 73].

Cell-Seeded Engineered Urethral Tissues

Prior investigations into synthetic and naturally-derived matrices had only shown efficacy as patch grafts and acellular scaffolds. Challenged by the need of tubularized urethral segments, the concept of engineering urethral tissue with scaffolds seeded with expanded urothelium and smooth muscle cells became an area of inquiry. Additional challenges surrounded maintaining urethral patency without the development of strictures, diverticula, or other complications. Reports of successful tubularized urethral replacement were first demonstrated in a rabbit model in 2002, where investigators seeded tubularized, acellular bladder submucosa with autologous bladder urothelium that had been previously harvested from the animal and expended in culture [74]. Subsequent studies seeded biodegradable poly L-polylactic acid stents with rabbit urothelial cells, allowed them to expand in culture, and repaired urethral strictures in a rabbit model with the seeded scaffolds, which demonstrated complete regeneration of urothelium at 24 weeks [75]. While regeneration was eventually demonstrated, one of the limitations cited for these synthetic polymer scaffolds was the prolonged time required for complete urothelialization along the length of the graft.

The first use of an engineered urethra in patients, constructed with a scaffold and cells, was in 2005. Polyglycolic acid:poly(lactide-co-glycolide acid) scaffolds were utilized clinically in human patients to repair urethral defects of traumatic origin. Urothelium and bladder-derived smooth muscle cells were harvested from five male pediatric patients and scaffolds were co-cultured with these autologous cells; specifically, the luminal surface was seeded with patient-derived urothelial cells, while the outer surface was seeded with patient-derived bladder smooth muscle cells [76]. After expansion in culture, seeded scaffolds were used to repair urethral defects.

Serial post-operative biopsies demonstrated organized layers of smooth muscle and urothelium starting at 3 months following scaffold placement. Functionally, urethras were patent and without strictures or diverticula, and uroflowmetry studies demonstrated adequate flow rates over a median follow-up time of 71 months (Fig. 25.1).

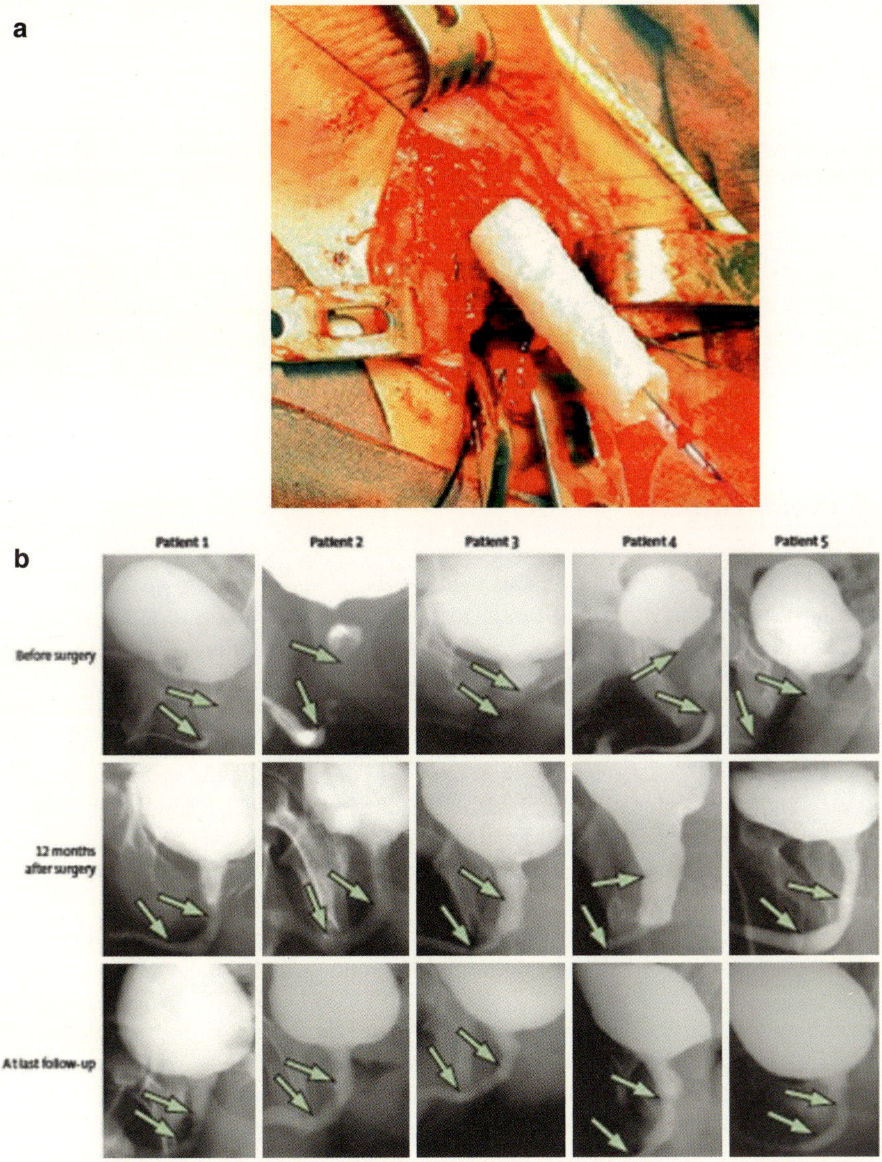

Fig. 25.1 Neo-urethra implantation and clinical outcome. (**a**) A cell-seeded graft sutured to the normal urethral margins from the first patient. (**b**) Voiding cystourethrograms of all five patients before surgery (*arrows* show the abnormal margins), 12 months after surgery (*arrows* show margins of tissue engineered urethras), and at last follow-up (*arrows* show margins of tissue engineered urethras)

Recognizing the unique advantages for each of the aforementioned biomaterials, studies investigating the utility of scaffolds comprised of both synthetic polymers and natural collagen-based materials, so-called hybrid scaffolds, as potential acellular or seeded grafts, are currently under evaluation in animal models [77, 78].

Tissue Engineering of Urinary Bladders

Surgical removal or replacement of the urinary bladder may be indicated for a variety of etiologies, including congenital abnormalities and subsequent end-stage bladder disease, pelvic trauma, or genitourinary malignancy. The oldest, and still today, most commonly utilized source of tissue for bladder repair or replacement are segments of bowel. However, reconstruction of the genitourinary tract with gastrointestinal tissues is associated with substantial morbidity, including excessive mucous production, development of nephrolithiasis, an increased risk of neoplasia, and the onset of metabolic abnormalities owing to the absorptive nature of gastrointestinal mucosa [79, 80].

Acellular Grafts

The earliest known surgical replacement of the bladder was reported in 1917 by Neuhoff, who used a graft of fascia for bladder augmentation in a canine model [81]. Since then, a variety of sources for tissue grafts, including skin, bladder submucosa, and small intestinal submucosa, along with multiple synthetic materials, such as plastic molds, polyvinyl sponge, tetrafluoroethylene, and collagen matrices have been evaluated for bladder replacement [82]. These substrates ultimately proved to be inadequate, as they were unable to demonstrate the mechanical, functional, and/or biocompatibility properties needed for bladder reconstruction. More recently, tissue engineering and regenerative medicine strategies have been applied towards the bladder, including the use of biomaterials derived from collagen matrices and synthetic polymers as scaffolds for regeneration.

One of the earliest reports of the use of collagen as a bladder substitution material consisted of a collagen/vicryl composite membrane to repair defects [83]. SIS was also used for augmentation cystoplasty in rat and canine models [84, 85]. The investigators reported histologic evidence of regeneration of urothelium, smooth muscle, and serosa along the implanted scaffold. Canine bladders demonstrated similar functionality to control animals on urodynamics studies. In 1997, Probst and colleagues used a rat model to perform partial cystectomy and grafting with homologous acellular bladder matrix, demonstrating neovascularization of the graft and regeneration of bladder urothelium and smooth muscle cells at 8 weeks [86].

The ability to successfully regenerate both the luminal urothelial and smooth muscle layers of the bladder on an acellular naturally-derived scaffold is somewhat variable in the literature. Investigations as recent as 2008 report successful regeneration of bladder urothelium, but incomplete or absent regeneration of the smooth muscle layer when using natural collagen-based scaffolds [87, 88]. Moreover, limitations in maximum scaffold size have been suggested, as investigators who have used both acellular and seeded SIS to replace the bladder in a canine model that has undergone subtotal cystectomy reported severe graft shrinkage, minimal regeneration of urothelium, and inflammatory infiltrate and smooth muscle hypertrophy on histological examination [89]. In a clinical investigation, five exstrophic pediatric patients presenting with poor bladder function underwent augmentation cystoplasty with an acellular SIS scaffold [90]. Although functional parameters, such as bladder capacity and compliance, increased by upwards of 30% compared to the pre-operative state, this did not translate to a clinically meaningful improvement in the duration of dry intervals reported by patients. Moreover, histological analysis of grafts following implantation revealed diminished presence of bladder smooth muscle. Due to the challenges encountered with acellular matrices, several modifications to enhance their preparation have been proposed, including incubating scaffolds in bioreactors that simulate physiological stretch of the bladder wall or exposing three-dimensional urothelial cultures to cyclical increases and rapid decreases of pressure to simulate physiological bladder filling and rapid emptying [91, 92].

Tissue Engineered Bladders

Harvesting autologous urothelium, expanding cells in culture, and then seeding those cells onto a biodegradable polymer scaffold for eventual replacement of genitourinary tissues was first described in 1992 [93]. In this proof of concept study, culture-expanded rabbit urothelial cells were seeded onto nonwoven PGA mesh and implanted into mice. This model was further expanded on by demonstrating the ability of harvested human urothelium and bladder smooth muscle cells to be expanded *in vitro*, seeded onto biodegradable PGA scaffolds, and implanted *in vivo* to create urological structures consisting of both cell types [94]. Subsequent studies in the canine model demonstrated improved regenerative capacity of allogenic acellular bladder matrix scaffolds when grafts were seeded with autologous cells prior to implantation. Specifically, investigators harvested bladder urothelium and smooth muscle cells, isolated each cell type and expanded them separately in culture, and seeded the luminal surface of the scaffolds with urothelium and the outer surface with smooth muscle [95]. Additionally, when compared to animals receiving unseeded acellular matrices, augmentation with seeded matrices resulted in a significantly greater increase in bladder capacity (99% vs. 30% for acellular matrices). Seeded matrices also retained their size compared to acellular matrices, which demonstrated graft contraction and shrinkage. In another study, culture-expanded autologous urothelial and smooth muscle cells were seeded on the luminal and exterior surfaces, respectively, of biodegradable PGA scaffolds molded into the shape of a bladder [96]. These scaffolds were then implanted into a canine model after animals

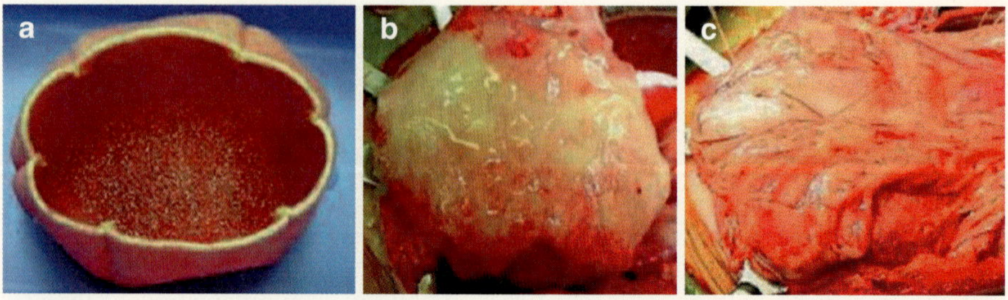

Fig. 25.2 Construction of engineered bladder. Scaffold seeded with cells (**a**) and engineered bladder anastomosed to native bladder with running 4–0 polyglycolic sutures (**b**). Implant covered with fibrin glue and omentum (**c**)

underwent trigone sparing cystectomy. At 11 months following implantation, organs demonstrated filling capacities of upwards of 95% of the baseline, pre-cystectomy bladder volume, physiological properties of elasticity, and normal bladder histology consisting of organized urothelium, muscle fiber, and submucosal layers, making this the first report of a successfully tissue-engineered autologous hollow organ.

This technology was eventually translated into the clinical setting when seven patients with myelomeningocele were identified to undergo cystoplasty with tissue-engineered autologous bladders [97]. Autologous bladder urothelium and smooth muscle were harvested and individually expanded *in vitro*. Scaffolds fashioned from a combination of collagen and PGA were molded into the shape of a bladder; the luminal surface and outer surface were seeded with patient-derived urothelium and smooth muscle cells, respectively. Constructs used for reconstruction cystoplasty with the addition of an omental wrap resulted in increased bladder volume and compliance, along with decreased LPP at an average of 46 months post-operative follow-up (Fig. 25.2). Moreover, the cellular phenotype and structural architecture of the implanted constructs resembled that of histologically normal bladder tissues. The most frequently encountered complications of cystectomy, including mucous production, metabolic abnormalities, neoplasia, or nephrolithiasis, were absent in this cohort, demonstrating the safety and feasibility of using tissue engineering technologies for the structural and functional regeneration of human bladders. Although phase II trials, which utilized cell expansion and manufacturing scale-up methods, did not show functional differences long term, the phase I patients continue to do well and Phase III trials are currently in preparation with a modified scale-up protocol [98, 99].

Tissue-Engineered Urinary Conduits

Patients who undergo cystectomy and urinary diversion face exceptionally high rates of perioperative complications (50–70%), 90-day hospital readmission (25%), intensive care unit admission (20%), and perioperative mortality (5%) [100]. To this end, tissue engineered urinary conduits (TEUC) have been proposed with the goal of obviating the need for elective surgical manipulation of the gastrointestinal tract, arguably one of the most morbid aspects of this surgery. One of the earliest descriptions of TEUCs was made in 2007 by Drewa, who constructed a conduit in a rat model using SIS seeded with culture-expanded fibroblasts [101]. In another preclinical study using a porcine model, conduits were created from tubularized constructs of type I bovine collagen and a synthetic polymer mesh and subsequently seeded with porcine urothelial cells [102]. While implanted conduits demonstrated growth of luminal urothelium and neovascularization on histological analysis, the rates of animal survival and creation of a functional urostomy was only 80% and 50%, respectively. Additional work using a porcine model was performed by seeding biodegradable polymer scaffolds with autologous adipose- and peripheral blood-derived smooth muscle cells [103]. Histological analysis of tubular conduits following their implantation revealed *de novo* regeneration of "urinary-like neotissue" with similar morphologic appearance to native bladder.

TEUCs have also been evaluated in a phase I open label clinical trial in nine patients with bladder cancer undergoing radical cystectomy and urinary diversion. Biodegradable PGA polymer mesh constructs coated with a PLGA copolymer were tubularized to create a 20 cm long conduit, which was subsequently seeded with autologous adipose-derived smooth muscle cells and implanted at the time of surgery [104]. Investigators utilized the omental pedicle for vascularization of the TEUC and optimized surgical techniques for ureteral implantation and stoma creation. Histologically, the implanted conduits demonstrated regeneration of urothelium and smooth muscle along the tract. Long-term follow-up detailing the patency and structural integrity of these TEUCs, along with rates of complications, are pending.

Tissue Engineered Female Genital and Reproductive Tissues

A variety of conditions may result in either absence or loss of female genital and reproductive tissues. Congenital disorders, such as Mayer-Rokitansky-Kuster-Hauser syndrome (MRKHS), cloacal malformations, or intersex disorders, may result in vaginal aplasia, while acquired disorders, such as malignancies or trauma, may lead to substantial structural and/or functional organ damage. Patients requiring vaginal reconstruction commonly undergo McIndoe vaginoplasty, where a pelvic canal is created from the potential space posterior to the urethra and urinary bladder and anterior to the rectum. In creating this neovagina, a tissue substitute is needed to line the wall of this cavity and aid in its functionality. Multiple sources of tissue have been previously evaluated, including skin grafts, buccal mucosa, vaginal epithelium, acellular dermal matrix, and acellular porcine SIS [105–109]. While some of these tissues have demonstrated satisfactory take to native tissue beds, they have typically only resulted in epithelial regeneration with an absence of an adequate muscle layer resulting in eventual graft stenosis or contracture and need for dilation. Reconstruction of vaginal structures has also been attempted using segments of bowel; however, similar to what has been previously reported in the setting of urinary diversions or bladder reconstruction, use of intestine to reconstruct female genital tissues has also been associated with complications, such as excessive mucous production, poor hygiene, and risk for onset of neoplasia [110, 111]. To attempt to overcome these challenges, tissue engineering strategies have been applied towards the regeneration of vaginal organs, with the objective to provide patients with both structural and functional organ replacement and an improved quality of life over currently available options.

The first report of successfully engineering vaginal tissues with cells was published in 2003. In this proof of concept study, vaginal epithelial and smooth muscle cells were harvested from female rabbits and individually expanded in culture [112]. These cells were then seeded onto biodegradable PGA scaffolds and constructs were implanted into female mice. At 4 weeks post-implantation, grafted cell seeded scaffolds demonstrated neovascularization and tissue-level organization of vaginal epithelium and smooth muscle; additionally, regenerated vaginal tissues demonstrated functional contractile properties similar to that of control tissues when subjected to electrical stimulation. In a follow up study, the feasibility of engineering a functional autologous vagina was demonstrated using a rabbit model [113]. Harvested and culture-expanded vaginal epithelial cells and smooth muscle cells were seeded onto the inner surface and outer surface, respectively, of PGA scaffolds constructed to resemble a vaginal canal. At 6 months following implantation, histological examination of constructs demonstrated neovascularization and organized epithelial and smooth muscle. Moreover, vaginal canals remained patent without the development of strictures and tissue functionality testing demonstrated appropriate physiological responses to either stimulation with electrical currents or an adrenergic agonist.

This technology was further developed with the first report of successful tissue engineered autologous vaginal organs in human patients in 2014. Four patients with vaginal aplasia secondary to MRKHS underwent vulvar tissue biopsy, followed by isolation of epithelial and smooth muscle cells and expansion in culture [114]. SIS scaffolds were molded to the unique pelvic anatomy for each patient and subsequently seeded with autologous epithelial cells on the inner surface of the vaginal canal and autologous smooth muscle cells on the outer surface. Following growth and maturation of these constructs in an incubator, tissue engineered neovaginas were surgically implanted into patients. At 8 years follow up, annual vaginal biopsies consistently demonstrated organized vaginal histology consisting of epithelial, submucosal, and smooth muscle layers. Before and after pelvic cross-sectional imaging demonstrated the severity of vaginal aplasia pre-operatively and the durability of regenerated tissues post-operatively (Fig. 25.3). Moreover, adequate functional outcomes were reported based on the Female Sexual Function Index questionnaire. Certainly, the use of seeded constructs for female genital organ regeneration is promising and necessitates further investigation.

Investigations directed at engineering uterine tissue have also been performed [115]. In a similar fashion as described above, uterine epithelial cells and smooth muscle were harvested from female rabbits, individually expanded in culture, and

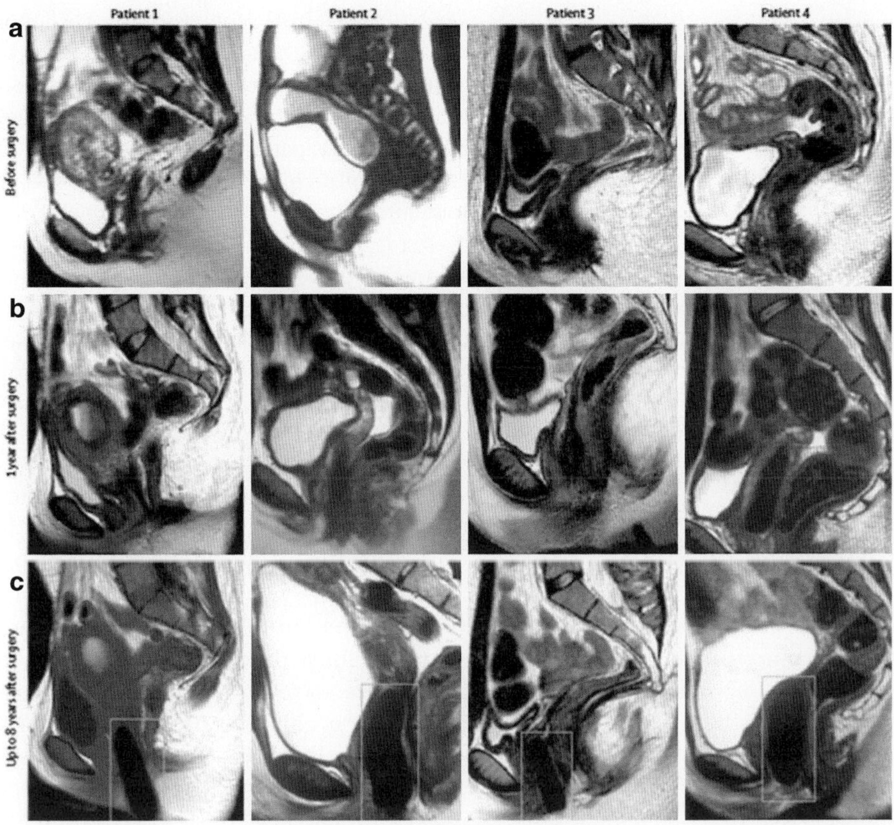

Fig. 25.3 Preoperative and Postoperative MRI images. (**a**) Preoperative MRI images show absence of vaginal organs. (**b**) MRIs 1 year after surgery show engineered vaginal organs. (**c**) Latest MRI images up to 8 years after surgery (boxes within the MRIs show engineered vaginal organs)

seeded onto biodegradable polymer scaffolds which were constructed to resemble a uterine cavity. Seeded scaffolds were implanted into corresponding autologous animals. Histologic, molecular, and biomechanical studies at 6 months following implantation demonstrated the presence of normal uterine tissue components and normal uterine functionality.

Tissue Engineering of Renal Structures

Perhaps one of the greatest medical achievements over the past half-century has been the development of surgical techniques that have made renal transplantation feasible. First reported in 1955, renal transplantation is the gold standard and only curative therapy available for end-stage renal disease [116]. However, a severe donor organ shortage for renal transplantation exists and, although substantial advancements have been made, immunosuppressive pharmacology regimens are still associated with significant morbidity and mortality. Transplant recipients are also at risk of rejection or loss of graft function over time. Currently, patients with renal failure are most commonly treated with dialysis as a renal replacement therapy, but, this too, is highly morbid. Given its highly complex architecture and cellular heterogeneity, the kidney is arguably the most difficult organ to regenerate in the genitourinary system. Efforts in renal tissue engineering have sought to create tissues or whole organs capable of regenerating diminished renal function, with the ultimate objective of providing an alternative therapy to dialysis or transplantation. Towards this goal, investigators have proposed several concepts for renal tissue regeneration, ranging from therapies derived from stem cells and embryologic precursors to total functional renal replacement with decellularized naturally-derived scaffolds.

Cell-Based Therapies

The complexities of renal stromal architecture and the heterogeneous cell types which comprise the kidney make developing cellular therapies for renal disease inherently challenging. Many investigations have revolved around mesenchymal stem cells (MSC) for tissue engineering with the objective of harnessing their capacity to differentiate into one of many different cell types as a therapeutic option. The restorative capabilities of MSCs are often studied in the setting of acute kidney injury (AKI) or chronic kidney disease (CKD), where the number of primary renal cells remaining may be inadequate to achieve proper renal function.

Bone marrow-derived MSCs have been demonstrated to be capable of differentiating into, and ultimately regenerating, several cell lineages, including glomerular endothelial cells in the setting of significant damage [117]. Bone marrow-derived MSCs also have a role in renal development, specifically in nephron formation, when stimulated by a variety of nephrogenic signals following injection into an embryologic rat metanephros [118]. However, this report generated controversy as to whether the primary cell type responsible for kidney regeneration in the setting of AKI is intrarenal versus extrarenal. Additional experimentation using a renal ischemia-reperfusion injury mouse model demonstrated a majority of regenerated cells arose from renal tubular epithelial cells originating from the host [119].

Multiple animal models have been utilized to determine the renoprotective capabilities of systemically administered bone marrow-derived MSCs in the setting of renal injury [120, 121]. In a mouse model for renal injury induced by cisplatin administration, injected MSCs honed to the damaged kidney and differentiated into tubular epithelial cells [122]. Evidence of MSC induced restoration of renal structure and function were observed with enhanced rates of renal tubular proliferation and significant reductions in serum urea following MSC administration. In a rat model for ischemia-reperfusion AKI, early administration of fluorescently labeled

MSCs following injury resulted in their localization to the basement membranes of glomeruli, as identified by *in vivo* two-photon laser confocal microscopy [123]. Several renoprotective effects, including recovery of renal function, high rates of proliferation, and low rates of apoptosis, were reported following MSC administration. Human cord blood MSCs have also been delivered to a mouse model of cisplatin-induced renal injury, resulting in production of pro-regenerative growth factors and inhibition of inflammatory mediators [124].

Mesenchymal stem cells as a renoprotective therapeutic have been translated into the clinic for evaluation in a variety of settings. The immunomodulatory effects of MSCs were first evaluated in a clinical trial of eight patients with steroid-resistant graft versus host disease (GVHD), resulting in resolution of disease in six patients and significantly improved survival compared to a matched cohort not receiving MSCs [125]. A subsequent multi-center, phase II clinical trial evaluating MSCs for treatment of steroid-refractory, acute GVHD treated 55 patients with culture expanded MSCs [126]. Overall, a complete response was achieved in 30 patients and nine additional patients demonstrated clinical improvement; there were no reported side effects or toxicities associated with infusion of MSCs. In a randomized, controlled clinical trial, living-related kidney transplant recipients who received pre-transplant induction therapy with autologous MSCs had a significantly lower rate of acute graft rejection, a significantly higher rate of recovery of renal function (eGFR) at 1 month post-operatively, and a significantly lower rate of opportunistic infection within the first year post-operatively compared to patients who underwent induction therapy with standard anti-IL2 receptor antibodies [127].

Other investigations have sought to isolate renal cell types of certain functionality as a targeted therapeutic towards a specific aspect of renal dysfunction. Whereas currently available therapies for anemia secondary to end-stage renal disease (ESRD) necessitate regular administration of recombinant erythropoietin (Epo), cell-derived therapies could potentially be used to treat anemia in this setting. Investigators first isolated and expanded in culture renal cells from mice that stably expressed Epo and later demonstrated these cells were capable of regulating expression of Epo in response to their environmental oxygen tension [128, 129]. This concept was further developed using a model for chronic kidney injury and human primary kidney cells enriched with renal cells expressing Epo [130]. These cells were introduced following injury, resulting in significant improvement of renal function and reduction of renal injury markers, such as urinary albumin, urinary kidney injury molecule-1 (a tubular injury marker), and 8-hydroxy-deoxyguianosine (an oxidative DNA marker). As a mechanism for delivery of cell-based therapies, a three-dimensional collagen-based culture system was developed to enable *in vitro* generation of renal structures comprised of primary renal cells [131]. Glomeruli and renal tubules, identified by positive Tamm-Horsfall protein staining, developed as early as 1 week in culture. Further studies involved expanding isolated human primary renal cells in culture and constructing *in vitro* three-dimensional renal cell cultures [132]. These functional three-dimensional cultures were subsequently implanted in a rat kidney model, surviving *in vivo* for up to 6-weeks post-implantation.

Transplantation of Metanephroi

Another potential mechanism for regeneration of renal function is through transplantation of embryological precursors, such as the metanephros. Metanephroi were first transplanted into cortical tunnels in a mouse model by Woolf et al. in 1990 and subsequent investigations demonstrated development of new nephrons, neovascularization, and glomerular and tubular cytodifferentiation when metanephroi were implanted subcapsularly in a mature rat host [133, 134]. In another investigation, embryologic day 15 (E15) metanephroi were transplanted either subcapsularly or into the omentum of adult rats, demonstrating renal differentiation, cortical and meduallary architecture, neovascularization, and production of urine [135]. The same group later reported implanted metanephroi into rat omentum are viable for upwards of 32 weeks [136]. Further studies transplanted E15 metanephroi from rats into an adult rat omentum, with investigators performing unilateral nephrectomy at the time of the initial implantation and contralateral nephrectomy 20 weeks later to create a model of end-stage renal disease [137]. Animals that received transplanted metanephroi and underwent ureteroureterostomy to create a continuous urinary tract demonstrated significantly prolonged survival. This was the first report to illustrate transplanted metanephroi were capable of prolonging survival.

Eventually, human embryologic metanephroi were utilized as a renal precursor and transplanted into kidneys of a mouse model [138]. These implants differentiated into functional nephrons that produced dilute urine, but did not generate ureters. Further work in this area involved *in vitro* culturing of isolated metanephric mesenchyme and ureteric bud tissues derived from rat metanephroi [139]. When cultured individually, both mesenchymal- and ureteral-derived tissues were successfully propagated and grew to the approximate size of their progenitors; moreover, combining propagated ureteric buds with fresh-harvested mesenchymal tissues *in vitro* generated a contiguous neokidney with identical morphology to the whole rat kidney rudiment. This same group later developed a stepwise technique for inducing budding of an epithelial tubule and then combining it with mesenchymal tissues *in vitro* [140]. When implanted into an adult rat model, the recombined tissue demonstrated evidence of early neovascularization and development of glomeruli. These studies have proven the feasibility of developing a metanephros-like structure by culturing ureteral buds and mesenchymal tissues, indicating the potential for propagation of the metanephros under these conditions as a technique for engineering renal tissues for substitution.

As techniques for developing and culturing renal precursors advanced, investigators sought to further elucidate the functional benefits which could potentially be acquired through transplantation of metanephroi. In 2012, a group from Japan published multiple reports describing the effect of metanephroi transplantation in a rat models. Specifically, transplanted metanephroi expressed increased levels of renin, increased plasma renin activity, and maintained mean arterial blood pressures in a rat hypotension model [141]; expressed increased levels of Epo in a rat anemia model [142]; and prevented progression of vascular calcification in a rat chronic renal failure model [143]. Cumulatively, these experiments indicate the potential for transplanted renal precursors to not only promote neovascurization and nephrogenesis in renal tissues, but to also regenerate lost renal function in a diseased kidney.

In Situ Development of Renal Units

In vitro renal units have also been proposed as a potential renal replacement therapy. These scaffolds could ideally be seeded with autologous cells to prevent complications associated with immune system rejection or immunosuppression seen in transplant recipients. The realization of tissue engineered renal units was not only dependent on the development of techniques for growth and expansion of renal cells in culture, but also the development of biomaterials scaffolds to serve as adequate vehicles for the eventual delivery of these regenerative therapies. Early advancements in this area were made by successfully culturing individual populations of renal cells harvested from rabbits, including proximal tubules, glomeruli, and distal tubules [144]. Cells were expanded in culture, seeded both individually and as mixed cultures on biodegradable PGA scaffolds, and subsequently implanted into a mouse model. Seeded cells were able to successfully attach to the polymer scaffold and histologic examination demonstrated progressive organization of nephrons. However, it could not be concluded whether the observed tubular structures within polymer fibers regenerated *de novo* from previously dissociated renal elements or whether they were remnants of intact tubular structures that survived harvesting and expansion in culture. To this end, renal cells were harvested from mice, culture-expanded, and individually isolated cells were seeded on biodegradable polymer scaffolds for implantation into immune-competent syngenic hosts [145]. Histological analyses of the implants demonstrated renal epithelial cells developed into tubules over time by first generating a solid, cord-like structure and then canalizing to create a hollowed core. Further examination of cell types confirmed the ability of these individually isolated cells to reconstitute renal tubular structures comprised of proximal tubules, distal tubules, loop of Henle, collecting tubules, and collecting ducts.

In another investigation, a tubular polycarbonate device was used as a scaffold for renal cells which had been harvested from mice and culture-expanded [146]. The device was subcutaneously implanted in a mouse model, while the other end was fed into a Silastic catheter that entered into a reservoir. When the device was evaluated histologically, well-organized glomeruli and tubular structures, including proximal and distal tubular cells and loop of Henle, were observed in the setting of widespread neovascularization. Osteopontin and fibronectin were identified on immunohistochemistry staining of tubular cells and regions of extracellular matrix, respectively. Analysis of fluid collected from the reservoir revealed significantly elevated mean concentrations of uric acid (66 mg/dL, vs. 2 mg/dL in serum) and creatinine (27.91 mg/dL, vs. 4.49 mg/dL in serum) compared to those found in serum. Overall, results from this investigation proved single renal cells are able to form complex, multicellular structures and functional renal units, which demonstrate unidirectional secretion of solutes and concentration of uric acid in the form of a urine-like fluid.

An extracorporeal renal tubular assist device (RAD) has also been developed which functions in a complementary fashion to hemodialysis units. The RAD is comprised of a multi-fiber bioreactor in which a confluent monolayer of proximal tubule cells are seeded. In the setting of hemodialysis, blood is first processed through a conventional hemofilter and is then directed towards the RAD for filtration across the fibers of the device as a means to provide supplemental cellular metabolic functionality to hemofiltration. Using porcine renal tubular cells in a canine model in which acute uremia was induced, the RAD resulted in increases in both ammonia excretion and plasma 1,25-dihydroxyvitamin D_3 [147]. A RAD comprised of monolayers of human-derived proximal tubule cells was evaluated clinically in a phase I/II trial in ten patients admitted to the ICU with AKI [148]. Although these patient's likelihood of pre-treatment survival was low secondary to comorbidities and multiple organ failures in an intensive care setting, 60% of the patients who used the RAD survived past 30 days. A follow-up randomized, controlled phase III clinical trial was performed comparing RAD with hemofiltration ($n = 40$) versus hemofiltration alone ($n = 18$) for patients admitted to the ICU with AKI [149]. Those who were randomized to treatment with the RAD and hemofiltration had significantly improved survival at 180 days and demonstrated earlier recovery of renal function, although this outcome was non-significant.

Renal Tissue Regeneration Through Therapeutic Cloning

While prior strategies for renal tissue regeneration have relied on stem cells, embryologic precursors, or allogenic renal cells as a biologic starting material, somatic cell nuclear transfer has also been evaluated as a potential cell source for regenerative therapies. Nuclear material was extracted from harvested bovine fibroblasts and subsequently transferred into unfertilized bovine oocytes that had undergone enucleation [150]. From these cloned embryos, renal cells were isolated, culture-expanded, and seeded onto three-dimensional biodegradable scaffolds, which were then implanted into the exact animal from which the original cells were harvested. Twelve weeks following implantation, these functioning renal units were capable of secreting solutes unidirectionally, concentrating urea nitrogen and creatinine, and producing urine (Fig. 25.4). Additionally, glomerular architecture and tubular structures were identified on histological examination and the tissues regenerated in this setting were genetically identical to the animal from which the cells were originally harvested. Results from this investigation were the first to demonstrate therapeutic cloning techniques can produce viable cells for *in vitro* expansion and subsequent seeding onto biodegradable scaffolds for implantation and regeneration of tissues *in vivo*.

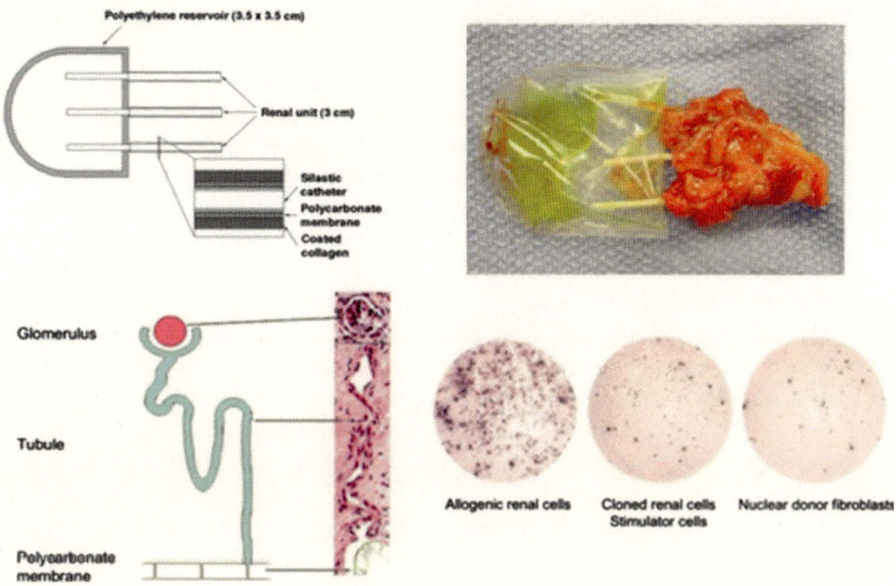

Fig. 25.4 Illustration of tissue engineered renal unit (*top left*); Unit seeded with cloned cells and retrieved 3 months after implantation demonstrating accumulation of urine-like fluid (*top left*); Renal explants demonstrated a clear unidirectional continuity between the mature glomeruli, their tubules, and the polycarbonate membrane (*bottom left*); and ELISpot analyses of the frequencies of T cells that secrete IFN-gamma after primary and secondary stimulation with allogenic renal cells, cloned renal cells, or nuclear donor fibroblasts (*bottom right*)

Total Renal Function Replacement

Development of natural collagen-derived acellular kidney matrices would allow for transplantation of large volumes of renal cells. Such grafts are created through extensive whole organ decellularization protocols, which utilize specific combinations of detergents and enzymes for removal of renal cellular material and maintenance of vascular and stromal architecture for subsequent recellularization. Advancements in the area of total renal function replacement began with the development of an acellular collagen-based matrix mimicking renal stromal architecture [151]. The surface of such scaffolds was capable of receiving a large quantity of cells, allowing for adhesion, proliferation, and differentiation into renal tubular and glomerular structures as early as 8-weeks post-implantation. The technique of organ decellularization arose from the necessity to deliver larger volumes of renal tissue within structures that closely resemble the highly complex stromal and vascular architecture of the kidney. One of the earliest reports of this technology involved decellularization of rat kidneys and subsequent seeding with pluripotent murine embryonic stem cells, which eventually proliferated and differentiated into various renal cell types under the suggested guidance of the extracellular matrix [152]. Further studies using this model demonstrated evidence of the aforementioned hypothesis, as signaling from 'matrix-to-cell' produced endothelialization of vascular cells and basement membrane remodeling [153].

Decellularization methods were applied to rhesus monkey kidneys, which served as adequate scaffolds for cell adhesion and migration [154]. Acellular renal extracellular matrix scaffolds have also been generated from porcine kidneys, which investigators subsequently seeded and re-implanted in pigs [155]. While explanted scaffolds revealed maintenance of renal ultrastructure, further pathologic analysis revealed pericapsular inflammatory infiltrate and widespread vascular thrombosis. Additional experimentation with the porcine kidney scaffold sought to determine optimal conditions through the design of a high-throughput system for rapid decellularization [156]. Investigators concluded a 0.5% sodium dodecyl sulfate solution produced the most effective removal of porcine renal cells, while maintaining the vascular and stromal architecture of the scaffold and enabling subsequent seeding with human primary renal cells. Further optimization of methods have been proposed involving use of non-ionic detergents to accelerate the decellularization process, physiological infusion of stem cells through the renal artery, and pressure-controlled perfusion to promote seeding and differentiation towards vascular and glomerular cell types [157].

In another study, rat, porcine, and human kidneys underwent decellularization to generate an acellular stromal scaffold with a collecting system and ureters [158]. While incubated in a bioreactor, epithelial and endothelial cell seeded rat scaffolds were perfused through their native vasculature and demonstrated the ability to generate rudimentary urine. Moreover, orthotopic transplantation of these scaffolds in rats yielded graft urine production *in vivo*. Additional developments in cell culture and seeding methods have been reported, which enable culture-expansion of porcine primary renal cells with preserved phenotype and efficient repopulation of scaffolds, respectively [159]. Functionally, these renal proximal tubular cells reabsorbed electrolytes, demonstrated hydrolase activity, and produced erythropoietin.

References

1. Hutch J. Vesico-ureteral reflux in the paraplegic: cause and correction. J Urol. 1952;68:457–69.
2. Lich R, Howerton L, Davis L. Recurrent urosepsis in children. J Urol. 1961;86:554.
3. Hawkins K, Pernarelli J, Ozminkowski R. The prevalence of urinary incontinence and its burden on the quality of life among older adults with medical supplemental insurance. Qual Life Res. 2011;20:723–32.
4. Gersuny R. Uber eine subcutane prosthese. Zeutscrift f Heilkd Wein u Leipzig. 1900;21:199.
5. Murless B. The injection treatment of stress incontinence. J Obs Gynaecol Br Emp. 1938;45:67–73.
6. Sachse H. Treatment of urinary incontinence with sclerosing solutions. Indications, results, complications. Urol Int. 1963;15:225–44.
7. Bubanz H, Truss F, Zimmermann A. Ureterstenosis after periurethral injection of granugenol oil. Urol A. 1980;19:143–4.
8. Berg S. Polytef augmentation urethroplasty. Correction of surgically incurable urinary incontinence by injection technique. Arch Surg. 1973;107:379–81.

9. Politano V, Small M, Harper J, Lynne C. Periurethral teflon injection for urinary incontinence. Trans Am Assoc Genitourin Surg. 1973;65:54–7.
10. Matouschek K. Die Behandlung des vesikorenalen refluxes durch transueterale Einspritzung von polytetrafluoroethylenepaste. Urol A. 1981;20:263–4.
11. Geiss S, Alessandrini P, Allouch G, et al. Multicenter survey of endoscopic treatment of vesicoureteral reflux in children. Eur Urol. 1990;17:328–9.
12. Puri P, Ninan G, Surana R. Subureteric Teflon Injection (STING). results of a European survey. Eur Urol. 1995;27:71–5.
13. Malizia A, Reiman H, Myers R, et al. Migration and granulomatous reaction after periurethral injection of Polytef (Teflon). JAMA. 1984;251:3277–81.
14. Aaronson I, Rames R, Greene W, et al. Endoscopic treatment of reflux: migration of teflon to the lungs and brain. Eur Urol. 1993;23:394–9.
15. Merguerian P, McLorie G, Khoury A, et al. Submucosal injection of polyvinyl alcohol foam in rabbit bladder. J Urol. 1990;144:531–3.
16. Buckley J, Scott R, Aitchison M. Periurethral microparticulate silicone injection for stress incontinence and vesicoureteric reflux. Minim Invasive Ther. 1991;1:72.
17. Walker R, Wilson J, Clark A. Injectable bioglass as a potential substitute for injectable polytetrafluoroethylene. J Urol. 1992;148:645–7.
18. Shortliffe L, Freiha F, Kessler R, et al. Treatment of urinary incontinence by the periurethral implantation of Glutaraldehyde cross-linked collagen. J Urol. 1989;141:538–41.
19. Leonard M, Canning D, Peters C, et al. Endoscopic injection of glutaraldehyde cross-linked bovine dermal collagen for correction of vesicoureteral reflux. J Urol. 1991;145:115–9.
20. Khullar V, Cardozo L, Abbott D, Anders K. GAX collagen in the treatment of urinary incontinence in elderly women: a two year follow up. Br J Obstet Gynaecol. 1997;104:96–9.
21. Cross C, English S, Cespedes R, McGuire E. A follow up on transurethral collagen injection therapy for urinary incontinence. J Urol. 1998;159:106–8.
22. Herschorn S, Radomski S. Collagen injections for genuine stress urinary incontinence: patient selection and durability. Int Urogynecol J Pelvic Floor Dysfunct. 1997;8:18–24.
23. Monga A, Robinson D, Stanton S. Periurethral collagen injections for genuine stress incontinence: a 2-year follow-up. Br J Urol. 1995;76:156–60.
24. Haferkamp A, Contractor H, Möhring K, et al. Failure of subureteral bovine collagen injection for the endoscopic treatment of primary vesicoureteral reflux in long-term follow-up. Urology. 2000a;55:759–63.
25. Haferkamp A, Mohring K, Staehler G, et al. Long-term efficacy of subureteral collagen injection for endoscopic treatment of vesicoureteral reflux in neurogenic bladder cases. J Urol. 2000b;163:274–7.
26. Stenberg A, Lackgren G. A new bioimplant for the endoscopic treatment of vesicoureteral reflux: experimental and short-term clinical results. J Urol. 1995;154:800–3.
27. Kirsch A, Perez-Brayfield M, Scherz H. Minimally invasive treatment of Vesicoureteral reflux with endoscopic injection of dextranomer/hyaluronic acid copolymer: the Children's hospitals of Atlanta experience. J Urol. 2003;170:211–5.
28. Puri P, Chertin B, Velayudham M, et al. Treatment of vesicoureteral reflux by endoscopic injection of Dextranomer/hyaluronic acid copolymer: preliminary results. J Urol. 2003;170:1541–4.
29. Stenberg A, Larsson G, Johnson P. Urethral injection for stress urinary incontinence: long-term results with dextranomer/hyaluronic acid copolymer. Int Urogynecol J. 2003;14:335–8.
30. Dewan P. Evaluation of polydimethylsiloxane as an alternative in the endoscopic treatment of vesicoureteral reflux. J Urol. 1995;153:1644–5.
31. Harriss D, Iacovou J, Lemberger R. Peri-urethral silicone microimplants (macroplastique) for the treatment of genuine stress incontinence. BJU Int. 1996;78:722–8.
32. Ghoniem G, Miller C. A systematic review and meta-analysis of macroplastique for treating female stress urinary incontinence. Int Urogynecol J. 2013;24:27–36.
33. Elder J, Diaz M, Caldamone A, et al. Endoscopic therapy for vesicoureteral reflux: a meta-analysis. Reflux resolution and urinary tract infection. J Urol. 2006;175:716–22.

34. Lightner D, Calvosa C, Andersen R, et al. A new injectable bulking agent for treatment of stress urinary incontinence: results of a multicenter, randomized, controlled, double-blind study of Durasphere. Urology. 2001;58:12–5.
35. Chrouser K, Fick F, Goel A, et al. Carbon coated zirconium beads in β-Glucan gel and bovine Glutaraldehyde cross-linked collagen injections for intrinsic sphincter deficiency: continence and satisfaction after extended followup. J Urol. 2004;171:1152–5.
36. Mevorach R, Hulbert W, Rabinowitz R, et al. Results of a 2-year multicenter trial of endoscopic treatment of vesicoureteral reflux with synthetic calcium hydroxyapatite. J Urol. 2006;175:288–91.
37. Mayer R, Dmochowski R, Appell R, et al. Multicenter prospective randomized 52-week trial of calcium hydroxylapatite versus bovine dermal collagen for treatment of stress urinary incontinence. Urology. 2007;69:876–80.
38. Santiago Gonzalez de Garibay A, Castro Morrondo J, Castillo Jimeno J, et al. Endoscopic injection of autologous adipose tissue in the treatment of female incontinence. Arch Esp Urol. 1989;42:143–6.
39. Santarosa R, Blaivas J. Periurethral injection of autologous fat for the treatment of sphincteric incontinence. J Urol. 1994;151:607–11.
40. Lee P, Kung R, Drutz H. Periurethral autologous fat injection as treatment for female stress urinary incontinence: a randomized, double-blind, controlled trial. J Urol. 2001;165:153–8.
41. Atala A, Cima L, Kim W, et al. Injectable alginate seeded with chondrocytes as a potential treatment for vesicoureteral reflux. J Urol. 1993a;150:745–7.
42. Atala A, Kim W, Paige K, et al. Endoscopic treatment of vesicoureteral reflux with a chondrocyte-alginate suspension. J Urol. 1994b;152:641–4.
43. Diamond D, Caldamone A. Endoscopic correction of vesicoureteral reflux in children using autologous chondrocytes: preliminary results. J Urol. 1999;162:1185–8. doi:10.1016/S0022-5347(01)68124-2.
44. Caldamone A, Diamond D. Long-term results of the endoscopic correction of vesicoureteral reflux in children using autologous chondrocytes. J Urol. 2001;165:2224–7. doi:10.1016/S0022-5347(05)66170-8.
45. Bent A, Tutrone R, McLennan M, et al. Treatment of intrinsic sphincter deficiency using autologous ear chondrocytes as a bulking agent. Neurourol Urodyn. 2001;20:157–65.
46. Atala A, Cilento B, Paige K, Retik A. Injectable alginate seeded with human bladder muscle cells as a potential treatment for vesicoureteral reflux. J Urol. 1994a;151:362a.
47. Cilento B, Atala A. Treatment of reflux and incontinence with autologous chondrocytes and bladder muscle cells. Dial Pediatr Urol. 1995;18:11.
48. Chancellor M, Yokoyama T, Tirney S, et al. Preliminary results of myoblast injection into the urethra and bladder wall: a possible method for the treatment of stress urinary incontinence and impaired detrusor contractility. Neurourol Urodyn. 2000;19:279–87.
49. Yokoyama T, Pruchnic R, Lee J, et al. Autologous primary muscle-derived cells transfer into the lower urinary tract. Tissue Eng. 2004;7:395–404.
50. Kwon D, Kim Y, Pruchnic R, et al. Periurethral cellular injection: comparison of muscle-derived progenitor cells and fibroblasts with regard to efficacy and tissue contractility in an animal model of stress urinary incontinence. Urology. 2006;68:449–54.
51. Strasser H, Marksteiner R, Margreiter E, et al. Autologous myoblasts and fibroblasts versus collagen for treatment of stress urinary incontinence in women: a randomised controlled trial. Lancet. 2007;369:2179–86.
52. Kajbafzadeh A, Elmi A, Payabvash S, et al. Transurethral autologous myoblast injection for treatment of urinary incontinence in children with classic bladder exstrophy. J Urol. 2008;180:1098–105.
53. Carr L, Steele D, Steele S, et al. 1-year follow-up of autologous muscle-derived stem cell injection pilot study to treat stress urinary incontinence. Int Urogynecol J. 2008;19:881–3.
54. Blaganje M, Lukanovic A. Ultrasound-guided autologous myoblast injections into the extrinsic urethral sphincter: tissue engineering for the treatment of stress urinary incontinence. Int Urogynecol J. 2013;24:533–5.

55. Peters K, Dmochowski R, Carr L, et al. Autologous muscle derived cells for treatment of stress urinary incontinence in women. J Urol. 2014;192:469–76.
56. Gras S, Klarskov N, Lose G. Intraurethral injection of autologous minced skeletal muscle: a simple surgical treatment for stress urinary incontinence. J Urol. 2014;192:850–5.
57. Jack G, Almeida F, Zhang R, et al. Processed lipoaspirate cells for tissue engineering of the lower urinary tract: implications for the treatment of stress urinary incontinence and bladder reconstruction. J Urol. 2005;174:2041–5.
58. Fu Q, Song X, Liao G, et al. Myoblasts differentiated from adipose-derived stem cells to treat stress urinary incontinence. Urology. 2010;75:718–23.
59. Zhao W, Zhang C, Jin C, et al. Periurethral injection of autologous adipose-derived stem cells with controlled-release nerve growth factor for the treatment of stress urinary incontinence in a rat model. Eur Urol. 2011;59:155–63.
60. Yamamoto T, Gotoh M, Kato M, et al. Periurethral injection of autologous adipose-derived regenerative cells for the treatment of male stress urinary incontinence: report of three initial cases. Int J Urol. 2012;19:652–9.
61. Kuismanen K, Sartoneva R, Haimi S, et al. Autologous adipose stem cells in treatment of female stress urinary incontinence: results of a pilot study. Stem Cells Transl Med. 2014;3:1–6.
62. Wessells H, McAninch JW. Use of free grafts in urethral stricture reconstruction. J Urol. 1996;155:1912–5.
63. Ehrlich R, Reda E, Koyle M. Complications of bladder mucosal graft. J Urol. 1989;142:626–7.
64. Provet J, Surya B, Grunberger I, et al. Scrotal island flap urethroplasty in the management of bulbar urethral strictures. J Urol. 1989;142:1455–8.
65. Atala A. Regenerative medicine and tissue engineering in urology. Urol Clin North Am. 2009;36:199–209.
66. Olsen L, Bowald S, Busch C, et al. Urethral reconstruction with a new synthetic absorbable device. An experimental study. Scand J Urol Nephrol. 1992;26:323–6.
67. Kropp BP, Ludlow JK, Spicer D, et al. Rabbit urethral regeneration using small intestinal submucosa onlay grafts. Urology. 1998;52:138–42.
68. Atala A, Guzman L, Retik A. A novel inert collagen matrix for hypospadias repair. J Urol. 1999;162:1148–50.
69. El-Kassaby A, Retik A, Yoo J, Atala A. Urethral stricture repair with an off- the-shelf collagen matrix. J Urol. 2003;169:170–3.
70. El-Kassaby A, AbouShwareb T, Atala A. Randomized comparative study between buccal mucosal and acellular bladder matrix grafts in complex anterior urethral strictures. J Urol. 2008;179:1432–6.
71. le Roux P. Endoscopic urethroplasty with unseeded small intestinal submucosa collagen matrix grafts: a pilot study. J Urol. 2005;173:140–3.
72. Palminteri E, Berdondini E, Colombo F, Austoni E. Small intestinal submucosa (SIS) graft urethroplasty: short-term results. Eur Urol. 2007;51:1695–701.
73. Palminteri E, Berdondini E, Fusco F, et al. Long-term results of small intestinal submucosa graft in bulbar urethral reconstruction. Urology. 2012;79:695–701.
74. De Filippo R, Yoo J, Atala A. Urethral replacement using cell seeded tubularized collagen matrices. J Urol. 2002;168:1789–93.
75. Fu W, Zhang X, Zhang B, et al. Biodegradable urethral stents seeded with autologous urethral epithelial cells in the treatment of post-traumatic urethral stricture: a feasibility study in a rabbit model. BJU Int. 2009;104:263–8.
76. Raya-Rivera A, Esquiliano DR, Yoo JJ, et al. Tissue-engineered autologous urethras for patients who need reconstruction: an observational study. Lancet. 2011;377:1175–82.
77. Horst M, Madduri S, Milleret V, et al. A bilayered hybrid microfibrous PLGA-acellular matrix scaffold for hollow organ tissue engineering. Biomaterials. 2013;34:1537–45.
78. Fu W, Xu Y, Wang Z, et al. New ureteral scaffold constructed with composite poly(L-lactic acid)-collagen and urothlial cells by new centrifugal seeding system. J Biomed Mater Res A. 2012;100:1725–33.

79. McDougal W. Metabolic complications of urinary intestinal diversion. J Urol. 1992;147:1199–208.
80. Soergel T, Cain M, Misseri R, et al. Transitional cell carcinoma of the bladder following augmentation cystoplasty for the neuropathic bladder. J Urol. 2004;172:1649–51.
81. Neuhoff H. Fascial transplantation into visceral defects: an experimental and clinical study. Surg Gynecol Obs. 1917;25:383.
82. Atala A. Tissue engineering for bladder substitution. World J Urol. 2000;18:364–70.
83. Monsour M, Mohammed R, Gorham S, et al. An assessment of a collagen/vicryl composite membrane to repair defects of the urinary bladder in rabbits. Urol Res. 1987;15:235–8.
84. Kropp B, Eppley B, Prevel C, et al. Experimental assessment of small intestinal submucosa as a bladder wall substitute. Urology. 1995;46:396–400.
85. Kropp B, Rippy M, Badylak S, et al. Regenerative urinary bladder augmentation using small intestinal submucosa: urodynamic and histopathologic assessment in long-term canine bladder augmentations. J Urol. 1996;155:2098–104.
86. Probst M, Dahiya R, Carrier S, Tanagho E. Reproduction of functional smooth muscle tissue and partial bladder replacement. Br J Urol. 1997;79:505–15.
87. Jayo M, Jain D, Wagner B, Bertram T. Early cellular and stromal responses in regeneration versus repair of a mammalian bladder using autologous cell and biodegradable scaffold technologies. J Urol. 2008;180:392–7.
88. Zhang Y. Bladder reconstruction by tissue engineering--with or without cells? J Urol. 2008;180:10–1.
89. Zhang Y, Frimberger D, Cheng E, et al. Challenges in a larger bladder replacement with cell-seeded and unseeded small intestinal submucosa grafts in a subtotal cystectomy model. BJU Int. 2006;98:1100–5.
90. Caione P, Boldrini R, Salerno A, Nappo S. Bladder augmentation using acellular collagen biomatrix: a pilot experience in exstrophic patients. Pediatr Surg Int. 2012;28:421–8.
91. Farhat W, Yeger H. Does mechanical stimulation have any role in urinary bladder tissue engineering? World J Urol. 2008;26:301–5.
92. Bouhout S, Gauvin R, Gibot L, et al. Bladder substitute reconstructed in a physiological pressure environment. J Pediatr Urol. 2011;7:276–82.
93. Atala A, Vacanti J, Peters C, et al. Formation of urothelial structures in vivo from dissociated cells attached to biodegradable polymer scaffolds in vitro. J Urol. 1992;148:658–62.
94. Atala A, Freeman M, Vacanti J, et al. Implantation in vivo and retrieval of artificial structures consisting of rabbit and human urothelium and human bladder muscle. J Urol. 1993b;150:608–12.
95. Yoo J, Meng J, Oberpenning F, Atala A. Bladder augmentation using allogenic bladder submucosa seeded with cells. Urology. 1998;51:221–5.
96. Oberpenning F, Meng J, Yoo J, Atala A. De novo reconstitution of a functional mammalian urinary bladder by tissue engineering. Nat Biotechnol. 1999;17:149–55.
97. Atala A, Bauer SB, Soker S, et al. Tissue-engineered autologous bladders for patients needing cystoplasty. Lancet. 2006;367:1241–6. doi:10.1016/S0140-6736(06)68438-9.
98. Atala A. Regenerative bladder augmentation using autologous tissue – when will we get there? J Urol. 2014;191:1204–5.
99. Joseph D, Borer J, De Filippo R, et al. Autologous cell seeded biodegradable scaffold for augmentation cystoplasty: phase II study in children and adolescents with spina bifida. J Urol. 2014;191:1389–95.
100. Shabsigh A, Korets R, Vora K, et al. Defining early morbidity of radical cystectomy for patients with bladder cancer using a standardized reporting methodology. Eur Urol. 2009;55:164–74.
101. Drewa T. The artificial conduit for urinary diversion in rats: a preliminary study. Transplant Proc. 2007;39:1647–51.
102. Geutjes P, Roelofs L, Hoogenkamp H, et al. Tissue engineered tubular construct for urinary diversion in a preclinical porcine model. J Urol. 2012;188:653–60.
103. Basu J, Jayo M, Ilagan R, et al. Regeneration of native-like neo-urinary tissue from nonbladder cell sources. Tissue Eng Part A. 2012;18:1025–34.

104. Kates M, Singh A, Matsui H, et al. Tissue-engineered urinary conduits. Curr Urol Rep. 2015;16:8.
105. Alessandrescu D, Peltecu G, Buhimschi C, Buhimschi I. Neocolpopoiesis with split-thickness skin graft as a surgical treatment of vaginal agenesis: retrospective review of 201 cases. Am J Obstet Gynecol. 1996;175:131–8.
106. Lin W, Chang C, Shen Y, Tsai H. Use of autologous buccal mucosa for vaginoplasty: a study of eight cases. Hum Reprod. 2003;18:604–7.
107. Panici PB, Bellati F, Boni T, et al. Vaginoplasty using autologous in vitro cultured vaginal tissue in a patient with Mayer-von-Rokitansky-Kuster-Hauser syndrome. Hum Reprod. 2007;22:2025–8.
108. Zhu L, Zhou H, Sun H, et al. Anatomic and sexual outcomes after vaginoplasty using tissue-engineered biomaterial graft in patients with Meyer-Rokitansky-Kuster-Hauser syndrome: a new minimally invasive and effective surgery. J Sex Med. 2013;10:1652–8.
109. Ding J, Zhang X, Chen L, Hua K. Vaginoplasty using acellular porcine small intestinal submucosa graft in two patients with Meyer-von-Rokitansky-Kuster-Hauser syndrome: a prospective new technique for vaginal reconstruction. Gynecol Obs Invest. 2013;75:93–6.
110. Hendren W, Atala A. Use of bowel for vaginal reconstruction. J Urol. 1994;152:752–7.
111. Schober J. Cancer of the neovagina. J Pediatr Urol. 2007;3:167–70.
112. De Filippo RE, Yoo JJ, Atala A. Engineering of vaginal tissue in vivo. Tissue Eng. 2003;9:301–6.
113. De Filippo RE, Bishop CE, Filho LF, et al. Tissue engineering a complete vaginal replacement from a small biopsy of autologous tissue. Transplantation. 2008;86:208–14.
114. Raya-Rivera AM, Esquiliano D, Fierro-Pastrana R, et al. Tissue-engineered autologous vaginal organs in patients: a pilot cohort study. Lancet. 2014;384:329–36.
115. Wang T, Koh C, Yoo J. Creation of an engineered uterus for surgical reconstruction. In: American academy of pediatrics section on urology. New Orleans; 2003.
116. Guild W, Harrison J, Merrill J, Murray J. Successful homotransplantation of the kidney in an identical twin. Trans Am Clin Clim Assoc. 1955;67:167–73.
117. Ikarashi K, Li B, Suwa M, et al. Bone marrow cells contribute to regeneration of damaged glomerular endothelial cells. Kidney Int. 2005;67:1925–33.
118. Yokoo T, Ohashi T, Shen J, et al. Human mesenchymal stem cells in rodent whole-embryo culture are reprogrammed to contribute to kidney tissues. Proc Natl Acad Sci. 2005;102:3296–300.
119. Lin F, Moran A, Igarashi P. Intrarenal cells, not bone marrow-derived cells, are the major source for regeneration in postischemic kidney. J Clin Invest. 2005;115:1756–64.
120. Humphreys B, Bonventre J. Mesenchymal stem cells in acute kidney injury. Annu Rev Med. 2008;59:311–25.
121. Lin F. Renal repair: role of bone marrow stem cells. Pediatr Nephrol. 2008;23:851–61.
122. Morigi M, Imberti B, Zoja C, et al. Mesenchymal stem cells are renotropic, helping to repair the kidney and improve function in acute renal failure. J Am Soc Nephrol. 2004;15:1794–804.
123. Togel F, Hu Z, Weiss K, et al. Administered mesenchymal stem cells protect against ischemic acute renal failure through differentiation-independent mechanisms. Am J Physiol Ren Physiol. 2005;289:F31–42.
124. Morigi M, Rota C, Montemurro T, et al. Life-sparing effect of human cord blood-mesenchymal stem cells in experimental acute kidney injury. Stem Cells. 2010;28:513–22.
125. Ringden O, Uzunel M, Rasmusson I, et al. Mesenchymal stem cells for treatment of therapy-resistant graft-versus-host-disease. Transplantation. 2006;81:1390–7.
126. Le Blanc K, Frassoni F, Ball L, et al. Mesenchymal stem cells for treatment of steroid-resistant, severe, acute graft-versus-host disease: a phase II study. Lancet. 2008;371:1579–86.
127. Tan J, Wu W, Xu X, et al. Induction therapy with autologous mesenchymal stem cells in living-related kidney transplants: a randomized controlled trial. JAMA. 2012;307:1169–77.
128. AbouShwareb T, Egydio F, Straker L, et al. Erythropoietin producing cells for potential cell therapy. World J Urol. 2008;26:295–300.

129. Gyabaah K, Aboushwareb T, Guimaraes Souza N, et al. Controlled regulation of erythropoietin by primary cultured renal cells for renal failure induced anemia. J Urol. 2012;188:2000–6.
130. Yamaleyeva L, Guimaraes-Souza N, Krane L, et al. Cell therapy with human renal cell cultures containing erythropoietin-positive cells improves chronic kidney injury. Stem Cells Transl Med. 2012;1:373–83.
131. Joraku A, Stern K, Atala A, Yoo J. In vitro generation of three-dimensional renal structures. Methods. 2009;47:129–33.
132. Guimaraes-Souza NK, Yamaleyeva LM, AbouShwareb T, et al. In vitro reconstitution of human kidney structures for renal cell therapy. Nephrol Dial Transplant. 2012;27:3082–90.
133. Woolf A, Palmer S, Snow M, Fine L. Creation of a functioning chimeric mammalian kidney. Kidney Int. 1990;38:991–7.
134. Abrahamson D, St John P, Pillion D, Tucker D. Glomerular development in intraocular and intrarenal grafts of fetal kidneys. Lab Investig. 1991;64:629–39.
135. Rogers S, Lowell J, Hammerman N, Hammerman M. Transplantation of developing metanephroi into adult rats. Kidney Int. 1998;54:27–37.
136. Rogers S, Powell-Braxton L, Hammerman M. Insulin-like growth factor I regulates renal development in rodents. Dev Genet. 1999;24:293–8.
137. Rogers S, Hammerman M. Prolongation of life in anephric rats following de novo renal organogenesis. Organogenesis. 2004;1:22–5.
138. Dekel B, Burakova T, Arditti F, et al. Human and porcine early kidney precursors as a new source for transplantation. Nat Med. 2003;9:53–60.
139. Steer D, Bush K, Meyer T, et al. A strategy for in vitro propagation of rat nephrons. Kidney Int. 2002;62:1958–65.
140. Rosines E, Sampogna R, Johkura K, et al. Staged in vitro reconstitution and implantation of engineered rat kidney tissue. Proc Natl Acad Sci. 2007;104:20938–43.
141. Yokote S, Yokoo T, Matsumoto K, et al. Metanephros transplantation inhibits the progression of vascular calcification in rats with adenine-induced renal failure. Nephron Exp Nephrol. 2012b;120:e32–40.
142. Matsumoto K, Yokoo T, Matsunari H, et al. Xenotransplanted embryonic kidney provides a niche for endogenous mesenchymal stem cell differentiation into erythropoietin-producing tissue. Stem Cells. 2012;30:1228–35.
143. Yokote S, Yokoo T, Matsumoto K, et al. The effect of metanephros transplantation on blood pressure in anephric rats with induced acute hypotension. Nephrol Dial Transplant. 2012a;27:3449–55.
144. Atala A, Schlussel R, Retik A. Renal cell growth in vivo after attachment to biodegradable polymer scaffolds. J Urol. 1991;153:4.
145. Fung L, Elenius K, Freeman M, et al. Reconstitution of EGFr-poor renal epithelial cells into tubular structures on biodegradable polymer scaffold. Pediatrics. 1996;98(Suppl):S631.
146. Yoo J, Ashkar S, Atala A. Creation of functional kidney structures with excretion of kidney-like fluid in vivo. Pediatrics. 1996;98S:605.
147. Humes H, Buffington D, MacKay S, et al. Replacement of renal function in uremic animals with a tissue-engineered kidney. Nat Biotechnol. 1999;17:451–5.
148. Humes H, Weitzel W, Bartlett R, et al. Initial clinical results of the bioartificial kidney containing human cells in ICU patients with acute renal failure. Kidney Int. 2004;66:1578–88.
149. Tumlin J, Wali R, Williams W, et al. Efficacy and safety of renal tubule cell therapy for acute renal failure. J Am Soc Nephrol. 2008;19:1034–40.
150. Lanza RP, Chung HY, Yoo JJ, et al. Generation of histocompatible tissues using nuclear transplantation. Nat Biotechnol. 2002;20:689–96.
151. Amiel G, Yoo J, Atala A. Renal therapy using tissue-engineered constructs and gene delivery. World J Urol. 2000;18:71–9.
152. Ross E, Williams M, Hamazaki T, et al. Embryonic stem cells proliferate and differentiate when seeded into kidney scaffolds. J Am Soc Nephrol. 2009;20:2338–47.

153. Ross E, Abrahamson D, St John P, et al. Mouse stem cells seeded into decellularized rat kidney scaffolds endothelialize and remodel basement membranes. Organogenesis. 2012;8:49–55.
154. Nakayama K, Batchelder C, Lee C, Tarantal A. Decellularized rhesus monkey kidney as a three-dimensional scaffold for renal tissue engineering. Tissue Eng Part A. 2010;16:2207–16.
155. Orlando G, Farney A, Iskandar S, et al. Production and implantation of renal extracellular matrix scaffolds from porcine kidneys as a platform for renal bioengineering investigations. Ann Surg. 2012;256:363–70.
156. Sullivan D, Mirmalek-Sani S, Deegan D, et al. Decellularization methods of porcine kidneys for whole organ engineering using a high-throughput system. Biomaterials. 2012;33:7756–64.
157. Bonandrini B, Figliuzzi M, Papadimou E, et al. Recellularization of well-preserved acellular kidney scaffold using embryonic stem cells. Tissue Eng Part A. 2014;20:1486–98.
158. Song J, Guyette J, Gilpin S, et al. Regeneration and experimental orthotopic transplantation of a bioengineered kidney. Nat Med. 2013;19:646–51.
159. Abolbashari M, Agcaoili S, Lee M, et al. Repopulation of porcine kidney scaffold using porcine primary renal cells. Acta Biomater. 2016;29:52–61.

Chapter 26
A Physician's Guide to Navigating the Patent Process

Hannah Koyfman

Introduction

The first patent statute can be traced to Renaissance Italy, and since then the requirements for obtaining a patent have changed surprisingly little [1]. A patent is a government-granted right to be the exclusive maker, user, and seller of the new composition of matter or method. Today, the patent law system is a key engine for translating new inventions into broadly adopted advances in medicine.

This chapter provides an introduction to the patent system for medical practitioners. It begins with an example of a historically interesting medical device patent. It then describes the process of obtaining a patent, starting with actions to take while the invention is being made, progressing through filing a patent application and prosecuting it until it grants, and finishing with ways to monetize a granted patent. Each country has a slightly different set of requirements for patentability, and this chapter emphasizes US law while noting differing approaches in other countries.

Lessons from a Case Study

In the 1930s, Frederic Foley was one of several inventors competing to make the first effective self-retaining balloon catheter. The balloon catheter had been envisioned as early as 1853, when J.F. Reybard introduced a device made of oil-dipped fabric attached to a balloon [2]. In 1927, Dr. Vincent Oddo tested a catheter design with a 5 cc rubber balloon attached to a two-way woven catheter [3]. However, Oddo's approach proved unsuccessful because the rubber available at the time

H. Koyfman, Ph.D., J.D.
Lando and Anastasi LLP, Cambridge, MA 02142, USA
e-mail: hkoyfman@jd13.law.harvard.edu

S.R. Patel et al. (eds.), *The History of Technologic Advancements in Urology*,
DOI 10.1007/978-3-319-61691-9_26

disintegrated upon contact with urine [3]. In the 1930s, Foley was a urologist in St. Paul Minnesota. His key innovation to the catheter was making the balloon and catheter from a single piece of rubber, resulting in a device that was stronger and cheaper to manufacture than earlier catheters. Foley presented his improved catheter at the 1935 meeting of the American Urological Association [2]. He did not patent it.

After settling on the catheter design, Foley struggled to find a commercially viable way to manufacture it, and ultimately filed for a patent on such a method in 1936 [4]. This method relied on a new manufacturing technology: dipping a form into latex rubber, pulling the latex-coated form out, and allowing the latex to dry on the form [2]. However, as often happens, a competitor had been developing the idea concurrently. Paul Raiche, working for the Davol Rubber Company, had independently developed the form-dipping method for manufacturing a wide range of rubber products, including balloon catheters. He applied for a patent on this method a few months before Foley did [4].

Despite a legal challenge by Foley, the patent office awarded a patent to Raiche and none to Foley. As a result, while the recognition for the Foley catheter went to Frederic Foley, the financial reward accrued to Raiche and his employer. Had Foley obtained a patent to the catheter or a method of using it, by filing the patent application before he publically disclosed the invention, he would have been in a position to obtain a royalty from the Davol Rubber Company, or even block them from manufacturing the catheter altogether. This example illustrates the importance of filing promptly on a new invention.

Step 1: Factors to Consider While Making the Invention

The first step towards obtaining a patent is recognizing that your invention can be patented. Almost any type of invention is eligible for patent protection. US law allows you to patent "any new and useful process, machine, manufacture, or composition of matter, or any new and useful improvement thereof" but prohibits patents on laws of nature, natural phenomena, and abstract ideas [5]. More concretely, eligible inventions include new medical devices, diagnostic devices, new drugs, a new use of an old drug (e.g., to treat a different disease), or a use of an old drug at a new dosage or frequency. It is even possible to patent diagnostic methods, surgical procedures, and radiological procedures, although several countries make it difficult or impossible to patent these types of inventions. An unpatentable idea akin to a law of nature might be a discovery about the underlying mechanism of a disease, or a discovery about why a preexisting treatment actually works. However, when an inventor makes a "law of nature" discovery, she often makes a patentable invention at the same time, for instance, by inventing a way to improve a preexisting treatment based on an understanding of how the treatment works.

A question that arises with every invention is: when is the invention ready to patent? The answer is that it's ready to patent when you can describe the invention well enough so that a person skilled the relevant art (for example, in the case of a urological device, a urologist or a surgical equipment manufacturer) can make and use the invention [6]. This moment often comes earlier than an inventor might think. If the invention is a surgical device, it's not necessary to have made the device. If the invention is a method of treatment, it's not necessary to have used it on a patient. That said, if you have tested the invention, it is useful to describe the test results in your patent application. For instance, it's useful to include results of a clinical study (even a small one), a test in an animal model, an *in vitro* model, or a computer simulation. A patent office generally requires much less experimental proof than a scientific journal does.

While developing a new invention, many inventors find it productive to share their ideas with colleagues. However, the patent laws of most countries impose severe confidentiality requirements on an inventor. In most countries, if the inventor publically discloses an enabling description of the invention (for instance, in an article or a seminar) before filing a patent application, the inventor is considered to have dedicated the invention to the public, and the invention is no longer patentable. For that reason, it's important to keep the invention confidential until a patent application is filed. Confidential discussions between co-inventors are not considered public disclosures. If you need to discuss the idea with someone who is not an inventor, e.g., a collaborator at another institution, it is useful to have a confidentiality agreement in place before you discuss the substance of the idea.

Working with collaborators, such as university researchers or contract research organizations, raises additional questions. One is: who owns the idea? If you are in private practice, you generally own your invention. On the other hand, if you are an employee at a university or hospital, your employment agreement may give your employer ownership of any of your inventions that are related to your job. That's not necessarily a drawback. If the institution owns the invention, they generally cover the cost of getting a patent and help find a licensee to commercialize it. Many institutions pay an inventor a flat fee per patent or a percentage of license royalties.

When there are co-inventors, each inventor (or their employer) is a joint owner of the patent application or patent. If you hire a contract research organization (CRO) to test or refine your invention, you probably don't want them to become an owner of your patent. Many inventors negotiate a contract with the CRO that requires, if the CRO invents an improvement to the invention, the CRO assigns ownership of that improvement to the inventor. While questions of ownership can sometimes be sorted out after the patent application is filed, it is better to get a clear understanding of ownership early in the process.

Step 2: What to Do Once the Invention Is Made

Once the invention is made, you should file a patent application as soon as possible. Most countries use a "first to file" patent system rather than a "first to invent" system, meaning that if two people independently make the same invention, the patent generally goes to the one who first filed for a patent, regardless of which person actually made the invention first.

While it is technically possible to write and file a patent application yourself, it's extremely advantageous to have a patent lawyer do it. A patent lawyer can phrase the description of the invention in a way that maximizes the strength and breadth of your intellectual property. Inventors who work at a university or research hospitals can usually take advantage of the technology licensing office. There, lawyers who represent the institution and can prepare patent applications for employees' inventions. In contrast, a physician in private practice will generally need to engage their own patent lawyer. For patent drafting and prosecution, it is important to hire a lawyer who is registered to practice before the patent office.

The patent application will contain several sections. The heart of the application is the claim set. The claims define the scope of exclusivity that the inventor is seeking. A competitor is prohibited from making or using a device or performing a method as described in the claims, but is permitted to work outside the claims. As an example, the first claim from the Raiche catheter manufacturing patent reads, "The method of forming articles by dipping, comprising dipping a form in a coating solution of rubber to form an initial coat, treating a local area of the initial coat with surface curing means to obtain a local curing of the treated area, and again dipping the coated treated form in the coating solution, whereby an integral article with a recess is obtained" [7].

The claims should be written in a way that foresees what competitor, or group of competitors, might practice the invention. It is much easier to assert a patent against a unitary infringer – a single party that practices each element of your claim—than if infringement is divided between multiple parties. As an example, consider an invention of a method of (1) collecting cells from a patient, (2) inducing the cells to become pluripotent and then differentiate into a desired cell type, and (3) administering the cells to a patient to treat a disease. In this scenario, a clinic performs step 1, a laboratory performs step 2, and a hospital performs step 3. If the claim recited steps 1–3, none of the parties would be a unitary infringer. In contrast, if the patent claims a method of performing step 2, then the laboratory would be a unitary infringer of that claim. The patent could also claim a method of performing step 3. This claim would be infringed by the hospital. The patent could also claim the type of cell generated in step 2 (assuming the *in vitro* differentiated cell has some difference from its natural counterpart). The clinic would infringe this claim by making the cell, and the hospital would infringe the claim by using the cell. A well thought-out patent application contains a variety of claims with overlapping scope, for maximum coverage of the invention.

The function of the rest of the patent is to support the claims. For instance, a patent application claiming a device should also include enough detail to enable one of skill in the art to make and use the device. The patent application can also contain data you generated from testing your invention. Finally, with an eye to the future, the patent application can also contain language for claims that you would like to pursue later. A patent attorney can help develop a strategy for when to pursue the different claims.

Step 3: The Lifecycle of a Patent from Filing to Grant

Once the patent application is drafted, the applicant must choose one country's patent office in which to file the application. The appropriate patent office depends on the citizenship of the inventors, the residence of the inventors, the nationality of the inventor's company or institution, and the place the invention was made. Several countries insist on performing a national security review on a patent application invented in that country or by a citizen of that country before allowing it to be filed in another country. A patent attorney, advised by associates in the relevant countries, can make this determination.

There are two main types of patent application relevant to medical inventions under the U.S. system. Most commonly, a new invention is filed as a provisional application. A provisional has several advantages: relatively low filing fees, delaying the cost of prosecuting the application through the patent office, the opportunity to add improvements and data during the year after filing, and a later expiration date. As an alternative, a utility application can appropriate when the invention is fully fledged and is not expected to change substantially in the year after filing, the applicant wants to accelerate grant of the patent (for example, to sue a competitor as soon as possible), and most of the patent value comes during the beginning of its 20-year term (for example, in technology areas with rapid obsolescence).

If a provisional application is filed, the inventor has 1 year after its filing date to decide whether the idea is commercially valuable and refine the invention further. At the one-year date, the inventor can either abandon the provisional application, or file a corresponding nonprovisional application (for example, a U.S. utility application as described above). This utility "claims priority to" the provisional application, meaning that the utility is considered to have been filed on the date that the provisional was filed. Being entitled to the earlier priority date is a key advantage for the inventor, because the inventor is immune to any third party publications made after that earliest priority date (at least with respect to the disclosures present in the inventor's provisional filing).

At the same 1-year mark, the inventor may file an international application called a PCT (patent cooperation treaty) application. Before international applications were created, an inventor needed to file an application in every country in which they wished to pursue a patent. This made for an enormous up-front expense of government filing fees and translation costs. An international application defers the decision and costs, allowing the inventor time to explore the commercial value of the invention. Briefly, the international application gives the inventor an additional 18 months to decide on the countries in which to pursue patents. Importantly, an international application never grants as a patent and never confers any patent rights to the applicant; it must be followed by national stage applications which confer rights in the specified countries. At the time of writing, 148 regions can be entered through a PCT application; these include the US, Japan, China, India, Canada, Australia, and the European Patent Office. A few countries do not recognize the

PCT framework and require directly-filed applications by the one-year mark; these include Taiwan, Argentina, and Venezuela. The choice of which countries to enter is highly individualized. It depends on where the inventor intends to produce or market the invention, where competitors might produce or market an infringing product, the expense of obtaining a patent in a country, and the likelihood of obtaining a patent in the country.

After the patent application is filed, it typically remains pending from months to years, depending on the patent office backlog in the country where it was filed. Next, in the vast majority of countries, the patent office substantively examines the application for patentability. Most countries share the same broad outlines of patent law thanks to several intellectual property treaties, though differences certainly exist. The application is assigned a patent examiner, who usually holds a graduate degree in the same general technology area as the application. The Examiner reads the application, searches the prior art (meaning all public disclosures available before the earliest priority date), and reaches a conclusion on whether the claims meet the country's requirements for patentability. If the claims are acceptable, the Examiner will allow the patent. If the Examiner finds that the claims do not meet one of the requirements for patentability, she will issue a rejection. The requirements differ by country, and change rapidly as the courts interpret them. However, overall, they fall into four main categories.

Patentable subject matter, discussed above, refers to what type of invention can be patented. For instance, some countries do not allow patents on methods of treating a patient. For some countries, merely rewording the claim into the preferred local phrasing overcomes this rejection.

The novelty requirement calls for the patent to be new relative to the state of the art at the time of the application's earliest priority date. Generally, the prior art contains all publications made in any country and in any language. The prior art also contains oral public disclosures, public use of an item, sale of the item, and offers for sale. An Examiner issues a novelty rejection when one piece of prior art (such as a journal article or an earlier patent) describes even one embodiment of an invention that falls within the claims of the patent application under exam.

The non-obviousness requirement, called inventive step in many countries, states that even if an invention is new over the prior art, it is not patentable if it is only an obvious variant of the prior art. An Examiner generally makes an obviousness rejection over two pieces of prior art, saying that it would have been obvious to combine the teachings of the first piece of art with those of the second, to arrive at the applicant's claimed invention.

The final category of patentability requirements includes the enablement requirement and the written description requirement. Briefly, the application as filed must disclose the invention in sufficient detail to enable a person of skill in the relevant art to make and use the invention [6]. The courts have held that an application that is merely a wish or a plan (e.g., a screen to identify a drug molecule having desired properties) does not meet this requirement [8]. To meet the written description requirement, the application as filed must demonstrate that the applicant was in possession of the invention as claimed at the time of filing [9].

Separately from the main four categories above, the US and a few other countries impose on the inventor a duty of candor and good faith in dealings with the patent office. In the US, the duty of candor includes the duty to provide the patent office with any piece of prior art of which the inventor is aware, that makes the claimed invention non-novel or obvious. To comply, an inventor should provide to their patent attorney all such pieces of prior art so that the attorney can submit them to the patent office. This duty does not require the inventor to search for prior art.

Once the Examiner issues a rejection, the applicant can respond. While most interaction with the patent office is in writing, interviews with the Examiner (by phone or in person) are also allowed. In the response, the applicant can argue that the rejection is incorrect, amend the claims to overcome the argument, or both. Often, the Examiner identifies a new piece of prior art of which the applicant was not aware. In that circumstance, the applicant can narrow the claims so that the prior art falls outside the claims. Crucially, when the applicant amends the claims, they must do so using only the disclosures that were in the application as it was originally filed. This underscores the importance of having a thoughtfully-drafted application as of the filing date.

There are often one or more iterations of rejection and response. This process is called patent prosecution. Typically, after a few rounds of prosecution, the Examiner will allow the claims, and the patent can proceed to issue. Once the patent issues, it confers on the patentee the right to exclude others from making, using, and selling the invention described in the claims, in the country that issues the patent. These rights last until the patent's expiration date, typically 20 years after its earliest non-provisional priority date. The US Patent and Trademark Office grants additional term—sometimes several years' worth—when there was patent office delay in issuing the patent. This is called patent term adjustment (PTA).

Most of the time, the claims in the granted patent do not cover every conceivable competing product. This can be because the claims were narrowed during prosecution, the inventor launches a second generation product, or a competitor designs a product to fall just outside the claims. In these situations, the applicant can keep the granted patent and get a second (or third, or fourth) bite at the apple by filing a continuing application. A continuing application (sometimes called a child application) is a newly filed, identical copy of the earlier application (the parent application), and claims priority to the parent application. The continuing application must be filed while the prior application is pending, i.e., before it issues or goes abandoned. The continuing application is entitled to the parent application's earliest priority date. A continuing application is truly an applicant's chance to have their cake and eat it too, by accepting the claims that grant in the parent, while preserving the ability to amend claims in the continuing application to cover second generation products and competing products. It is a good practice to keep a child application pending in each commercially important country to cover these evolving products.

Stepping back, the two most important attributes of a patent are its breadth and its strength. A broad patent has claims that cover not just an applicant's exact device, but even competing products with different designs. A strong patent is one that is resistant to an invalidity challenge when the patent is asserted against an infringer.

Often, narrow claims are stronger than broad ones, because narrow claims are not as vulnerable to being found non-novel over a newly discovered piece of prior art. Accordingly, a well-balanced patent portfolio contains a mix of broad, intermediate, and narrow claims.

Step 4: Monetizing the Patent

The two main ways to monetize your patent are to license it to third parties, or to produce your own product and use the patent exclusivity to prevent generic competition.

A license is an agreement, negotiated between two parties, that the licensee (often a company) can make and sell the patented product without being liable for patent infringement to the licensor (often the inventor). In exchange, the company makes a series of payments to the inventor. A license often includes an up-front payment to the inventor, payments when milestones are reached (e.g., a clinical trial is completed), and royalties from sales of the patented item.

A license can be exclusive, meaning all the rights are assigned to one licensee. This is most common when the patent covers a commercial product and the licensee wants to be the sole distributor. In other cases, a license is non-exclusive, meaning the licensor grants rights to any number of licensees. This is most common when the patent covers a platform technology with many uses. A license can also be geographically limited. For instance, an inventor might grant a U.S. company the right to distribute in the U.S., and a European company the right to distribute in Europe.

Whether you license the patent or produce a product with your own company, at some point you may wish to assert your patent against a competitor who is infringing your claims. While a detailed look at patent litigation is outside the scope of this chapter, two points relevant to medical patent litigation are discussed here.

It is important to carefully consider which entity to sue. Patent-holders generally prefer to sue a manufacturer or diagnostic services company rather than a doctor. This preference can spring from ethical reasons and practical ones, including the fact that U.S. law grants a narrow scope of immunity against patent infringement liability to medical practitioners in their performance of certain medical or surgical procedures on a patient [10]. For this reason, patent claims that the manufacturer or diagnostic company would infringe are extremely valuable. However, even if your claims cover a method that a doctor would perform, these can often be asserted against an entity besides the doctor. For example, consider a claim of treating disease X by implanting a certain medical device in a patient. If a manufacturer produces the device and markets it as effective against disease X, the manufacturer can be liable to the patent-holder because, by selling the product, the manufacturer is inducing doctors to infringe the patent claims. Induced infringement is especially easy to show when a patented product has FDA approval for the very use claimed in the patent, because the manufacturer is clearly producing the device to be used for the FDA-approved purpose. Thus, it is valuable for inventors to pursue patent claims mirroring the FDA approved use of a drug or device.

Patent protection is crucial for commercializing most inventions. This is especially true in medicine, where the cost of inventing and testing an innovative product is vastly greater than the cost of producing a generic equivalent. A carefully thought-out patent strategy can protect the inventor's rights while promoting commercialization and broad adoption of the invention.

References

1. Dutfield and Suthersanen, Global Intellectual Property Law. Edward Elgar Publishing; 2008.
2. Patel SR, Caldamone AA. The history of urethral catheterization. Med Health RI. 2004;87:240–2.
3. Herman JR. A journey through the retrospectroscope. Hagerstown, MD: Harper & Row Publishers; 1975. p. 35–40.
4. Raiche v. Foley F.2d 497 (C.C.P.A., 1940).
5. U.S.C. § 101.
6. U.S.C. § 112(a).
7. US Patent 2,043,630, issued June 9, 1936.
8. MPEP § 2164 II(A)3(a).
9. MPEP § 2163 I.
10. U.S.C. 287 (c).

organs. However, bioprinting is still in its early stages of development. Many challenges will still need to be overcome and much testing done, before it can be used in urology patients [9].

Further advances in robotics have led to more widespread application for robotic technologies for other surgical procedures. The flexible Sensai® robotic catheter system (Hansen Medical System, Mountain View, CA), initially used for cardiac and vascular procedures, has been applied for robotic flexible ureteroscopy [11, 12]. The Avicenna Roboflex™, a robotic external manipulator that can be used to stabilize any commercially available flexible ureteroscope, has been used clinically to perform flexible ureteroscopy where the surgeon manipulates the ureteroscope using a joystick at a console [13]. Robotic ultrasound and needle guidance for prostate biopsy as well as an MRI-safe robot has also been developed for targeted transrectal prostate biopsy [14, 15].

Ultrasonic propulsion is a new technology using focused ultrasound waves applied transcutaneously to reposition renal calculi in the collecting system [16]. The acoustic pressure and energy for this technique are lower than those used currently for SWL and have been shown in a clinical trial to successfully reposition stones and facilitate passage of fragments in humans [17].

Despite the excitement and promise of many of the new technologies that we see today, we still have to temper our enthusiasm until clinical trials are performed to establish and validate their future role. We hope that our text has helped you appreciate the history of many of the technologic innovations that have and continue to shape urology today and inspire you to make your own contributions to urology.

Albert Einstein, on his own genius stated "I have no special talent. I am only passionately curious." It is that curiosity that is the spark for the creativity to invent and innovate. However, it must also be coupled with one's perseverance as Einstein would also state "It's not that I'm so smart, it's just that I stay with problems longer."

References

1. Sohn W, Clayman RV, Lee J, Cohen A, Mucksavage P. Low-dose and standard computed tomography scans yield equivalent stone measurements. Urology. 2013;81:231–4.
2. Pooler BD, Lubner MG, Kim DH, Ryckman EM, Sivalingam S, Tang J, Nakada SY, Chen GH, Pickhardt PJ. Prospective trial of the detection of urolithiasis on ultralow dose (sub nSv) noncontrast computerized tomography: direct comparison against routine low dose reference standard. J Urol. 2014;192:1433–9.
3. Rosenkranz AB, Verma S, Choyke P, et al. Prostate magnetic resonance imaging and magnetic resonance imaging targeted biopsy in patients with a prior negative biopsy: a consensus statement by AUA and SAR. J Urol. 2016;196:1613–8.
4. Schoots IG, Roobol MJ, Nieboer D, et al. Magnetic resonance imaging-targeted biopsy may enhance the diagnostic accuracy of significant prostate cancer detection compared to standard transrectal ultrasound-guided biopsy: a systematic review and meta-analysis. Eur Urol. 2015;68:438–50.
5. Valerio M, Donaldson I, Emberton M, et al. Detection of clinical significant prostate cancer using magnetic resonance imaging-ultrasound fusion targeted biopsy: a systematic review. Eur Urol. 2015;68:8–19.

6. Ukimura O, Gill IS. Image-fusion, augmented reality and predictive surgical navigation. Urol Clin North Am. 2009;36:115–23.
7. Ukimura O, Aron M, Nakamoto M, Shoji S, Abreu AL, Matsugasumi T, Berger A, Desai M, Gill IS. Three-dimensional surgical navigation model with TilePro display during robot-assisted radical prostatectomy. J Endourol. 2014;28:625–30.
8. Rassweiler J, Rassweiler MC, Muller M, Kenngott H, Meinzer HP, Teber D, ESUT Expert Group. Surgical navigation in urology: European perspective. Curr Opin Urol. 2014;24:81–97.
9. Youssef RF, Spradling K, Yoon R, et al. Applications of three-dimensional printing technology in urological practice. BJU Int. 2015;116:697–702.
10. Soliman Y, Feibus AH, Baum N. 3D printing and its urologic applications. Rev Urol. 2015;17:20–4.
11. Desai MM, Aron M, Gill IS, et al. Flexible robotic retrograde renoscopy: description of novel robotic device and preliminary laboratory experience. Urology. 2008;72:42–6.
12. Desai MM, Grover R, Aron M, et al. Robotic flexible ureteroscopy for renal calculi: initial clinical experience. J Urol. 2011;186:563–8.
13. Saglam R, Muslumanoglu AY, Tokath Z, et al. A new robot for flexible ureteroscopy: development and early clinical results (IDEAL stage 1-2b). Eur Urol. 2014;66:1092–100.
14. Kaye DR, Stoianovici D, Han M. Robotic ultrasound and needle guidance for prostate cancer management: review of contemporary literature. Curr Opin Urol. 2014;24:75–80.
15. Srimathveeravalli G, Kim C, Petrisor D, Exeli P, Coleman J, Hricak H, Solomon SB, Stoianovici D. MRI-safe robot for targeted transrectal prostate biopsy: animal experiments. BJU Int. 2014;113:977–85.
16. May PC, Bailey MR, Harper JD. Ultrasonic propulsion of kidney stones. Curr Opin Urol. 2016;26:264–70.
17. Harper JD, Cunitz BW, Dunmire B, Lee FC, Sorensen MD, His RS, Thiel J, Wessells H, Lingeman JE, Bailey MR. First human clinical trial of ultrasonic propulsion of kidney stones. J Urol. 2016;195:956–64.

Index

S.R. Patel et al. (eds.), *The History of Technologic Advancements in Urology*,
DOI 10.1007/978-3-319-61691-9

Printed by Printforce, the Netherlands